HEARING AND DEAFNESS

An Introduction for Health and Education Professionals

Peter V. Paul
Professor
School of Teaching and Learning
College of Education and Human Ecology
The Ohio State University

Gail M. Whitelaw
Director of Clinical Instruction and Research
Department of Speech and Hearing Science
College of Arts and Sciences
The Ohio State University

D1369583

JONES AND BARTLETT PUBLISHERS
Sudbury, Massachusetts
BOSTON   TORONTO   LONDON   SINGAPORE

World Headquarters

Jones and Bartlett Publishers
40 Tall Pine Drive
Sudbury, MA 01776
978-443-5000
info@jbpub.com
www.jbpub.com

Jones and Bartlett Publishers
Canada
6339 Ormindale Way
Mississauga, Ontario L5V 1J2
Canada

Jones and Bartlett Publishers
International
Barb House, Barb Mews
London W6 7PA
United Kingdom

Jones and Bartlett's books and products are available through most bookstores and online booksellers. To contact Jones and Bartlett Publishers directly, call 800-832-0034, fax 978-443-8000, or visit our website, www.jbpub.com.

Substantial discounts on bulk quantities of Jones and Bartlett's publications are available to corporations, professional associations, and other qualified organizations. For details and specific discount information, contact the special sales department at Jones and Bartlett via the above contact information or send an email to specialsales@jbpub.com.

Production Credits

Publisher: David Cella
Associate Editor: Maro Gartside
Production Manager: Julie Bolduc
Associate Production Editor: Jessica Steele Newfell
Marketing Manager: Grace Richards
Manufacturing and Inventory Control
  Supervisor: Amy Bacus

Cover Design: Scott Moden
Cover Image: © Jan Carbol/ShutterStock, Inc.
Composition: Publishers' Design and Production
  Services, Inc.
Printing and Binding: Malloy, Inc.
Cover Printing: Malloy, Inc.

Library of Congress Cataloging-in-Publication Data
Paul, Peter V.
  Hearing and deafness : an introduction for health and education professionals / Peter V. Paul, Gail M. Whitelaw.
      p. ; cm.
  Includes bibliographic references and index.
  ISBN 978-0-7637-5732-8
  1. Deafness.   2. Hearing.   I. Whitelaw, Gail M.   II. Title.
  [DNLM: 1. Hearing.   2. Deafness.   3. Rehabilitation of Hearing Impaired. WV 270 P324h 2011]
  RF290.P33 2011
  617.8—dc22
                                                                          2010002936

6048

Printed in the United States of America
14 13 12 11 10   10 9 8 7 6 5 4 3 2 1

BRIEF CONTENTS

CONTENTS

PREFACE

We, the authors, feel that it is appropriate and necessary to begin this preface with the timeless passage by Alexander Pope. Although reading and understanding this basic text, *Hearing and Deafness*, might be analogous to "a little learning," we sincerely hope that the contents motivate you to do further reading and thinking, and perhaps a little research and writing on your own. For us, intensive and extensive "thinking, reading, and writing" clears much of the debris on the path to adequate knowledge. Occasionally, we drink "largely" and become "sober"; however, this is only an ephemeral state of mind. We admit that we have to continue the knowledge-seeking process to minimize the "intoxication" of limited understanding.

It is our experience that part of the intoxication, warned by Pope above, is due to misinformation and negative attitudes—indeed *stigmas*—associated with terms such as *speech* and *hearing*, especially for a number of professionals who work with d/Deaf or hard of hearing children, adolescents, and adults. We clearly do not mean to denigrate the dedication and accomplishments of our colleagues and those who will become our colleagues in deaf education or educational interpreting. We value and believe that there is a place for American Sign Language (ASL) and Deaf culture in the schools.

Specifically, for our colleagues and future colleagues in audiology, speech/language pathology, and otolaryngology, who may view hearing loss only from a disease/disorder perspective, it is our hope that this book provides a broader perspective of hearing loss for your consideration. The explosion of technology for people who are d/Deaf or hard of hearing is exciting; however, one must be cautious of the old adage that "if your tool is a hammer, everything looks like a nail." We hope that it becomes clear that there is no "one size fits all" approach to addressing hearing loss and that many aspects must be considered, including family dynamics, cultural issues, etiology of hearing loss, and educational options.

The crux of our contention is this: we have made considerable progress in our understanding of hearing and hearing-related technology that it is pertinent to explore and utilize the fruits of our labor with d/Deaf or hard of hearing individuals. Essentially, this means a collaborative approach among professionals to develop auditory, spoken, and written language abilities. We implore that you, the reader, do not misconstrue this as favoritism toward *oralism* and as antagonistic toward signing, ASL, or Deaf culture. Here's one way to frame it: this is a basic text about the articulatory–auditory foundations of *hearing* for the development of English—both spoken and written.

Let's proceed to the discussion of the contents of *Hearing and Deafness*. In Chapter 1, our introductory chapter, we provide background on the notion of hearing acuity and the importance of hearing and speech (especially for a language such as English). We attempt to create an integrative roadmap for the major constructs covered in this text; that is, we want to show how each chapter coheres or is related to the major theme of hearing with respect to development, technology, intervention, and professional collaboration. Also included is a brief rendition of our research and theoretical perspectives so that readers can understand our integrative conceptual framework. In essence, we present an overview on the impact of hearing on the development of speech, language, and literacy in English.

To render faithfully the articulatory–auditory foundations of hearing, it becomes relevant to discuss the anatomy and physiology of the auditory mechanism—the focus of Chapter 2. This also entails a discussion of the nature and perception of sounds and the nature of hearing impairment. Hopefully, our readers appreciate the efforts we expended in explaining a few of the concepts of sounds such as frequency, intensity, phase, and recruitment as well as types of impairment, such as conductive, sensorineural, and central.

After exposure to and understanding of the basic information in Chapter 2, the reader is ready to interpret and use an audiogram or, namely, to understand the essentials of a hearing screening and an audiologic evaluation—the purview of Chapter 3. Although we do not expect you to become a virtual audiologist (or even a real one!), we do expect an understanding of the relation of the audiogram to speech, language, and literacy development, to functional listening abilities, and to the decisions regarding appropriate technology options. After reading this chapter, we even anticipate that there might be a clearer picture of the value of hearing and the need to assess it at birth (i.e., universal newborn hearing screening) and periodically throughout life.

Having a solid understanding of an audiologic evaluation and the anatomy and physiology of the ear should provide a background for the later chapters in this book. Of course, the fun begins (well, for us anyway...) with the next two chapters on hearing aids, cochlear implants, and other amplification devices—Chapters 4 and 5. A number of breathtaking (and colorful!) advances have been made with digital hearing aids and cochlear implants, and this warrants adequate treatment for preservice (and, perhaps, inservice) professionals. Professionals such as teachers, educational interpreters, and speech-language pathologists should know the basics of how these devices work, including their limitations and benefits.

In general, educators and other professionals working with children, adolescents, and adults who are d/Deaf or hard of hearing might not have a strong grasp on how hearing development relates to speech, language, and reading development (of English). We attempt to shed some light (and hopefully not too much heat) on these interrelations in Chapters 6 and 7. Chapter 6 examines a range of topics, from the components and development of speech to those of language. We are confident that you will remember that speech does not equal language—among other tidbits of information.

In Chapter 1, we assert that phonology represents the building blocks of learning a language, especially a language based on sound. In Chapters 6 and 7, we demonstrate this principle and relate the component of phonology to the development of the other components of a spoken language such as English. Also, in Chapter 7, we introduce our readers to emerging perspectives on alternative techniques of developing phonological awareness, such as cued speech/language and visual phonics.

To put it in a nutshell, the rest of the book might best be viewed as an application of the contents in Chapters 2 through 7; albeit, we have certainly provided more information that should be useful and pertinent. The application aspect entails aural rehabilitation and intervention techniques as well as collaboration among professionals in schools and clinics. Chapter 8 focuses on the aural rehabilitation components of speechreading and auditory development (training/learning); Chapter 9 on the merits of early intervention; and Chapter 10 on interdisciplinary collaboration among professionals to enhance the development of children and adolescents.

We are aware that early intervention might be a hotly contested issue for some professionals, especially when the decision involves early amplification. Nevertheless, we feel that there is no more important issue, and we have little or no doubt that the growth and improvement in technology—discussed in Chapters 4 and 5—will minimize or resolve many of the conflicts associated with early identification and amplification. To paraphrase a popular news show in our area, it is critical to provide fair and balanced information in relation to how early intervention and educational options are delivered to families.

In Chapter 10, we argue that collaboration is a major key to success. Setting aside the politics of parity and power, we feel that professionals need to be willing to work together to ensure the most positive educational experience for the child. In short, we highlight that an interdisciplinary team approach entails the use of various ideas to provide the best outcomes for children and adolescents. We not only believe in the power and value of diversity—we celebrate it. Diverse viewpoints create a more productive framework for decision making. To put this succinctly: a diverse view is better than one view.

In the last chapter—the epilogue—we decided to have more fun by "summing up" briefly and presenting our view of the future. Nobody likes to know the ending to a good book ahead of time, so we shall spare you most of the details here. We do proffer a few recommendations for teacher education and clinical education programs in university settings. More important, we present an integrative view of our own perspectives about this controversial topic of *hearing* as it relates to *deafness*.

In closing, it is our desire that this book will inflame and inform your intellect—and that's no exaggeration (albeit, it might be a good metaphor). If we can stretch your learning beyond "a little learning," we can conclude that we have done our job. But, this little book should be a necessary first step of the long stairway. Perhaps, we can avoid a repeat of the situation described by Louise Tracy, who wrote the foreword to the first edition of *Hearing and Deafness* (Davis & Silverman, 1978) in August of 1947:

> There is no other subject that vitally affects the lives of so many people on which there is so little positive information and so much fuzzy and widespread misinformation and misunderstanding. I doubt if over 5 percent of our population has ever read anything authentic on the deaf or the hard of hearing. And yet the impression that the deaf have no vocal cords and so cannot speak is wide-spread. It might surprise you to know how many people ask if the deaf learn to read Braille. (p. xiii)

Finally, we are indebted to all of the researchers and scholars who contributed the findings on which this book is based. We thank our reviewers for providing valuable comments on earlier versions of the manuscript, and we thank those persons who have contributed to the production and provision of photos in this book (acknowledgments are listed in the relevant places; specifically, we would like to acknowledge Landa McGinnis of *Cochlear Americas*, Maureen Doty-Tomasula of *Oticon*, and Brad Ingrao of *e-Audiology*). We appreciate the assistance of the staff at Jones and Bartlett—including their tolerance for the corny, eccentric humor of the first author via emails. Last, and certainly not least, we thank our spouses and family for bearing with our ups and downs throughout the intensive and extensive thinking, reading, and writing process for this book.

 Reference

Davis, H., & Silverman, S. R. (1978). *Hearing and deafness*. New York: Holt, Rinehart, & Winston.

CONTRIBUTORS

Karen S. Engler, MA, BS
Clinical Associate Professor
Communication Sciences and Disorders
Missouri State University

Ye Wang, PhD, MA
Assistant Professor
Communication Sciences and Disorders
Missouri State University

REVIEWERS

Shalini Arehole, PhD
Associate Professor
University of Louisiana at Lafayette

Susan M. Brandner, AuD, CCC-A/FAAA
Newark Public Schools
Audiology Associates of Freehold
East Windsor, NJ

Rebecca Crowell, AuD, CCC-A
Assistant Professor
St. Cloud State University

Maria C. Hartman, MA
Instructor, Student Teaching Coordinator
Teachers College, Columbia University

Chad E. Smith, PhD
Director of Deaf Education
Texas Woman's University

Jim Steiger, PhD
Associate Professor
Northeast Ohio AuD Consortium
The University of Akron

Brenda Stephenson, BS, MS
Lecturer/Intern Supervisor
Education of the Deaf and Hard of Hearing Program
The University of Tennessee

Claudia D. Updike, PhD, CCC-A, FAAA
Professor of Audiology
Ball State University

Deborah R. Welling, AuD, CCC-A, FAAA
Chair, Associate Professor
Department of Speech-Language Pathology
Seton Hall University

Introduction to Hearing and Deafness

What really is deafness? Is it a number on a decibel scale that describes the severity of hearing impairment? Is it a disease like mumps or measles or meningitis? Is it an ankylosed stapes? Is it a piece of tissue in the auditory system that would be judged to be abnormal if viewed under a microscope? Is it an affliction to be conquered by the ingenious scientist? Is it the burden of a child whose parent hopes persistently and fervently that the scientist will be successful and soon? Is it a special mode of communication? Is it something that is encountered occasionally in the man or woman whose fingers fly and whose utterances are arrhythmic and strident? Is it a cause to which diligent, skillful, and patient teachers have committed themselves for generations? Is it the agony of isolation from a piece of the real world? Is it the joy of accomplishment that mocks the handicap? Is it the bright mind and the potentially capable hands for which the economy has no use because they are uncultivated? Is it a crystallization of attitudes of a distinctive group whose deafness, modes of communication, and other associated attributes . . . that they have in common cause them to band together to achieve social and economic self-realization? Of course, it is all of these and more, depending on who ask the question and why.

—Davis & Silverman (1978, p. v)

Key Concepts

After completing this chapter, readers should have a basic understanding of:

- Audiologic descriptions of hearing acuity
- The importance of hearing and speech

- Major concepts in the book
- Perspectives of the authors

Despite the use of a few outdated words and phrases, the passage by Davis and Silverman (1978) at the beginning of this chapter continues to be awe inspiring, perhaps prophetic even, more than 30 years since its publication. One can see the precursors to the major perspectives on deafness, often characterized—on a superficial level—as the clinical–cultural dichotomy (e.g., Baker & Cokely, 1980; Paul, 2009; Paul & Jackson, 1993). Clinically, deafness, in its broadest meaning, includes all degrees of hearing loss, from slight to profound, and is viewed as a disease; a disability; something that causes problems; something to eradicate, overcome, or prevent. Culturally, deafness (i.e., mostly individuals with severe-to-profound hearing loss, who are members of a culture) is a natural condition, which should be preserved and revered, especially because it is often accompanied by the use of the language of signs. It can be argued that categorizing perspectives as either *clinical* or *cultural* is most likely an oversimplification that undermines the complexity of the manner in which humans develop their attitudes, mores, and belief systems.

Most likely, Davis and Silverman did not have a crystal ball that would have illustrated graphically and strongly the varying implications of what they wrote. Viewing deafness as a natural, cultural condition in which individuals are often associated with members of a sociological group has resulted in an extension of effective methods used in the education and rehabilitation of children and adolescents. Educators, clinicians, and other professionals have been (or should be) exposed to ideas and positions pertaining to the rights of Deaf individuals (capitalized D refers to members of the culture).

It is important also to be introduced to, to understand, and to respect the terminology reflecting the empowerment of minorities, in this case the terms Deafhood, Deaf Identity, DEAF-WORLD, and Deaf Epistemologies (similar to Feminist or African American Epistemologies, which is the basis for Feminist [or Women] or African American Studies, respectively. Note: epistemology refers to the nature, extent, and perspective on knowledge.). This awareness has led to the call and need for the involvement of Deaf teachers, administrators, and researchers and for the right of every d/Deaf person to learn to communicate effectively. Within this perspective, some scholars might add that effective communication is most likely via the use of a sign language, particularly American Sign Language in the United States (e.g., see discussions in Bauman, 2008; Ladd, 2003; Lane, 1992; Lane, Hoffmeister, & Bahan, 1996).

However, Davis and Silverman (1978) could not foresee our deeper, current understanding of the effects of any level of hearing loss on the development of speech, language, and literacy in English (in our case). Just think of the impact of conditions such as unilateral (one ear) hearing loss, fluctuant hearing loss, and chronic otitis media (middle ear infections). In one sense, to put it mildly, and perhaps metaphorically, hearing is or might be important for the development of speech, language, and literacy in English. We shall expound on this proclamation periodically throughout this text.

Our goal is not to promote one perspective over the other. We feel that there is a place for both in the education and/or rehabilitation of children, adolescents, and adults who are d/Deaf or hard of hearing. In essence, both views should be valued and respected, and the decision to adhere to or apply one or the other or some combination of the two frameworks might best be left up to educators and parents and, ultimately, to children who are d/Deaf and hard of hearing as they become older and more mature.

Nevertheless, the tensions and controversies engendered by these dichotomous, albeit limited, perspectives may have resulted in the downplaying of the importance of the variables of hearing and speech in the developmental stages of most individuals who have severe-to-profound hearing losses and—from a radical standpoint—even in those with less severe hearing losses. More often than not, the concepts of hearing and speech have become, or can become, negative, perfunctory terms and/or are deemed to be, for the most part, inaccessible to or inappropriate for many individuals who are d/Deaf or hard of hearing (e.g., see discussions in Lane, 1992; Lane et al., 1996; cf., Paul, 1996, 1997; Trezek, Wang, & Paul, 2010; Wang, Trezek, Luckner, & Paul, 2008).

In our view, professionals who work in fields such as deaf education, audiology, speech and language pathology, educational interpreting, and in other related fields need an adequate understanding of the contribution and rehabilitation of hearing (and speech). A strong case for developing such an understanding can be made given the advent of advanced amplification systems and the emerging focus on the importance of phonemic and phonological awareness for both English language and literacy development (e.g., National Reading Panel, 2000; Paul, 2009; Snowling & Hulme, 2005; Trezek et al., 2010).

It might come as a surprise that this also applies to learning English either as a first or second language. In fact, the interrelations among hearing, speech, language, and literacy are so incredibly complex that research has not teased out the major contributions of their various aspects (e.g., McGuinness, 2004, 2005). Nevertheless, the interrelations cannot be ignored by educators and professionals.

In this text, our major focus is to provide up-to-date information on an array of critical areas in speech and hearing, such as hearing aids, cochlear implants, speechreading, aural rehabilitation, and the necessary constructs for developing English language and literacy. We want professionals not only to posses such current knowledge, but also to develop skills that can be used in their work settings. With our backgrounds (speech and hearing science and education), we feel that we are in a position to illustrate clearly the connections between knowledge and practice, particularly from an interdisciplinary framework. We aim to produce a text that is solid with respect to theory and research and that also contains demonstrations of practice.

As you read this chapter, we encourage you to think of questions that you expect to be answered or at least addressed. For example, you might consider questions related to the *Key Concepts*:

- What are the audiologic dimensions of a hearing loss? Is this important to know for the development of speech and language?

- Why is audition (hearing) important for speech and language development? Will this be related to the development of English? Will this be related to the development of English literacy? What about English as a second language?

- What are the major concepts to be discussed in this text? What will this chapter discuss with respect to these concepts?

- What are the theoretical/research orientations of the authors? Why is this important for me to know as a reader?

We shall return to these questions and more (hopefully, some of yours!) in the summary section of this chapter.

Audiologic Descriptions of Hearing Acuity

Hearing impairment is a generic term referring to all types, causes, and degrees of hearing loss. To delineate the impact of a hearing loss on the development of English speech, language, and literacy, a number of descriptive variables have been identified, including degree of hearing impairment; age at onset; age at identification; etiology; presence of additional disabilities; and hearing status, level of involvement, communication mode, socioeconomic status of the parents or caregivers. In this chapter, our goal is to provide some introductory information and to focus mainly on the degree of hearing loss and age at onset—two critical traditional variables for habilitation and rehabilitation purposes. These two variables have had a pervasive effect on the development of speech, language, and literacy in English. Age at identification, another critical variable, is discussed in the chapter on early intervention (Chapter 9).

An individual's hearing threshold level is indicated on the audiogram across a range of octave frequencies between 250–8000 Hz. The individual's audiogram results are often reflected in one number, known as a *pure tone average* (PTA). It is the average unaided threshold across three frequencies (500, 1000, and 2000 Hz) and is thought to reflect an individual's abilities to detect speech information. The PTA is designed to chart hearing sensitivity from 0 to 110 dB (see discussions in Ross, 1986; Schow & Nerbonne, 2007). Much of the emphasis in describing hearing loss has been placed on the degree of hearing loss. Although all of the factors mentioned previously should be considered concomitantly, degree of impairment has assumed the most weight in determining the educational placement of children who are d/Deaf or hard of hearing, rehabilitation procedures, and even the selection of amplification systems (e.g., Karchmer, Milone, & Wolk, 1979; Paul & Quigley, 1990).

To simplify matters, here we group hearing loss into five categories: slight, mild, moderate, severe, and profound (see **Table 1-1**). Traditionally, students in the first three categories have been referred to as *hard of hearing*, whereas those in the last one are labeled as *deaf*. Students in the category of *severe hearing loss* can constitute a mixed bag, so to speak. Historically, these students have been labeled as either hard of hearing or deaf, depending on their use of residual hearing (i.e., remaining or usable hearing).

It is possible for an individual in the severe category, for example, to *function* like a hard of hearing person in the areas of speech, language, and literacy even though she or he may be audiometrically deaf (Paul, 2001, 2009; Schow & Nerbonne, 2007). Our contention is that with early intervention and early amplification many individuals with severe-to-profound hearing losses can perform like *hard of hearing* individuals, which essentially means that they are connected to the world of sound (or audition). Being connected to the world of sound facilitates the development of spoken language and its written equivalent.

Table
1-1

Categories of Hearing Loss

Degree of Hearing Loss in dB	Description	Implications
Up to 26	Normal	No special class or treatment is necessary, but professionals should monitor language and academic progress.
27–40	Slight	Typically, special class or treatment is not required. Some individuals might need instruction in speechreading and speech. May need amplification and/or assistance in language and literacy development.
41–54	Mild	A number of individuals need special class and/or school placement. Most of these individuals will require targeted instruction in speechreading and in certain aspects of speech. Typically, most individuals in this area need specialized assistance in language and/or literacy development.
55–69	Moderate	Many individuals in this category require special class and/or school placement. A large number might need instruction in speechreading and in the development of speech. Almost invariably, these individuals will need specialized instruction in language and literacy.

(*continues*)

Table
1-1

Categories of Hearing Loss (continued)

Degree of Hearing Loss in dB	Description	Implications
70–89	Severe	Most individuals in this category require a full-time special education program with specialized, targeted instruction in language and literacy. An array of support services should be provided, as well as training in speechreading, speech, and the use of residual (i.e., usable or remaining) hearing.
>90	Profound or extreme	Most individuals require a full-time special education program with specialized instruction in language and literacy development. Comprehensive support services are needed. Training in speechreading, speech, and the use of residual hearing is mandatory. A number of individuals might require the use of sign communication.

Note: A few scholars (e.g., Schow & Nerbonne, 2007) assert that there should be two sets of categories for slight and mild—one for children and one for adults; however, research has not documented substantial differences between these two sets. Others argue that the slight impairment category should begin at 15 or 16 dB, instead of 27 dB (e.g., Ross, 1986).

Sources: Adapted from Paul (2009), Ross (1986), and Schow & Nerbonne (2007).

What might be surprising to most professionals and other interested individuals is that limited research exists on the relationship between a specific category of hearing loss (i.e., slight, mild, etc.) and educational achievement. Nevertheless, professionals need to be aware of and attend to children with *any* level of hearing loss, from slight to profound. Even a slight hearing loss can affect the development of language and literacy.

With respect to Table 1-1, scholars have offered general educational implications with regard to degrees of hearing loss (e.g., Paul & Quigley, 1990; Schow & Nerbonne, 2007). These implications (e.g., effects on speechreading, educational placement, etc.) are affected by individual differences, especially when age at onset and age at identification are considered in conjunction with degree of impairment.

Age at onset refers to the age at which the loss is sustained. It is often examined in relation to the optimal period for the acquisition of a spoken language, usually from birth to about 2 years. The more severe the hearing loss, the more crucial age at onset becomes for the development of a spoken language. When degree of impairment is considered in conjunction with age at onset, research has shown a significant effect on the development of spoken and written English skills (e.g., King & Quigley, 1985; Paul, 2009; Trezek et al., 2010). For example, children who acquire a severe-to-profound hearing loss at age 5 years may exhibit the same level of loss as those who incur this loss at birth; however, their language and communication skills are very different (e.g., Paul, 2009; Quigley & Kretschmer, 1982). As is discussed later in this text, the effects of age at onset can be minimized or reduced if the age at identification occurs early; that is, by early intervention at as early an age as possible.

Importance of Hearing and Speech

It seems axiomatic to discuss the importance of hearing and speech for language and literacy development in English. There is little debate that the loss of hearing affects the communication process with respect to the use of a spoken language. The root of the problem, however, resides in the pervasive impact of the hearing loss on the acquisition of oral or spoken foundational symbols; that is, the experiential and meaningful stimuli deemed necessary for the development of spoken language.

Let us illustrate this point another way with a passage that is still applicable, albeit with some updates that are discussed later in this text (Lovinger, Brandell, & Seestedt-Stanford, 1991):

> Stop for a moment and listen. What do you hear?...How did we learn to discriminate these sound differences, associate sound to experience, and then give them meaning? How did we learn to understand sound, to form words to communicate?
>
> The role of the ear in the normal course of speech development cannot be overemphasized. The ear serves as the main feedback mechanism in the development and production of speech. Sound is received by the ear, is interpreted by the brain and a reaction is expressed by the use of words. Input of sound to the brain for storage, analysis, and association is done through the ear. Not to hear the human voice is not to develop the ability to speak. It is well established that individuals born with significant hearing loss are unable to develop oral communication naturally. Whereas normal hearing children learn language first, later applying rules, deaf children learn the rules of language first in order for linguistic competencies to be obtained. (p. 17)

The conservation and rehabilitation of hearing (and speech and language) become necessary tasks for educators, audiologists, and speech-language pathologists. We can drive home the point by noting (again) that it is not always obvious that even a relatively slight hearing loss can negatively affect the development of spoken language, literacy, and academic achievement (e.g., Ross, Brackett, & Maxon, 1982; see also, the discussions in Paul, 2009; Spencer & Marschark, 2006). *Audition*, the meaningful use of hearing (or residual hearing), plays a critical role in the internalization, storage, and retrieval of spoken-language information by individuals, which becomes evident during a variety of cognitive and linguistic functions (e.g., answering questions, drawing conclusions, reciting a poem, writing a paper, presenting on a topic, reading).

With respect to typical language development, the production and comprehension of speech occur after a reasonable growth of inner (or internalized) spoken-language structures (i.e., structures related to phonology, morphology, syntax, etc.). Inner language results from the process of relating incoming, meaningful auditory stimuli to appropriate kinesthetic, tactual, and visual images (e.g., Ling, 1989, 2002; Ross, 1986). The individual internalizes these stimuli via the use of auditory perceptual abilities. In other words, individuals possess the ability to attend to, discriminate, recognize, and retain sensory input.

In order to develop adequate auditory perceptual abilities, individuals need reasonably intact peripheral mechanisms of hearing. The peripheral mechanisms involve the outer, middle, and inner structures of the ear (see Chapter 2). Also critical is the proper functioning of the central nervous system mechanisms and the auditory cortical structures of the brain, which results in the transmission, integration, assimilation, and interpretation of incoming auditory stimuli.

In essence, the development of spoken-language structures requires, at the very least, the exploitation of reliable, consistent auditory/articulatory experiences at as early an age as possible. To prevent or minimize the condition of auditory sensory deprivation, educators and other professionals should promote and utilize early detection and intervention (e.g., see related discussions in Harrison, 2006a, 2000b; Spencer & Marschark, 2006). To understand the underlying components of intervention, professionals need knowledge of and skills in amplification systems (e.g., see Chapters 4 and 5); speech, language, and literacy (Chapters 6 and 7); and speechreading and auditory development (Chapter 8).

Speech, Hearing, and Literacy

Since the seminal work of Vickie Hanson (1989), there has been a growing awareness that the connections among speech, hearing, and the development of English literacy skills are often overlooked by many current speech-language pathologists, and even by those who become teachers/educators of d/Deaf and hard of hearing children. Consequently, a great deal of attention in speech and language intervention or therapy for d/Deaf and hard of hearing students in their formative educational years is placed on producing intelligible speech, rather than on relating the elements of speech (i.e., via phonemes, sounds) to the conditions of print (e.g., phoneme–grapheme relationships).

There is no question that intelligible speech is desirable; however, it is becoming clear that a *cognitive knowledge* (i.e., representation) *of speech sounds*, particularly as it relates to the alphabet, is a critical factor for the development of literacy skills. This cognitive knowledge requires adequate or reliable access to the sounds of speech (actually, the sound system of a language) either via the peripheral mechanisms of hearing or through alternative mechanisms based on vision and touch. However this is accomplished, it is crucial for children to access the phonological level of a spoken language in order to develop language proficiency.

Phonology represents the building blocks of a language, whether spoken or signed. Phonological access is also critical for acquiring other components of the English language, such as morphology (e.g., word parts), syntax (word order), and aspects of semantics (meaning). A good rendition of the above discussion can also be found in other texts on language development (e.g., Catts & Kamhi, 2005; Owens, 2004; Pence & Justice, 2008).

Before becoming too enamored with the importance of speech and hearing skills for English language and literacy development, keep in mind that phonological and phonemic awareness are not the same as speech perception. *Speech perception* is the ability to detect and discriminate sounds. Because of the overlap of processing between speech perception and hearing ability, children with severe-to-profound hearing loss may also have poor speech discrimination skills. Even some children with otherwise typical intact hearing may have difficulty discriminating among speech sounds. For a number of reasons, children who possess poor speech discrimination skills have difficulty acquiring phonological awareness.

All of this does not mean that we should not work on the development of speech awareness, perception, and discrimination; we need to keep in mind that something more is needed for phonological and phonemic awareness. In any case, a deep awareness of phonology is important for developing both English speech, language, and literacy skills. This may become even more apparent when one considers the strong relations between phonology and short-term memory (peripheral memory) (discussed in Chapter 7).

The link between the conversational and written forms of English is also important for students learning English as a second language. Second-language students, including ASL-using d/Deaf students, typically do not begin English literacy development possessing the same level of proficiency of the English language and culture as native first-language learners (e.g., see discussions in Bernhardt, 1991; Horwitz, 2008; Paul, 2009). In addition, most second-language students have difficulty understanding the linguistic aspects of written English, for example, vocabulary, syntax, and the alphabetic principle.

Thus, if we hope to improve the English language and literacy levels of students who are d/Deaf and hard of hearing, then we need to find more effective methods (technological and educational) to assist them in learning the connections between the phonemes of speech and the graphemes of print (as well as other components related to English literacy). It should come as no surprise that this inevitably means that professionals need to understand the underpinnings of the development of language, speech, and audition and the accompanying amplification aspects (e.g., hearing aids, cochlear implants, etc.).

Major Concepts

By now, you might have figured out all or most of the major concepts that are discussed in this text. We present a brief description of these concepts in the following paragraphs. We also show how the chapters are connected.

If we intend to make a case for hearing, as accomplished eloquently by Davis and Silverman (1978) more than 30 years ago, then it is relevant to discuss the anatomy and physiology of the auditory mechanism (in Chapter 2). We shall present introductory information on the nature and perception of sounds and the nature of hearing loss.

After exposure to and understanding of the basic information in Chapter 2, you will be ready to interpret and use an audiogram and to understand hearing evaluations and hearing losses—the focus of Chapter 3. Professionals need knowledge of the development and characteristics of the audiogram from start to finish or, metaphorically and literally, from top to bottom. Relating the audiogram to the selection of a hearing aid or other amplification device is a given. However, a clearer picture of the value of hearing and the presence of an audiogram should shed light on the challenges of developing speech and language, especially a phonemic language such as English.

Having a solid background of the audiogram and hearing evaluation should facilitate the understanding of issues in the next two chapters (Chapters 4 and 5) on hearing aids and cochlear implants. The basic information on hearing aids should definitely not go into one hearing aid and out the other!

With respect to knowledge about hearing aids, it is important for professionals to know how to troubleshoot these systems (e.g., check for problems; provide basic maintenance, such as changing a battery, etc.). Troubleshooting is absolutely mandatory for teachers of the d/Deaf and hard of hearing and speech-language pathologists given the potential for breakdowns and situations that are bound to occur during a typical school day, especially with young children.

Research and development on digital hearing aids has benefited from advances in cochlear implantation research. Nothing causes more controversy (actually lots of heat and not much light!) than this topic, especially research on cochlear implants and the development of speech, language, and literacy. Like it or not, in our view there is no turning back—which is often the case for assistive technological innovations. During the 1980s, cochlear implants were like the early Ford Model T—and there were only a few of them. Now, more and more children are having cochlear implantations, and the devices have become more sophisticated.

With universal newborn hearing screening in place and the improvement in technology, cochlear implants have become more accepted and useful for individuals with severe-to-profound hearing losses. Educators, clinicians, and other professionals not only need to know the structure and function of a cochlear implant, but also, like a hearing aid, they need to know how to troubleshoot the instrument. We present a synthesis of the salient research findings on cochlear implants in Chapters 5 and 6.

We then move on to an examination of the development of speech and language (Chapter 6). Readers are introduced to the production of speech and the stages of language development, including specific components such as phonology, morphology, syntax, semantics, and pragmatics. We also focus on the nature or pattern of speech errors in children who are d/Deaf or hard of hearing.

It might be an understatement to assert (actually, repeatedly in our case) that *hearing*, or audition, contributes to the development of English language and literacy (i.e., reading and writing skills). We have argued that phonology represents the building blocks of learning a language, especially a language based on sound. In Chapters 6 and 7, we intend to demonstrate this principle and to relate the component of phonology to the development of the other components of English and to English literacy.

We emphasize that phonological (as well as phonemic) awareness assists children in understanding the relations between sounds and letters for beginning reading acquisition. Professionals should understand that to master the alphabetic system, the system upon which English writing is based, children need a working knowledge of phonology, phonemic awareness, and phonics skills, as well as other reading-related competencies.

Another important concept, examined in Chapter 7, is that of working memory and its relation to reading. Finally, Chapter 7 presents alternative techniques of developing phonological awareness. This entails a discussion of techniques such as cued speech/language and visual phonics.

After completing Chapters 1 through 7, readers should have a sufficient background to understand the major concepts in Chapter 8; that is, the development of aural rehabilitation techniques or procedures, such as speechreading and auditory learning/training. Speechreading (also known as lip reading) refers to the process of understanding a spoken message by observing a speaker's face. Auditory learning/training refers to the use of techniques to assist children in their development of audition or the use of residual hearing. Both speechreading and auditory learning/training are critical for the development of speech production and speech reception abilities. In addition, both can contribute, indirectly, to the development of English literacy skills.

One of the most important areas for the habilitation and rehabilitation of hearing is age at identification, especially for the development and use of early intervention techniques (Chapter 9). In our view, universal newborn hearing screening should truly be universal; that is, for everyone on earth. In Chapter 9, we cover some of the basic tenets of early intervention, for example, tasks of early identification of hearing loss, early amplification, the involvement of parents, and the educational preparation of professionals (e.g., see Harrison, 2006a, 2006b; see also Yoshinaga-Itano, 2006).

We are aware that early amplification is a hotly contested issue, especially when the decision involves cochlear implants. Nevertheless, we feel that there is no greater important issue than early intervention, and we have little or no doubt that the growth and improvement in technology will minimize or resolve many of the conflicts associated with early identification and amplification.

In Chapter 10, we argue for a team approach involving the collaboration of professionals working with children and adolescents who are d/Deaf and hard of hearing. At the very least, we are concerned with this process for educators, educational audiologists, speech-language pathologists, and educational interpreters. Other professionals, such as those who provide occupational or physical therapy and other ancillary services, can be involved as needed.

Collaboration is the key to success. School professionals need to be willing to work together to ensure the most positive education experience for the child. Chapter 10 outlines the different professional roles that are involved in a d/Deaf or hard of hearing child's education. It also discusses how professionals can work together and what they should be offering to each other to foster an effective working relationship. No person is an island when it comes to serving the wide variety of needs of children and adolescents in the schools.

In Chapter 11, we reexamine the ongoing controversy on the development and use of speech and hearing for individuals who are d/Deaf and hard of hearing. In fact, after getting out our crystal ball, we present a few—perhaps, bold—surprises with our own reflections! Finally, the chapter offers a few recommendations for teacher education and clinical education programs in university settings.

Perspectives of the Authors

Our backgrounds are in education, both elementary education for typical children and deaf education, and audiology. We both favor the use of a traditional scientific approach, which involves some version of the scientific method (generating and testing hypotheses, analyses, etc.). We believe that there is such an entity as objectivity and that an adequate understanding of the world is possible via a dispassionate objective synthesis—similar to our attempts within the current text. We know that there is a bias in our integrative conceptual framework. Most likely, the bias cannot be removed completely, but it can and should be minimized via the use of the traditional scientific method.

We certainly have faith in the application of different research methods (e.g., quantitative as in the use of statistics or qualitative as in the use of case studies, ethnography, or critical analyses) as long as the undertaking of the study is rigorous and systematic. Whatever approach is used to develop theory and conduct research is acceptable as long as there is a reciprocal relation between theory and research; that is, theory building needs to yield to new research findings, which either support or refute aspects of the theory, and research thrusts should be guided, eventually, by well-grounded and well-developed theories. We also acknowledge that practice can inform theory and research as well as vice versa.

We are driven by our theoretical perspectives (e.g., cognitive and social theories), which guide our discussions of research, practice, and issues related to the development of speech, hearing, language, and literacy in English. We should emphasize that our heads are not only in the clouds (so to speak), but also in the classrooms and clinics. We are passionate about the desire to improve the educational and social welfare of children and adolescents who are d/Deaf and hard of hearing. Thus, we want to create a text that is useful and usable for students and perhaps reinvigorating for inservice professionals. Not only do we discuss research, but we also provide what we hope to be helpful examples and exercises related to the major concepts in this book. Our strongest bias is this: hearing is important if the goal is to acquire a spoken language such as English, including the ability to read and write in this language.

Summary of Major Points

Now that you have completed this chapter, we hope that you have found some possible answers to the questions that you developed at the beginning of the chapter. It might be that you need to read further in this text. If your questions did not get answered, then we encourage you to do additional reading and/or to dialogue with your instructor. The overall intent of this chapter was to provide a brief introduction to the major themes and concepts that are discussed in the rest of the text. The *Key Concepts* were as follows:

- Audiologic description of hearing acuity

- The importance of hearing and speech

- Major concepts in the book

- Perspectives of the authors

With respect to audiologic descriptions of hearing acuity, we remarked that

- Clinical descriptions employ the use of audiologic and linguistic dimensions such as degree of hearing loss, age at onset, etiology, location, presence of additional disabilities, and hearing status of parents/caregivers.

- Two of the long-standing factors that have influenced educational placement and other issues are degree of hearing loss and age at onset. Both were described in detail in this chapter.

With respect to the importance of hearing and speech, the following points were made

- Audition plays a critical role in the internalization, storage, and retrieval of spoken-language information by individuals, which becomes evident during a variety of cognitive and linguistic functions.

- With respect to typical language development, the production and comprehension of speech occur after a reasonable growth of inner (or internalized) spoken-language structures. Inner language results from the process of relating incoming, meaningful auditory stimuli to appropriate kinesthetic, tactual, and visual images. The individual internalizes these stimuli via the use of auditory perceptual abilities.

- The development of spoken-language structures requires, at the very least, the exploitation of reliable, consistent auditory/articulatory experiences at as early an age as possible. To prevent or minimize the condition of auditory sensory deprivation, educators and other professionals should promote and utilize early detection and intervention.

- It is becoming clear that a *cognitive knowledge* (i.e., representation) *of speech sounds*, particularly as it relates to the alphabetic system of English, is a critical factor for the development of literacy skills. This cognitive knowledge requires adequate or reliable access to the sounds of speech.

In our review of major concepts, it was highlighted that

- Professionals who work in fields such as deaf education, audiology, speech pathology, educational interpreting, and in other related fields need an adequate understanding of the contribution and rehabilitation of *hearing (and speech)* to the development of English, including English literacy skills.

■ With the advent of advanced amplification systems, early intervention, and the emerging focus on the importance of phonemic and phonological awareness for both English language and literacy development, there needs to be a reconceptualization of the contributions of hearing (i.e., audition) in the lives of professionals who serve children and adolescents, especially those with hearing losses.

■ Rehabilitation and alternative means are also important. These include speechreading, auditory learning/training, and the use of visual phonics and cued speech/language.

■ Increased collaboration is needed among the various professionals working with individuals who are d/Deaf and hard of hearing.

In the section on the authors' framework, it was remarked that the authors

■ Favor the use of the traditional scientific method, particularly for building upon previous research and for offering generalizations.

■ Believe in the concept of objectivity, especially via the use of an integrative conceptual framework (i.e., synthesis). Such scholarly endeavors—indeed, all scholarly endeavors—should continually be debated and tested in a scientific and/or logical manner.

Now that you have finished the first chapter, we think that you are ready for more. All of the major topics and themes introduced in this chapter are elaborated upon in the rest of the book. In the next chapter, we focus on the anatomy and physiology of the hearing mechanism.

Chapter Questions

Note: *Some answers to the questions can be found in the chapter; however, others have a variety of possible responses based on the students' backgrounds and experiences.*

1. What do you think is the significance of Davis and Silverman's passage at the beginning of the chapter? Does this passage provide a perspective on the question "What is deafness"? Do you think there is a God's-eye view (an all-encompassing description) of deafness that would satisfy all professionals? Why or why not?

2. List and describe, briefly, the two major views of deafness.

3. From this chapter, can you glean the authors' purpose for writing this text? Do you or your instructor agree with the need for current and preservice professionals to be more knowledgeable in these areas? Is this really a problem?

4. Describe, briefly, the five categories of hearing loss. What are the two most important factors in the audiologic description of deafness? Do you think it is important to be aware of these categories? Why or why not?

5. According to the authors, why are speech and hearing important? Can you relate this to the development of English literacy skills? Was the connection between hearing and speech and reading new for you?

6. In this chapter, we mentioned that phonology represents the building blocks of a language. What does this mean?

7. Select and describe three major concepts that are discussed in this text.

8. How would you describe the authors' framework for discussing the contributions of speech and hearing to the development of English? Is this similar to or different from your own mental framework? How is it similar or different?

9. If you had an opportunity to converse with the authors, what burning questions would you ask them? Share and discuss these questions with your instructor and classmates.

Challenge Questions

Note: *Complete answers are not in the text. Additional research/reading is required. In some cases, reading further or elsewhere in the text might provide some information to guide a response to a particular question.*

1. The authors mention that phonology represents the building blocks of any language. Does this mean that this can serve as the litmus test for all invented language/communication systems for d/Deaf and hard of hearing students (e.g., signed English; signing exact English; seeing essential English; cued speech/language, etc.)?

2. What are your current views on cochlear implants? Can you support your views with theoretical and/or research data? Do you think that advances in technology such as digital hearing aids or cochlear implants will eradicate the Deaf culture? Why or why not? Should d/Deaf children (younger than age 18) of hearing parents have the opportunity to benefit from such technology? Why or why not? Who should make this decision? [Note: We will ask this question or a related question a couple of times in this text!]

3. It has often been remarked that "there is no God's-eye view of deafness." What does this statement mean? Do you agree or disagree? Why? Do you think that this statement applies to all aspects of deafness, for example, the development of speech, hearing, language and literacy development, and so on? Why or why not?

Suggested Activities

1. If possible, plan a visit to the following locations:

   ■ A residential school for d/Deaf or hard of hearing students

   ■ Special classes in a public school for d/Deaf or hard of hearing students

   ■ A speech and hearing clinic

For the school placements, list the similarities and differences with respect to communication methods, instructional techniques, and approaches for developing speech, language, and hearing skills. Interview a few teachers and a few clinicians (in the speech and hearing clinic). Ask about their views on the development of speech, language, and hearing skills. Share your findings with your instructor and the rest of your class.

2. Make a list of the major journals in deaf education, Deaf studies, and speech and hearing science. Select a few recent journal issues and list the range of topics discussed in these publications. How many of the articles (i.e., what percentage) are related to the development of speech, language, or literacy skills? Share your findings with your instructor and the rest of your class.

References

Baker, C., & Cokely, D. (1980). *American Sign Language: A teacher's resource text on grammar and culture*. Silver Spring, MD: T. J. Publishers.

Bauman, H-D. (Ed.). (2008). *Open your eyes: Deaf studies talking*. Minneapolis, MN: University of Minnesota Press.

Bernhardt, E. (1991). *Reading development in a second language*. Norwood, NJ: Ablex.

Catts, H., & Kamhi, A. (2005). *Language and reading disabilities* (2nd ed.). Boston: Pearson/Allyn & Bacon.

Davis, H., & Silverman, S. R. (1978). *Hearing and deafness* (4th ed.). New York: Holt, Rinehart, & Winston.

Hanson, V. (1989). Phonology and reading: Evidence from profoundly deaf readers. In D. Shankweiler & I. Lieberman (Eds.), *Phonology and reading disability: Solving the reading puzzle* (pp. 69–89). Ann Arbor, MI: University of Michigan Press.

Harrison, M. (Ed.). (2006a). Early hearing detection and intervention: Trends, progress, and challenges. *The Volta Review, 106*(3).

Harrison, M. (2006b). Forward. *The Volta Review, 106*(3), 233–235.

Horwitz, E. (2008). *Becoming a language teacher: A practical guide to second-language learning and teaching*. Boston: Pearson/Allyn & Bacon.

Karchmer, M., Milone, M., & Wolk, S. (1979). Educational significance of hearing loss at three levels of severity. *American Annals of the Deaf, 124*, 97–109.

King, C., & Quigley, S. (1985). *Reading and deafness*. San Diego, CA: College-Hill Press.

Ladd, P. (2003). *Understanding Deaf culture: In search of Deafhood*. Buffalo, NY: Multilingual Matters.

Lane, H. (1992). *The mask of benevolence: Disabling the Deaf community*. New York: Vintage.

Lane, H., Hoffmeister, R., & Bahan, B. (1996). *A journey into the DEAF-WORLD*. San Diego, CA: DawnSign.

Ling, D. (1989). *Aural habilitation: The foundation of verbal learning in hearing-impaired children* (2nd ed.). Washington, DC: Alexander Graham Bell Association for the Deaf.

Ling, D. (2002). *Speech and the hearing-impaired child: Theory and practice* (2nd ed.). Washington, DC: Alexander Graham Bell Association for the Deaf.

Lovinger, S., Brandell, M., & Seestedt-Stanford, L. (1991). *Language learning disabilities: A new and practical approach for those who work with children and their families*. New York: Continuum.

McGuinness, D. (2004). *Early reading instruction: What science really tells us about how to teach reading*. Cambridge, MA: MIT Press.

McGuinness, D. (2005). *Language development and learning to read: The scientific study of how language development affects reading skill.* Cambridge, MA: MIT Press.

National Reading Panel. (2000). *Report of the National Reading Panel: Teaching children to read—An evidence-based assessment of the scientific research literature on reading and its implications for reading instruction.* Jessup, MD: National Institute for Literacy at EDPubs.

Owens, R. (2004). *Language disorders: A functional approach to assessment and intervention* (4th ed.). Boston: Pearson Education.

Paul, P. (1996). Is there a psychology of deafness? A critical metaanalysis. *BRIDGE: Bridging Research in Deaf and General Education, 15*(3).

Paul, P. (1997). A final reply to Harlan Lane. *BRIDGE: Bridging Research in Deafness and General Education, 15*(3), 8–11

Paul, P. (2001). *Language and deafness* (3rd ed.). San Diego, CA: Singular/ThomsonLearning.

Paul, P. (2009). *Language and deafness* (4th ed.). Sudbury, MA: Jones & Bartlett.

Paul, P., & Jackson, D. (1993). *Toward a psychology of deafness: Theoretical and empirical perspectives.* Needham Heights, MA: Allyn & Bacon.

Paul, P., & Quigley, S. (1990). *Education and deafness.* White Plains, NY: Longman.

Pence, K., & Justice, L. (2008). *Language development from theory to practice.* Upper Saddle River, NJ: Pearson/Merrill Prentice Hall.

Quigley, S., & Kretschmer, R. E. (1982). *The education of deaf children: Issues, theory, and practice.* Austin, TX: Pro-Ed.

Ross, M. (1986). *Aural habilitation.* Austin, TX: Pro-Ed.

Ross, M., Brackett, D., & Maxon, A. (1982). *Hard of hearing children in regular schools.* Englewood Cliffs, NJ: Prentice-Hall.

Schow, R., & Nerbonne, M. (2007). *Introduction to audiologic rehabilitation* (5th ed.). New York: Pearson/Allyn & Bacon.

Snowling, M., & Hulme, C. (Eds.). (2005). *The science of reading: A handbook.* Malden, MA: Blackwell.

Spencer, P., & Marschark, M. (Eds.). (2006). *Advances in the spoken language development of deaf and hard of hearing children.* New York: Oxford University Press.

Trezek, B., Wang, Y., & Paul, P. (2010). *Reading and deafness: Theory, research, and practice.* Clifton Park, NY: Delmar/Cengage Learning.

Wang, Y., Trezek, B., Luckner, J., & Paul, P. (2008). The role of phonology and phonological-related skills in reading instruction for students who are deaf or hard of hearing. *American Annals of the Deaf, 153*(4), 396–407.

Yoshinaga-Itano, C. (2006). Early identification, communication modality, and the development of speech and spoken language skills: Patterns and considerations. In P. Spencer & M. Marschark (Eds.), *Advances in the spoken language development of deaf and hard of hearing children* (pp. 298–327). New York: Oxford University Press.

Further Readings

Boothroyd, A. (1976). *The role of hearing in the education of the deaf.* Northampton, MA: Clarke School for the Deaf.

Marschark, M., & Spencer, P. (Eds.). (2003). *Handbook of deaf studies, language, and education.* New York: Oxford University Press.

Martin, F. (Ed.). (1987). *Hearing disorders in children: Pediatric audiology.* Austin, TX: Pro-Ed.

Stark, R. (Ed.). (1974). *Sensory capabilities of hearing-impaired children.* Baltimore, MD: University Park Press.

THE AUDITORY SYSTEM: ANATOMY, PHYSIOLOGY, AND IMPAIRMENT

The mystery of the majesty of creation is abundantly evident in the structure and function of the human hearing mechanism. Originating as a simple extension of a pressure-sensing organ in primitive sea creatures, the human hearing mechanism is a product of evolution, resulting in the development of a highly complex sensory system. . . . Great strides have been made in recent years toward a more thorough understanding of how the auditory system translates physical acoustic energy into neural impulses that are interpreted by the brain. However, the truth is that many questions remain to be answered concerning the precise biologic, mechanical, neurochemical, and electrical mechanisms and relationships that operate at all levels within the auditory system.

—Northern & Downs (2002, p. 33)

Key Concepts

After completing this chapter, you should have a basic understanding of:

- Anatomy and physiology of the ear
- Nature and perception of sound
- Nature of hearing loss

A few students, especially those in deaf education and interpreting programs, actually wonder about the value of a course on the science and psychology of hearing. In some cases, you can hear the moans and groans in university classrooms. Students might ask what they think are tricky or sneaky questions. For example, the instructor might encounter inquiries, such as: What is the value of studying hearing if one is working with *deaf* children (the word, *deaf*, is typically emphasized with a strong, loud voice)? How will learning about anatomy and physiology help me become a better teacher or clinician? What is the purpose of understanding the nature of sound, or even hearing loss?

We have highlighted these questions, among others, because, as you might have noticed, they are specifically related to the major themes of this chapter. It will take us the rest of this book to justify the importance of hearing (and speech) to the development of a spoken language such as English and its secondary form; that is, the reading and writing of print. It is easy to argue that hearing affects the communication process, especially if one is referring to the development of a spoken language. It might be more complicated to show that hearing also affects the development of reading and writing of a spoken language such as English or another phoneme-based language.

In any case, we think that Plack (2005) provides a coherent, convincing argument on why we should study the science and psychology of hearing:

> We study hearing to understand how the ear and the brain make sense of these stimuli....If we understand how the auditory system responds to sounds, then we can use that knowledge to help design sound-producing devices, such as telecommunication systems, entertainment systems, and devices that produce auditory alerts and warnings. Furthermore, we can use our knowledge . . . to design artificial devices that mimic aspects of this system, such as speech recognition programs that enable us to talk to our machines. Last but not least, this knowledge helps us to understand and treat hearing disorders.... The design of hearing aids is dependent upon perceptual research. (p. 2)

In addition to the questions just discussed, occasionally, one of us (Paul) has been asked: Which is worse—deafness or blindness? If one has a bilateral profound hearing loss (Paul) and is dependent on *seeing*, then deafness is an easy choice. You might be surprised to learn the response by Helen Keller (1902/1961), who was both deaf and blind by the age of 19 months: she preferred blindness over deafness. Why? Her remarks are a reflection of the difficulty of her communications/interactions with other humans due to her deafness. Keller remarked that blindness separates individuals from things, whereas deafness separates individuals from other people.

Hearing and seeing are both distance senses, and both are critical for learning. In fact, it is not difficult to find textbooks that expound on the range of challenges of children and adolescents who are either deaf (e.g., Marschark, 2007; Moores, 2001; Paul, 2009) or blind (e.g., Corn & Koenig, 1996). However, Plack (2005) states that in most undergraduate psychology courses (in England), "the study of hearing is neglected in favor of the study of vision" (p. 1). He maintains that this neglect is not justified because hearing is just as important as seeing.

One of the most amazing aspects of hearing is that if you have normal or adequate hearing you are never shut off from the world, so to speak. Even when you go to sleep at night, you are still connected via your ears, but not your eyes. In fact, we bet that you would find it uncomfortable (and perhaps frightening) if you used earplugs designed for hearing protection and tried to perform your typical daily activities. You might even become slightly depressed because of the missing, comforting elements of sound, even though the use of earplugs, if placed properly, would only result in a mild hearing loss.

So now you are thinking that the evolution of your ears for hearing must be a survival condition. Well—yes and no. First of all, the primary (or original) responsibility of the ear is to maintain equilibrium. The second responsibility is to capture sounds for the purposes of hearing (e.g., Moore, 2003; Northern & Downs, 2002). In essence, the sense of hearing has evolved or developed from the structures for balance; thus, your ears perform two major duties: hearing and the maintenance of balance.

It is a fascinating story to learn about the evolution of the anatomical structures of the human ear and its concomitant physiology or function (e.g., for additional details, see Moore, 2003; Northern & Downs, 2002; Zemlin, 1998). It is equally fascinating to learn about the development of the ear from the embryonic stage to birth and beyond. The anatomy, or structure, of the ear is developed and completed at birth (the external ear does grow in size in tandem with the rest of the body as it grows to adulthood, but the anatomical structures are all there at birth). However, the physiology, or function, of the auditory system continues to evolve throughout adolescence and is amendable to educational and medical interventions.

In this chapter, we provide a basic introduction to the anatomy and physiology of the ear as well as to the nature and perception of sounds and the nature of hearing loss. You will discover that as we move from the outer ear to the inner ear and up to the auditory processing system in the brain, our knowledge regarding both the structures and functions diminishes. Or, to put it another way, we have a long way to go in our understanding of the central auditory system.

As you read, think of a few questions to which you hope to find answers. Your questions should be related to the major themes of the chapter. For example, you might ask: What are the critical components of the ear? How does each contribute to the function of hearing? What is the nature of sound? What does it mean to perceive sound? What is the nature of hearing loss? If you wonder about the importance of hearing for language and literacy, then you will have to wait until the later sections of this book (e.g., Chapters 6 and 7). Consider this chapter the first step along the way on learning why we should study hearing.

Anatomy of the Ear

We shall aim for simplicity and borrow the organizational scheme used in several books on audiology (e.g., Moore, 2003; Plack, 2005; Zemlin, 1998). The ear can be divided into four parts: outer, middle, inner, and central. The outer ear contains structures of the pinna (or auricle), the ear canal (external auditory meatus), and one side of the eardrum (tympanic membrane). The middle ear begins with the air-filled cavity that is beyond the eardrum. This cavity contains three tiny bones (ossicles), the malleus, incus, and stapes, which are also popularly known as the hammer, anvil, and stirrup, respectively. We should throw in the Eustachian tube, because it starts in the middle ear and extends inward and downward into the upper part of the throat, also called the nasopharynx. The inner ear contains the cochlea and the auditory nerve (eighth [VIIIth] nerve). The central part of the ear involves brain structures responsible for coding auditory information, including structures and pathways from the brainstem to the cortex. Other structures associated with the major ones mentioned here are also included in the relevant sections below. The basic divisions of the ear are shown in **Figure 2-1**.

In addition to maintaining equilibrium, the overall function of the ear is to capture sounds from the environment and to change them into a form that can be interpreted by the brain (Davis, 1978; Moore, 2003; Northern & Downs, 2002; Plack, 2005; Schow & Nerbonne, 2007; Zemlin, 1998). As sound energy proceeds through the various parts of the ear, from outer to inner, it is converted into mechanical energy, electrical energy, and finally neural impulses on its way to the brain. The conversion of energy is called *transduction*, and this process occurs in a relatively simultaneous manner. Nevertheless, we can trace the conversion journey from the outer ear to the brain.

Before we proceed further, consider the following question: If a tree falls down in the forest and there is no human around to hear it, does it make a sound? It is not difficult to imagine, but this little quip and others have engendered a number of philosophical debates. We are not academic philosophers, so we will not engage you in a debate on the perception of an entity called *sound*. Rather, we simply want to discuss what happens when the sound is emitted from the fall of the tree (of course, we do not want you to stand too close to that tree!). But first, we need to provide more details on the anatomy of the ear.

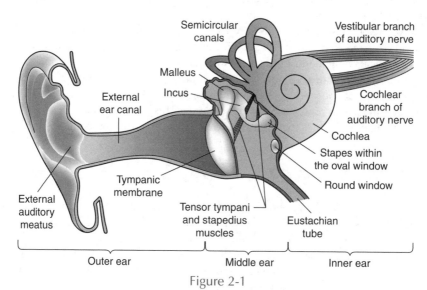

Figure 2-1

Basic Structures of the Ear

Image courtesy of Brad Ingrao, AuD.

OUTER EAR

As mentioned previously, the structures of the outer ear include the pinna (auricle), the ear canal (external auditory meatus), and the eardrum (tympanic membrane; however, some authors consider the eardrum as part of the middle ear). The pinna is the external flaplike structure (pliable cartilage framework) that is covered tightly with soft tissue (Davis, 1978; Maltby & Knight, 2000; Northern & Downs, 2002; Plack, 2005; Schow & Nerbonne, 2007; Zemlin, 1998). This is the structure upon which you hook your glasses, park your pencil, attach ear ornaments, and that is often the butt of a number of jokes (e.g., cauliflower ears; elephant ears, etc.). The pinna comes in a variety of shapes and sizes, often related to genetics.

In some animals, the pinna is highly developed and serves not only to gather and locate sounds, but also to keep foreign objects out of the ear canal (Davis, 1978; Northern & Downs, 2002; Plack, 2005; Schow & Nerbonne, 2007; Zemlin, 1998). One can marvel at animals in the rodent family or the feline family that can simply turn their pinnas without moving their heads to locate the source of a sound. Other animals (e.g., seals, moles) can actually manipulate their pinnas to close off their ear canal to prevent debris from entering.

In humans, the pinna plays a minor role with respect to hearing (Davis, 1978; Maltby & Knight, 2000; Northern & Downs, 2002; Plack, 2005; Schow & Nerbonne, 2007; Zemlin, 1998). It does help to localize and gather sounds and funnel them into the ear canal. However, this structure only contributes about 5 to 7 decibels (dB) for the perception of high frequencies (decibels and frequencies are discussed later in this chapter). We can do without our pinnas, for the most part, although we suspect that we might look a little odd. The artist Vincent Van Gogh certainly looked odd (or perhaps chic) with one pinna cut off, but it likely did not change his ability to hear.

The opening in the pinna, the concha, flows into the ear canal—the external auditory meatus. Like the pinna, the external auditory meatus varies from individual to individual in shape and size (Davis, 1978; Maltby & Knight, 2000; Northern & Downs, 2002; Plack, 2005; Schow & Nerbonne, 2007; Zemlin, 1998). The external auditory meatus is lined with skin.

The section of the canal nearest to the concha contains hair and glands. The glands secrete a substance called cerumen, also known as earwax. This cerumen is designed to moisturize and protect the ear canal. Both the hair and the wax combine to keep foreign objects out of the ear canal (albeit, a few young children manage to defy this natural process by putting things such as peas or beads in their ear canal). The ear canal extends and ends at the tympanic membrane (see Figure 2-1).

Because some authors (e.g., see discussions in Moore, 2003; Plack, 2005; Zemlin, 1998) consider the tympanic membrane to be part of the middle ear, we shall compromise: one side of the tympanic membrane is in the outer ear area and the other side is in the middle ear area. Or, if you like ambiguity, perhaps we should say that the eardrum divides the outer ear from the middle ear and is either a part of both or of neither. In any case, as is discussed later, the tympanic membrane is responsible, via a vibrating movement, for transmitting sound from the external ear canal to the three small bones (ossicles) in the middle ear.

MIDDLE EAR

Now we have arrived at the middle section of the ear. The middle ear includes the tympanic membrane, three tiny bones (ossicles), and an air-filled cavity. We should also include two tiny muscles that are attached to the malleus and the stapes, whose function we will explain later (Davis, 1978; Maltby & Knight, 2000; Northern & Downs, 2002; Plack, 2005; Schow & Nerbonne, 2007; Zemlin, 1998). Another structure that starts in the middle ear is the Eustachian tube.

The main function of the Eustachian tube is to ventilate the air-filled cavity. Ventilation equalizes pressures on both sides of the eardrum, which is often appreciated when traveling in an airplane or when trying to address the discomforts of a head cold. Typically, the Eustachian tube opens when an individual yawns or swallows.

Attached to the inner side of the tympanic membrane is the malleus (hammer), the first of the three tiny bones (ossicles). The malleus has a bulky upper end, which extends and fits into the socket of the incus (anvil), the second bone. The incus is connected to the head of the stapes (stirrup), the third bone. The ossicles are held in place—actually suspended in space so to speak—by two small muscles, the stapedius and tensor tympani, as well as by several ligaments (i.e., tough bands of tissue).

The base of the stapes is called the footplate, and this structure nestles into an opening called the oval window. As discussed later, sound enters the inner ear via the oval window. Just below the oval window is another membrane-covered opening called the round window. This window relieves the pressure of the fluid in the inner ear, which is set in motion by the vibrations of the oval window. Both the oval and round windows are "membrane-covered holes in the bony wall of the cochlea," a structure of the inner ear (Maltby & Knight, 2000, p. 3).

INNER EAR

One of the most interesting, complicated, and challenging parts of the ear is the inner ear. Let us label this component as all structures beyond the middle ear up to and including the auditory nerve (VIIIth nerve) (e.g., Moore, 2003; Northern & Downs, 2002; Plack, 2005; Zemlin, 1998). Salient structures of the inner ear are the cochlea, the semicircular canals, and the auditory nerve. In essence, the inner ear contains structures for hearing (e.g., cochlea) and balance (semicircular canals as part of the vestibular system; see Davis, 1978; Northern & Downs, 2002; Plack, 2005; Zemlin, 1998). The cochlea, from the Latin word for *snail*, which also describes the shape of this structure, is coiled for two and one-half turns and is about the size of a pea (Maltby & Knight, 2000). We can describe the cochlea as a thin coiled tube with the basal end next to the middle ear, specifically the oval window, and the apical end (peak of the coil) the farthest away.

The cochlea is divided along its length by two membranes; one of these is the basilar membrane. This creates three fluid-filled cavities with structures, as can be seen in **Figure 2-2**, which is a cross-sectional view of the cochlea. The scala media, the middle cav-

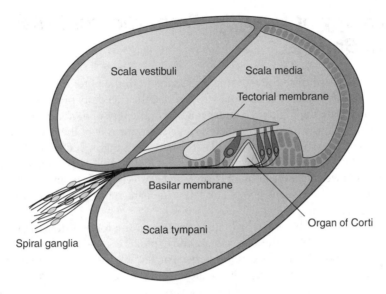

Figure 2-2
Cross-sectional View of the Cochlea
Image courtesy of Brad Ingrao, AuD.

ity, contains the basilar membrane and another important structure, the organ of Corti. The basilar membrane forms the floor of the scala media and the organ of Corti lies on top of it with the tectorial membrane just above it. The organ of Corti contains hair cells, which are crucial to the sensation of hearing. A more in-depth discussion of the cochlea and its intricate structures can be found elsewhere (e.g., Moore, 2003; Plack, 2005; Zemlin, 1998).

CENTRAL AUDITORY SYSTEM

Information flows through the auditory nerve via a chain of nuclei in the brainstem and then proceeds to the auditory cortex. The brain interprets the signal (frequency and intensity) based on the configuration (more on this later) sent from the cochlea and by the number of nerve impulses received. Needless to say, this interpretation is much more complicated than is presented here. Obviously, a better and deeper understanding of the structure and function of the cochlea (in the inner ear) should result in the development of a more efficient cochlear implant that can aid the brain in its interpretation of the electrical signal. In general, the implant is designed to bypass the damaged inner ear by sending electrical stimuli to the brain for interpretation. We explore cochlear implants in Chapter 5.

Physiology of Hearing: From the Outer Ear to the Brain

In this section, we trace the movement of sound from the outer ear to its interpretation by the brain. Of course, it is fairly easy to describe the trajectory from the outer ear to the inner ear. We are improving our understanding of the physiology of the inner ear, but we still have a long way to go to completely understand the role of the brain in the interpretation of auditory stimuli (see Davis, 1978; Maltby & Knight, 2000; Northern & Downs, 2002; Plack, 2005; Schow & Nerbonne, 2007; Zemlin, 1998). Tremendous progress has been made since the publication of *Hearing and Deafness* by Davis and Silverman (1978), which inspired the present book. The following paragraphs provide a basic tour of the physiology of hearing.

Let us return to the proverbial fall of the tree in the forest. After the tree slams the ground, the action causes the air to vibrate and to produce sound waves, which we can label as *acoustic energy*. The pinna, or the external ear, funnels the acoustic energy through the concha and into the external auditory meatus, which, in turn, amplifies the energy as it moves toward the tympanic membrane, or eardrum. The membrane of the eardrum oscillates; that is, it moves in and out in response to the changes in sound pressure. The movement of the eardrum changes the acoustic energy into mechanical energy as it enters the middle ear.

In the middle ear, the ossicles go to work. Basically, the three tiny bones amplify the sound pressure. For sounds of typical intensities (i.e., not too loud, such as normal conversational speech), the malleus and incus do their social dance by moving as a single unit in a rocking motion. Next, the stapes with its footplate comes into action by vibrating like a piston in and out of the oval window. This vibration causes the fluid in the inner ear to move, which is described as a hydraulic action.

Note that the tympanic membrane and the ossicles work together to transmit the acoustic energy into the inner ear, and this is not a trivial process. As aptly described by Plack (2005), the ossicles concentrate:

> the forces produced by the sound waves at the eardrum onto a smaller area (the *oval window* in the cochlea). Because pressure equals force divided by area, the effect of this transformation is to increase the pressure by a factor of about 20. The ossicles also act as a lever system, so that large, weak vibrations at the eardrum are converted into smaller, stronger vibrations at the oval window. Finally, the eardrum itself performs a buckling motion that increases the force of the vibrations and decrease the displacement and velocity. The overall effect of all these components is to increase the pressure at the oval window to around 20–30 times that at the eardrum. . . . (pp. 64–65)

Historically, it was believed that for sounds of high intensities (i.e., above 75 dB, such as very loud speech) and mostly below 1000 Hz (to be discussed later), the two small muscles in the middle ear—the stapedius and tensor tympani—collaborated to reduce the amount of sound energy in order to protect the ear. However, recent research suggests that this view is an oversimplification, because the reflex happens too slowly to actually be protective, particularly from impulsive sounds such as gunshots or explosions. Contraction of these two muscles may have a role in preventing acoustic overstimulation (Peng, Tao, & Huang, 2007). These muscles contract reflexively and stiffen the movements of the ossicles. This results in a less efficient transfer of energy to the inner ear because less fluid is being displaced.

The pathway that has been described for sound traveling through the auditory system is known as *air conduction* and is the most efficient method for sound transmission. There is a second route for sound transmission that requires sound to be transmitted to the inner ear via vibrations of the bony structures of the skull. This latter process is known as *bone conduction*, and it can be used to test hearing (as described in Chapter 3). Because bone conduction is extremely inefficient—it results in an enormous loss of energy—it does not contribute much to audition under typical hearing conditions. In other words, air conduction (the typical route) is most efficient and overrides any contributions from the other routes.

We are now in the inner ear, which houses the complex stages of hearing. Sound energy enters the cochlea through the oval window. The vibration of the stapes leads to a vibration of the basilar member (see Figure 2-2). Each section of the basilar membrane is responsive to a particular range of frequencies that are amplified as the sound wave rolls over the membrane. This selective responsiveness is known as *tonotopic organization* (a term that is discussed periodically in Chapter 5). At the basal end of the membrane, the higher frequencies are amplified, whereas the lower frequencies are amplified nearer the apical end. In general, the activity of the basilar membrane results in a shearing force that is applied to the hair cells in the organ of Corti. The shearing action produces neural impulses that are transmitted to the hearing center of the brain (see Northern & Downs, 2002; Plack, 2005; Zemlin, 1998 for a further discussion).

Nerve information leaves the cochlea through the nerve endings at the base of the hair cells and travels along a structure known as the auditory nerve (i.e., auditory pathway) to the brainstem (i.e., the central part of the ear). Nuclei between the auditory nerve and the auditory cortex in the brain process the auditory signals and transmit them to higher levels. The signals from each ear reach both hemispheres of the brain, but most information is transmitted to the opposite, or contralateral, side; that is, neural impulses from the right cochlea project predominantly to the left cortex and those from the left cochlea project predominantly to the right cortex. In general, the left hemisphere is considered to be specialized for language processing (see Northern & Downs, 2002; Plack, 2005; Zemlin, 1998).

The auditory cortex responds in an organized manner to the tones of the various frequency levels, again, having a tonotopic organization. After receiving and processing these impulses, the information is sent to other cortical areas and back to lower centers (even as far as back to the cochlea) for modulation purposes (see Moore, 2003; Northern & Downs, 2002; Plack, 2005; Zemlin, 1998).

As mentioned previously, the actions of the cochlea, including the basilar membrane, and the activity of the auditory cortex are not fully understood, and, indeed, are much more complicated than what has been described here. We shall borrow a few additional words again from Plack (2005) to end our physiology discussion:

> ...our degree of certainty about auditory processes declines from the peripheral to the central auditory system. We have a reasonable understanding of the transduction process, but we are still quite vague about how the auditory brainstem and the auditory cortex work. From a psychophysical perspective, as the stimuli and the processing become more complex, it becomes harder to relate our sensations to the characteristics of the sound waves entering our ears.... The difficulty is particularly acute with regard to high-level functions such as speech perception. (p. 238)

Nature of Sound

We promise not to become too philosophical in our discussion of the nature of sound (or even the perception of it). To obtain an adequate understanding of how hearing acuity is measured and evaluated, it is important to become familiar with some basic information. Let us begin with a question: What is sound?

Intuitively—and not to be funny—you probably think that sound means *noise*. Well, something can make a noise, but it might not be audible if the noise is not intense enough. It is better to think of sound, or rather the source of it, as movements from a vibrating body. In other words, a sound is produced by the vibrations of objects such as a guitar, a book hitting a wooden floor, a tree slamming the ground, and our voices. Each of the above objects vibrates, and the movement travels via a medium such as air (which is also caused to vibrate). Sound can travel via any type of medium—air, gas, liquid, or solid.

We may hear or feel these vibrations. Depending on our perceptions of the vibrations, we may interpret a particular sound as being high or low, loud or soft. If you stand near an amplifier at a rock concert, you can literally feel the sound pounding your body (and, yes, you may lose hearing from this experience, but we will save that for later). The word *vibration* is actually an interesting concept. Vibrations of objects produce sounds, and our hearing apparatus (eardrum, ossicles, cochlea, etc.) also vibrates in response to vibrations in order for us to hear and interpret the sounds. Sound is most intense at its original place of vibration, and it diminishes as it travels. [Question: How fast do you think sound travels in 1 second? Hint: It is a lot slower than the speed of light. Answer: Sound travels about 740 miles per hour; light travels about 186,000 miles per second, or 670 million miles per hour (Moore, 2003; Plack, 2005).]

Descriptions of sounds use objective terminology such as *waveform*, *frequency*, *intensity* or *pressure*, and *phase relations* (see Maltby & Knight, 2000; Northern & Downs, 2002; Plack, 2005). The simplest vibratory waveform is a sine wave, or sinusoid. Vibratory movements— oscillations or repetitive variations in time—are sinusoid in nature. We can label a simple sinusoid oscillation as a pure tone, as shown in **Figure 2-3**. Most sounds, such as speech, music, and environmental noises, are complex; that is, they vibrate in complicated recurring patterns. All complex sounds can be broken down into or analyzed by these simple

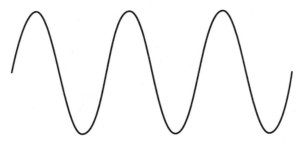

Figure 2-3
A Simple Sinusoid Oscillation (Pure Tone)
Image courtesy of Brad Ingrao, AuD.

component pure tones. Our focus here is on three physical terms: frequency, intensity, and phase.

FREQUENCY

Frequency refers to the number of recurring oscillations or cycles per unit of time, typically in 1 second (see Figure 2-3). The more vibrations (i.e., oscillations) per second, the higher the frequency. So, for example, if there is a movement of 2000 oscillations per second, then this movement is described as oscillating at 2000 cycles per second. The frequency is 2000. Because a frequency of 1 cycle per second is known as a hertz (Hz), a frequency of 2000 is oscillating at 2000 Hz per second. The term *hertz* is named in honor of the German physicist Heinrich Hertz, whose theoretical work in the area of electromagnetic waves eventually led to the development of the radio (Davis, 1978).

INTENSITY

Intensity refers to the pressure of the sound (remember the amplifier at the rock concert mentioned previously?). The vibration that produces pressure is the result of an applied force (i.e., *energy*) over a given area. Sound is an alternating pressure that exerts force in opposite directions (see Northern & Downs, 2002; Plack, 2005; Zemlin, 1998). In essence, the intensity of a sound represents the magnitude of the vibration in a sound wave.

Intensity is measured in decibels (dB), which is one-tenth of a bel. The unit *bel* is named after Alexander Graham Bell, the famous teacher of d/Deaf and hard of hearing children, whose research into electrical transmission of sound resulted in the development of the telephone (Davis, 1978; Northern & Downs, 2002). The decibel scale is a ratio scale; that is, it reflects whether a particular unit is greater or lesser than another unit. It is also a logarithmic scale. Each logarithmic unit represents a 10-fold increase (using a base 10).

When talking about measuring hearing, HL, or hearing level, is used to define the reference to the decibel. HL refers to decibel levels when compared to a large group of normal

7

hearing individuals. For sounds of similar frequency levels, a sound level of 10 dB HL has 10 times more intensity than a sound that is barely audible (i.e., 0 dB HL). Each 10 dB increment represents a 10-fold increase in intensity. A 20 dB HL sound is 100 times as intense as a barely audible sound, whereas a 30 dB HL sound is 1000 times as intense.

What is the intensity of a 40 dB HL sound compared to a barely audible sound (0 dB HL)? (Note this is 10^4, or 10,000 times, more intense than a barely audible sound. And you thought algebra was useless.). How about a 50 dB HL sound? (By now, you know this is 10^5, or 100,000 times, as intense as a barely audible sound). Have you wondered about the rock concert in which sound can be amplified to about the 120 dB HL level? The sound pressure levels of a few common sounds are presented in **Table 2-1**.

Table 2-1

Decibel (HL) Levels of a Few Common Sounds

Description	Decibels (dB HL)	Sound Source
Pain	140	Shotgun blast
Discomfort	130	Jet taking off
	120	Loud music
	110	
	100	Lawnmower
	90	
	80	Cocktail party
	70	
Conversational speech	60	
	50	
	40	
	30	Inside library
Whisper (5 feet)	20	
	10	
Threshold of hearing (1000 Hz)	0	

Source: Data based on Bess & McConnell (1981).

PHASE

Before moving on to a discussion of the perception of sound, we should briefly discuss one more concept—*phase*. We have described a simple sinusoid oscillation as a pure tone. Keep in mind that a sound wave consists of a series of compressions (i.e., points or areas of increased pressure) and rarefactions (i.e., points or areas of decreased pressure) (e.g., see Moore, 2003; Plack, 2005). Thus, the phase of a pure tone refers to the area or point of its progression in a cycle. The compression and rarefaction phases of a pure tone are depicted in **Figure 2-4**. Plack (2005) states that "The phase of a pure tone is the point reached on the pressure cycle at a particular time" (p. 11).

Now let us suppose that there are two pure tones, and we can consider two similar waveforms similar to the one illustrated in Figure 2-4. If these two pure tone waveforms have the same starting phase, amplitude, and frequency, we can state that they are in phase and will be heard at the same time (so to speak). As this occurs, the two waveforms combine in a constructive manner to produce "a larger amplitude waveform of the same frequency, i.e., perceived as louder than its constituents" (Maltby & Knight, 2000, p. 17; see also, Moore, 2003; Plack, 2005). We can illustrate this graphically, as shown in **Figure 2-5**.

An interesting situation occurs when two waveforms are out of phase. This can occur in an infinite number of scenarios; however, here we shall focus on when one pure tone waveform is delayed by half a cycle (actually, 180 degrees). The peak of one pure tone will

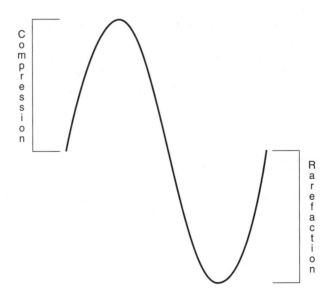

Figure 2-4
The Compression and Rarefaction Phases of a Pure Tone
Image courtesy of Brad Ingrao, AuD.

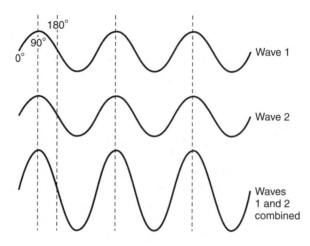

Figure 2-5
Two Waveforms in Phase

Image courtesy of Brad Ingrao, AuD.

coincide with the dip of another one, producing what is called a *phase cancellation* (e.g., Moore, 2003; Plack, 2005); that is, the peaks and dips will work together. The result of this phase cancellation is that there is no sound, as shown in **Figure 2-6**.

Phase cancellation can cause problems in free field testing with the use of pure tones (in a sound booth to test hearing) and is addressed by using a special modification of the pure tone called a *warble tone*. However, the principle is useful in that it can be used with digital hearing aids to minimize acoustic feedback (a whistling sound) or with headphones to cancel out background noises (e.g., Moore, 2003; Plack, 2005). Thus, the concepts of phase and phase cancellation are critical in the development of listening or amplification devices.

Perception of Sound

The human ear perceives frequency of sound as pitch and the intensity of sound as loudness (see Davis, 1978; Maltby & Knight, 2000; Northern & Downs, 2002; Plack, 2005; Schow & Nerbonne, 2007; Zemlin, 1998). With respect to frequency, there is a range from low (i.e., bass) to high (i.e., treble). The higher the frequency of a sound, the higher the perception of pitch. The ear is capable of perceiving fairly minute differences in frequency, and perception ranges from about 20 to 20,000 Hz.

Have you ever wondered about the frequency range of a dog whistle? Obviously, the frequency is above 20,000 Hz and cannot be perceived by the human ear. It must be an interesting philosophical moment to blow on this apparatus and hear nothing while your dog lets you know that he or she hears it quite clearly!

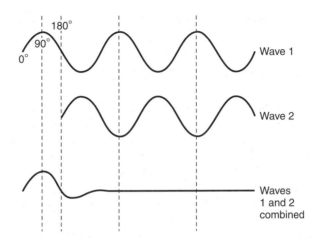

Figure 2-6
Phase Cancellation from Two Waveforms Not in Phase
Image courtesy of Brad Ingrao, AuD.

The ear cannot hear all frequency levels equally well. It is most sensitive to tones of 1000 Hz (i.e., 1000 cycles per second). Sound perceived at this frequency can be heard at a lower intensity than sounds presented at higher or lower frequencies. Most of the important information for speech occurs between 500 and 4000 Hz, and this is the range used to determine pure tone averages (see Northern & Downs, 2002; Zemlin, 1998).

With respect to loudness, the more intense the sound, the louder it is perceived. As indicated in Table 2-1, the upper comfortable level of intensity seems to be at the conversational speech range, albeit a few individuals are extremely sensitive to this level (i.e., typical speech is too loud for them). Anything more intense than conversational speech moves into the annoying stage, and anything higher than that moves into the discomfort and painful stages.

The hearing of sounds also involves perception of phase or time (temporal) relations (see earlier discussion of phases). The frequencies and intensities of sounds vary from moment to moment. The perception of these sounds is contingent on rhythm (i.e., ordered alternation of weak and strong stress patterns) and tempo (i.e., rate, or speed, of movements). Even more interesting and important are the contributions of rhythm and tempo to the development of the suprasegmentals of phonology, which is critical for the development of both language and literacy, as discussed later in this text (e.g., see Chapters 6 and 7).

Finally, as indicated previously, an adequate understanding of how the ear perceives and understands sounds is critical for our development of any kind of listening, assistive listening, or other auditory devices, such as amplifiers, hearing aids, entertainment devices, and cochlear implants (see Northern & Downs, 2002; Plack, 2005; Zemlin, 1998). One prominent scholar calls these amplification and listening devices *practical applications,* because they are based on our understanding of the psychology of hearing (e.g., Moore, 2003).

The Acoustics of the Environment

It is obvious that we live in a noisy world; nevertheless, it is extremely important to pay attention to the acoustics of the environment—especially classrooms in schools. Although standards that apply to new school buildings have been upgraded, most schools are not generally reflective of good listening situations. Walk down the hallway of any school building and you cannot help but notice the overall level of noise or reverberation, the persistence of the sound after the original sound has been presented, which might be perceived as an echo. Environmental noise can have a negative impact on listening for everyone, but it interferes the most with the listening and learning capabilities of children and adolescents (e.g., see discussions in Berg, 1993; Flexer, 1999).

Basically, we can divide noise into two areas: external and internal. *External noise* refers to those stimuli outside of the school and outside of the classroom. Depending on the location, a school may be affected by automobile or airplane traffic or by construction and other extraneous noises in the neighborhood. Stimuli outside the classroom include those resulting from the infrastructure of the school building, which may also reflect the infrastructure of the classroom. Our focus in this section is on two important conditions: signal-to-noise ratio and reverberation within the classroom.

SIGNAL-TO-NOISE RATIO

Every classroom has background noise, which may arise in the classroom (e.g., the heating system or the noise from children themselves) or outside of the classroom (even with the door closed). This background noise interferes with the teacher's voice and other students' voices, which are the important signals. Essentially, the classroom dialogue comprises the signal, but the teacher's voice should be considered as critical for instructional purposes.

The sound level difference between, for example, the teacher's voice and the background noise is labeled the *signal-to-noise ratio*, often abbreviated as SNR, and is referenced in decibels. A positive SNR suggests that the signal is more intense than the background noise; conversely, a negative SNR suggests that the background noise is more intense than the signal. So if the teacher's voice is at a 60 dB level and the background noise level is at 50 dB, then there is a +10 dB SNR (e.g., see discussions in Berg, 1993; Flexer, 1999). Suppose a teacher's voice is at 60 dB, and the background noise level is at 80 dB. Then, the SNR is –20 dB, which is definitely a problem, because the background noise is significantly more intense than the teacher's voice. There have been many discussions of children with normal hearing requiring a +6 to +10 dB SNR to maximize hearing in the classroom, with children with hearing loss requiring a +12 to +20 dB SNR in order to optimize auditory communication (e.g., see discussions in Berg, 1993; Flexer, 1999). However, this ratio is rarely accomplished in most school classrooms. In fact, research has indicated that school classrooms have a –7 to +5 dB SNR.

The use of hearing aids (see Chapter 4) does not resolve the problem, because many hearing aids amplify both background noise and speech. This means that the hearing aid amplifies all acoustic information equally. Some interesting new techniques and controls have been developed to address noise cancellation and control in hearing aids (see Chapter 4), but there are still limits to what a hearing aid can do.

REVERBERATION

Reverberation refers to the repetitions and extensions of reflected sounds (e.g., Berg, 1993; Flexer, 1999). As described by Mendel, Danhauer, and Singh (1999), reverberation is "the persistence of a sound in an enclosed space as a result of multiple reflections after the sound source has stopped; the amount of echo in the room; the more reverberatant the room, the poorer the speech-to-noise ratio and the less intelligible the speech" (p. 223).

Some reverberation in the environment is good, because it enhances sound quality. However, high levels of reverberation can interfere with understanding speech, particularly if there is a high level of background noise. In general, high-frequency sounds are absorbed by objects in the classrooms (e.g., carpets, etc.), whereas low-frequency sounds continue to be reflected (e.g., Plack, 2005). It is helpful to use carpets, curtains, and so on to absorb sounds in the classroom. Unfortunately, reverberation also occurs externally to the classroom, and closing the door may not help.

To create an environment conducive to learning, it is critical to reduce the noise level, both inside and outside the classroom. This becomes a critical issue for schools that house both children with typical hearing and those with hearing losses. It is axiomatic that noise can interfere with the development of speech and language for *all* children, not just for children with a hearing loss.

NATURE OF HEARING IMPAIRMENT

In Chapter 1, we discussed two major aspects of the nature of hearing impairment: degree of impairment and age at onset. The various levels and a few educational implications were presented in Table 1-1. In this section, we focus on the nature of hearing impairment with respect to location. Again, this is only a brief introduction, and the reader is referred elsewhere for more in-depth discussions (e.g., Bess & McConnell, 1981; Davis, 1978; Northern & Downs, 2002).

All hearing losses or disorders can be classified into two broad areas: exogenous and endogenous. *Exogenous disorders* are those caused by factors such as disease, toxicity, or accident or injury resulting from noise or damage to part of the auditory system. *Endogenous disorders* are conditions that occur as a result of genetics; for example, a hearing defect may be transmitted to a child as an inherited trait. Note that not all auditory disorders that are present at birth are hereditary. Conversely, not all hereditary disorders are present at birth (see Bess & Humes, 1995; Bess & McConnell, 1981; Davis, 1978; Northern & Downs, 2002).

In the following paragraphs, we briefly describe four types of hearing impairment with respect to location: conductive, sensorineural, mixed, and central. This discussion is extended further and related to the audiogram in Chapter 3. In Chapter 3, we also present information on commonly occurring hearing disorders (see Table 3-1).

CONDUCTIVE LOSSES

In general, conductive losses pertain to malfunctions or abnormalities of the outer and middle ear (see Bess & Humes, 1995; Bess & McConnell, 1981; Davis, 1978; Northern & Downs, 2002). Examples include the absence of a pinna or a pinna that is gathering sounds in an inefficient manner due to structural abnormalities of the pinna or the external auditory meatus. The external auditory meatus may be obstructed or filled with debris.

Hearing loss can result if the tympanic membrane or the ossicles experience restriction in their movements or are immobile (e.g., as in otitis media). This can cause an inefficient or an incomplete transfer of energy to the inner ear. It is even possible for the cochlea or the basilar membrane in the inner ear to experience physical changes, which result in an inefficient or incomplete transfer of information to the hair cells. Most conductive losses are medically treatable.

SENSORINEURAL LOSSES

We think Davis' (1978) description of a sensorineural loss is as accurate today as it was in 1978: sensorineural losses refer to damage to a "...sensory unit...; that is, an auditory nerve fiber plus the hair cell or cells that excite it" (p. 95). This type of damage may occur in the cochlea (and may or may not involve the hair cells), the auditory nerve, or, in most cases, a combination of both; it may even involve the central auditory system (Bess & McConnell, 1981; Meyerhoff, 1986). Sensorineural hearing impairments are generally not medically reversible. To remedy this condition, substantial improvements have been made in the development and use of amplification devices, such as hearing aids and cochlear implants, discussed in Chapters 4 and 5, respectively.

MIXED LOSSES

Sensorineural losses can occur concomitantly with conductive malfunctions or abnormalities, causing hearing loss involving both the outer or middle ear and the inner ear. This combination of conductive and sensorineural hearing impairments is considered as a *mixed hearing loss*. It can happen for a number of reasons, including a genetic hearing loss, which is generally permanent, or a sensorineural hearing loss that develops as a middle ear infection and results in a temporary decrease in hearing acuity.

CENTRAL LOSSES

One of the most challenging and still relatively poorly understood types of hearing loss is what might be characterized as a central loss, more commonly referred to as an *auditory processing disorder* (APD). This type of loss involves impaired perception of auditory information that occurs in the central auditory nervous system, involving the auditory nerve pathways from the brainstem to the auditory cortex. Central hearing disorders can occur concurrently with sensorineural losses; however, in most cases, they are defined by having normal peripheral hearing acuity in the face of auditory difficulties, such as difficulty hearing in less than optimal environments. Readers should consult others sources for more details on these types of disorders (e.g., Bellis, 2003; Parthasarathy, 2005).

Summary of Major Points

Now that you have survived this chapter—which should probably be renamed *Science and Psychology of Hearing 101*—we hope that we have stimulated your interest in this area and that you now understand why the study of hearing is important. In addition, we hope that you have obtained a few answers to questions that you had at the beginning of the chapter. If your questions did not get answered, then we encourage you to do further reading and/or to dialogue with your instructor.

Our goal in this chapter was to provide a brief introduction to the following *Key Concepts*:

- Anatomy and physiology of the ear
- Nature and perception of sound
- Nature of hearing loss

With respect to the anatomy of the ear, the following general points were made

- The outer ear includes the pinna (or auricle), ear canal (external auditory meatus), and eardrum (tympanic membrane; i.e., one side of the eardrum).
- The middle ear begins with the air cavity that is beyond the eardrum (one side) and contains three tiny bones (ossicles): the malleus, incus, and stapes, which are popularly known as the hammer, anvil, and stirrup, respectively.
- The inner ear contains the cochlea and involves the auditory (VIIIth) nerve.
- The central ear includes the auditory central processing system in the brain.
- In addition to maintaining equilibrium, the overall function of the ear is to capture sounds from the environment and to change them into a form that can be interpreted by the brain.

With respect to the physiology of the ear, it was remarked

- The pinna plays a minor role with respect to hearing. It helps to localize and gather sounds and funnel them into the ear canal. The pinna only contributes about 5 to 7 dB for the perception of high frequencies.
- The eardrum membrane oscillates in response to the changes in sound pressure and converts acoustical energy into mechanical energy as it enters the middle ear.

- The ossicles amplify the sound pressure. Eventually, the vibration from the stapes causes the fluid in the inner ear to move in a hydraulic action.

- In the inner ear, the activity of the basilar membrane results in a shearing force that is applied to the hair cells in the organ of Corti. The shearing action produces neural impulses that are transmitted to the hearing center of the brain.

- The auditory cortex responds in an organized manner to the tones of the various frequency levels. After receiving and processing these impulses, the information is sent to other cortical areas and even back to lower centers of the brain and the inner ear for modulation purposes.

With regard to the nature and perception of sound

- Sound is produced by the vibrations of objects. Each object vibrates, and the movements travel via a medium such as air (which is also caused to vibrate). Sound can travel via any type of medium—air, gas, liquid, or solid.

- Sound is most intense at its original place of vibration, and it diminishes as it travels.

- The simplest vibratory waveform is a sine wave, or sinusoid. Vibrations—oscillations, or up-and-down movements—are sinusoid in nature.

- Frequency refers to the number of recurring oscillations or cycles, per unit of time, typically in 1 second.

- Intensity refers to the pressure of the sound. The vibration that produces pressure is the result of an applied force (i.e., energy) over a given area. Intensity is measured in decibels (dB).

- The phase of a pure tone refers to the area or point of its progression in a cycle.

- The human ear perceives frequency of sound as pitch and the intensity of sound as loudness.

- The ear cannot hear all frequency levels equally well. It is most sensitive to 1000 Hz tones.

- Most of the important information for speech occurs between 500 and 2000 Hz, and this range is used to determine pure tone averages.

- The hearing of sounds involves perception of phase or time relations. The frequencies and intensities of sounds vary from moment to moment. The perception of these sounds is contingent on rhythm (i.e., ordered alternation of weak and strong stress patterns) and tempo (i.e., rate, or speed, of movements).

- The sound level difference between, for example, a teacher's voice and a background noise is the signal-to-noise ratio (SNR) and is recorded in decibels.

- Reverberation refers to the persistence of sound as a result of multiple reflections in an enclosed space after the original sound source has ended.

Considering the nature of hearing loss

■ Conductive losses pertain to malfunctions or abnormalities of the outer and middle ear.

■ Sensorineural losses refer to damage to a sensory or neural unit.

■ Sensorineural losses can occur concomitantly with conductive malfunctions or abnormalities, which occurs in the middle or inner ear or both. This combination of conductive and sensorineural hearing impairments is a mixed hearing loss.

■ One of the most challenging and still relatively poorly understood types of hearing losses is a central hearing loss, also known as an auditory processing disorder (APD). This type of loss involves problems in the central auditory nervous system.

Now that you have a good, basic understanding of the science and psychology of hearing, you are ready to learn about the measurement of hearing, which is the topic of Chapter 3. Do not forget what you have learned with respect to frequencies and decibels; more will be said about these terms and others in the next chapter.

Chapter Questions

Note: *Some answers to the questions can be found in the chapter; however, others have a variety of possible responses based on the students' backgrounds and experiences.*

1. At the beginning of this chapter, the authors attempted to make a case for the study of the science and psychology of hearing. What are their reasons? Is this case convincing to you as a preservice or inservice teacher, interpreter, or clinician? Why or why not? If not, what additional information do you think you need?

2. What are the primary and secondary functions of the ear with respect to evolution?

3. Discuss the anatomy of the ear in relation to four major parts or divisions. Be sure to discuss some of the salient structures in each part or division.

4. Discuss the physiology of the major structures of the ear; that is, what are the roles of the structures in the transfer and perception of sound? Take this from the outer ear to the auditory center in the brain.

5. The authors mentioned briefly one inefficient route for the transfer of sound in the ear. Describe the route.

6. Describe the following terms related to sound:

   a. Waveform

   b. Frequency

   c. Intensity

     d. Phase

     e. Phase cancellation

7. What are a few salient points in the section titled "Perception of Sound"?

8. With respect to the acoustics of the environment, describe the following terms:

     a. Signal-to-noise ratio

     b. Reverberation

9. Describe the four types of hearing impairment with respect to location.

10. If you had an opportunity to converse with the authors, what burning questions would you ask them? Share and discuss these questions with your instructor and classmates.

Challenge Questions

Note: *Complete answers are not in the text. Additional research/reading is required. In some cases, reading further or elsewhere in the text might provide some information to guide a response to a particular question.*

1. In this chapter, it was stated that a better and deeper understanding of the structure and function of the cochlea may result in the development of a more efficient implant that can aid the brain in its interpretation of the electrical signal. Why do you think this is the case?

2. The chapter mentions that hearing affects the development of reading and writing of a spoken language, such as English or other phoneme-based languages. Can you briefly discuss your views on this so far? [Note: Additional information can be gleaned from the contents of Chapter 7.]

3. In the section "Acoustics of the Environment," it was stated that the SNR is also critical for children with typical hearing for whom English is a second language; indeed, it is critical for all children. Why do you think this is true?

Suggested Activities

1. This is an activity to simulate hearing impairment or hearing loss. Use caution while engaging in activities (for some activities, you may want to bring someone along with you). Obtain a pair of earplugs used for hearing protection and place them in your ears as directed (often, these are small foam plugs that are rolled and then placed in the ear canal). Perform the following with the earplugs:

    ■ Watch television with and without captions.

    ■ Order a meal at a restaurant with friends or family members.

- Converse with friends and family members (more than three people).

- Purchase an item in a store and engage in a brief conversation with the clerk or cashier.

Share your findings and feelings with your instructor and the rest of your classmates.

2. Interview teachers of d/Deaf or hard of hearing children and ask them how they feel about courses in speech and hearing science (audiology, speech pathology, etc.). Did they take such courses as part of their educational program? Why or why not? Do they feel that such courses were helpful in their careers? Why or why not? Share your findings with your instructor and/or the rest of your classmates.

3. Research the literature or search the Internet to obtain the names of professionals (including medical professionals) in the area of speech and hearing science. List their major responsibilities. We shall start the list for you:

Audiologists: American Academy of Audiology (www.audiology.org)

Major responsibilities of audiologists:

- Prescribe and fit hearing aids.

- Assist in cochlear implant programs.

- Perform ear- or hearing-related surgical monitoring.

- Design and implement hearing conservation programs and newborn hearing screening programs.

- Provide hearing rehabilitation training, such as auditory training, speechreading, and listening skill improvement.

Speech-language pathologists: American Speech-Language-Hearing Association (www.asha.org)

Major responsibilities of speech-language pathologists:

- Evaluate and diagnose speech, language, cognitive-communication and swallowing disorders.

- Treat speech, language, cognitive-communication, and swallowing disorders in individuals of all ages, from infants to the elderly.

References

Bellis, T. J. (2003). *When the brain can't hear: Unraveling the mystery of auditory processing disorder*. New York: Atria.

Berg, F. (1993). *Acoustics and sound systems in schools*. San Diego, CA: Singular.

Bess, F., & Humes, L. (1995). *Audiology: The fundamentals* (2nd ed.). Baltimore: Williams & Wilkins.

Bess, F., & McConnell, F. (1981). *Audiology, education, and the hearing-impaired child*. St. Louis, MO: Mosby.

Corn, A., & Koenig, A. (Eds.). (1996). *Foundations of low vision: Clinical and functional perspectives.* New York: American Foundation for the Blind.

Davis, H. (1978). Anatomy and physiology of the auditory system. In H. Davis & S. R. Silverman, *Hearing and deafness* (4th ed., pp. 46–83). New York: Holt, Rinehart, & Winston.

Davis, H., & Silverman, S. R. (1978). *Hearing and deafness* (4th ed.). New York: Holt, Rinehart, & Winston.

Flexer, C. (1999). *Facilitating listening and hearing in young children* (2nd ed.). San Diego, CA: Singular.

Keller, H. (1902/1961). *The story of my life.* New York: Dell.

Maltby, M., & Knight, P. (2000). *Audiology: An introduction for teachers and other professionals.* London: David Fulton.

Marschark, M. (2007). *Raising and educating a deaf child: A comprehensive guide to the choices, controversies, and decisions faced by parents and educators* (2nd ed.). New York: Oxford University Press.

Mendel, L., Danhauer, J., & Singh, S. (1999). *Singular's illustrated dictionary of audiology.* San Diego, CA: Singular.

Meyerhoff, W. (1986). *Disorders of hearing.* Austin, TX: Pro-Ed.

Moore, B. C. J. (2003). *An introduction to the psychology of hearing* (5th ed.). Boston: Academic Press.

Moores, D. (2001). *Educating the deaf: Psychology, principles, and practices* (5th ed.). Boston: Houghton-Mifflin.

Northern, J., & Downs, M. (2002). *Hearing in children* (5th ed.). Baltimore, MD: Lippincott Williams & Wilkins.

Parthasarathy, T. K. (Ed). (2005). *An introduction to auditory processing disorders in children.* New York: Erlbaum.

Paul, P. (2009). *Language and deafness* (4th ed.). Sudbury, MA: Jones & Bartlett.

Peng, J. H., Tao, Z. Z., & Huang, Z. W. (2007). Long-term sound conditioning increases distortion product otoacoustic emission amplitudes and decreases olivocochlear efferent reflex strength. *Neuroreport, 18*(11), 1167–1170.

Plack, C. (2005). *The sense of hearing.* Mahwah, NJ: Erlbaum.

Schow, R., & Nerbonne, M. (2007). *Introduction to audiologic rehabilitation* (5th ed.). New York: Pearson/Allyn & Bacon.

Zemlin, W. (1998). *Speech and hearing science: Anatomy and physiology* (4th ed.). Boston: Allyn & Bacon.

Further Readings

Berg, F. (1972). *Educational audiology: Hearing and speech management.* New York: Grune & Stratton.

Boothroyd, A. (1982). *Hearing impairment in young children.* Englewood Cliffs, NJ: Prentice Hall.

Martin, F. (1986). *Introduction to audiology* (3rd ed.). Englewood Cliffs, NJ: Prentice Hall.

Stach, B. (2008). *Clinical audiology: An introduction.* San Diego, CA: Singular.

Audiologic Evaluation

*The purpose of testing hearing is to aid in the process of making deci-
sions regarding the type and extent of the patient's hearing loss.
Because some of these decisions may have profound effects on the
patient's medical, social, educational, and psychological status, accurate performance and careful interpretation of hearing tests are
mandatory. The reliability of any test is based on the interrelation-
ships among such factors as calibration of equipment, test environment, patient performance, and examiner sophistication. In the final
analysis, it is not hearing that we measure but, rather, responses to
a set of acoustic signals that we interpret as representing hearing.*

—Martin & Clark (2009, p. 77)

Key Concepts

After completing this chapter, readers should have a basic understanding of:

- Hearing screening
- Hearing evaluation
- Causes of hearing loss
- Interpreting results of a hearing evaluation

As suggested in the passage by Martin and Clark (2009), evaluating hearing is a complex
task that has broad-reaching implications. The purpose of a hearing, or audiologic, evaluation is to establish valid and reliable information regarding hearing and listening skills.
The basic information that can be obtained is type of hearing loss, degree of hearing loss,
and configuration of the hearing loss, which are discussed in detail in this chapter. In addition, results of the audiologic evaluation help to direct the diagnosis of hearing loss, to make
appropriate referrals, and to guide treatment and management decisions.

The impact of accurately and effectively testing hearing is critical, because hearing loss has a significant impact on the lives of those who experience it. More than 31 million Americans are estimated to have a hearing loss, which translates to 1 in 10 Americans (Kochkin, 2005). Of these, about a half million would be considered to be d/Deaf (Centers for Disease Control & Prevention, 2008). The incidence and prevalence of hearing loss in children is difficult to pinpoint, because there is no standard for reporting data. Thus, some studies report children with hearing loss in one ear (e.g., unilateral hearing loss), whereas others exclude these children. One estimate is that nearly 1.5 million children under the age of 18 have a hearing loss that impacts their language and literacy development (Kochkin, Luxford, Northern, Mason, & Tharpe, 2007).

Over 5 million children and teens between the ages of 6 and 19 years have been reported to have a hearing loss directly related to noise exposure. This number includes children with slight hearing losses (Niskar et al., 2001). As a point of perspective, 33 babies are born with a severe-to-profound hearing loss (1 to 3 in 1000 births) each day in the United States, with an estimated additional 33 babies born each day with a mild-to-moderate hearing loss (Petrak, 2000). These statistics demonstrate the need for access to a quality evaluation of hearing that can provide information necessary to direct diagnosis and treatment of a hearing loss.

As you proceed through this chapter, you should develop or think of a few questions to which you might want some answers. For example, you might develop questions related to the *Key Concepts* of the chapter, such as the following:

- What is a hearing screening?

- Is there a particular age at which one should have a hearing screening?

- What is a hearing evaluation?

- How is a hearing evaluation different from a hearing screening?

- What is an audiogram?

- How does one interpret an audiogram?

- What are the causes of hearing impairment?

These are just a few questions. We are confident that more will emerge during your reading. We hope that the above questions and others are answered in this chapter.

Hearing Screening

When the mention of a hearing test is made, you probably recall the experience of wearing headphones and raising your hand in response to a beep. Most people can relate to this experience, because it is a common screening administered to elementary school students. All tests of hearing start with the same basic premise: a stimulus (e.g., tone or word) is presented; and a response, such as a hand raise, is required to indicate that the stimulus has been heard. The "hearing a beep and raising the hand" experience most listeners describe as a hearing test is actually a hearing screening.

Although a hearing screening is an important first step in assessing a potential hearing loss, a hearing evaluation is *not* synonymous with a hearing screening. The purpose of a hearing screening is to identify those in the general population who have, or who are likely to have, a hearing loss. Hearing screenings quickly separate the population into two groups: those who pass the screening with normal results and those who do not pass the screening and who are referred either for rescreening or for more comprehensive testing. Because a loss of hearing is often classified as an invisible disorder, screening programs have been developed to find those most likely to have hearing losses that can be educationally, socially, or vocationally handicapping.

Hearing screening programs have been in public schools for many years. In a mass screening program, such as that conducted in a school setting, a number of factors must be considered, including the qualifications and training of the personnel administering the screening, the equipment, infection control, data management, and, most important, the environment in which the screening is performed. A hearing screening consists of the presentation of a limited range of tones (usually 500–4000 Hz) that are presented at one intensity level (usually 20 dB HL). The listener is instructed to respond by demonstrating some response behavior, such as raising a hand, when the tone is perceived. Although no standard for behavioral screenings has been established, both individual state departments of health and the American Speech-Language-Hearing Association provide guidelines for audiometric screenings (American Speech-Language-Hearing Association, 1997).

Recently, hearing screening programs have been applied to newborn infants as part of universal newborn hearing screening (UNHS) programs. Historically, screening of newborns was based on the presence of risk factors for hearing loss, such as low birth weight or maternal exposure to certain diseases during pregnancy. This risk-register approach generally missed about 60% of children born with a congenital hearing loss; that is, hearing loss that is present from birth. Most states have now implemented UNHS programs in which all babies receive a hearing screening at birth (see Chapter 9). It is estimated that 95% of all infants born in the United States have a hearing screening prior to discharge from the hospital (Wolfe & Rogers-Scholl, 2008).

Is it really possible to identify a hearing loss at birth? Remarkable progress has been made in this area. In fact, most people are surprised to learn that a hearing loss *can* be effectively and efficiently screened at birth. If a baby does not pass the newborn hearing screening, the goal is to have a comprehensive hearing test completed by 3 months of age. If a hearing loss is identified, treatment and management of the hearing loss should begin by 6 months of age. This treatment/management can span a range of options, from fitting with hearing aids to providing the family information about sign language or English sign systems (see Paul, 2009, for details on sign systems; see Chapter 9 of this text for early intervention issues).

Although hearing screening programs provide a foundation for identification of hearing loss, they have many limitations. Hearing screenings are often conducted at health fairs held in places such as malls, churches, or community centers, where the noise levels are too high to get valid screening results. Screenings may be timed at intervals where a hearing loss is missed, such as with a child who passes a kindergarten screening but develops a hearing loss in second grade.

Most important, a hearing loss is often described as *insidious*, sneaking up on the listener. The first indications that a person may have a hearing loss can be easily ignored, because they are subtle and can be explained in other ways, such as believing that the speaker is mumbling and so on. It is easy to miss the early signs of a hearing loss. This is particularly important with older adults, who generally do not have access to valid hearing screening programs despite research that suggests that undetected and untreated hearing loss can have a significant impact on the physical and emotional well-being of older adults.

Audiologic Evaluation

Let's assume that you do not pass a hearing screening. If so, then you should have a hearing test, which is also known as an audiologic evaluation. This evaluation is made up of a battery of tests, many of which are discussed later. Audiologic testing is performed by an audiologist. According to the American Academy of Audiology (2004), an audiologist is a professional who:

> by virtue of academic degree, clinical training, and license to practice...is uniquely qualified to provide a comprehensive array of professional services related to...the audiologic identification, assessment, diagnosis, and treatment of persons with impairment of auditory and vestibular function, and to the prevention of impairments associated with them. (p. 44)

The audiologic evaluation is composed of a number of tests that make up a comprehensive battery. This battery is designed to measure—to quantify—hearing and listening skills. The basic information is designed to look at hearing acuity, or responses to a simple detection task of pure tone audiometry.

The process of listening should also be addressed. *Listening* is an individual's ability to detect, discriminate, identify, and comprehend auditory information (Crandall & Smaldino, 2002), or, more basically, how a person is able to use auditory information functionally (i.e., in the real world). As noted in this definition, listening is a complex task that taps a number of auditory skills, not just the basic detection task incorporated into pure tone audiometry. This beep test, known as pure tone audiometry, is the foundation for audiologic evaluation; however, it entails just one aspect of it.

Most audiologists have incorporated the *cross-check* principle into audiologic evaluation. This principle simply states that "the results of a single test are cross-checked by an independent test measure" (Jerger & Hayes, 1976, p. 619). Although initially recommended for the assessment of children, the cross-check principle has expanded to general audiologic assessments as the rationale for using a battery of tests. The basics of hearing testing have not changed in nearly a century; however, the test battery continues to expand with the development of new technologies and approaches.

Audiologists also use the cross-check principle as part of the site of lesion assessment, which refers to using patterns of audiometric results to help determine the location of an auditory pathology that may cause a specific type of hearing loss or auditory disorder. For example, certain results are consistent with disorders of the cochlea of the inner ear and, when this pattern of results is obtained, it supports the disorder as consistent with a sensorineural hearing loss.

STANDARDIZATION AND PRECISION IN THE AUDIOLOGIC EVALUATION

One of the cornerstones of an audiologic evaluation is the ability to standardize the process. Standardization is one of the hallmarks of an adequate testing process. You will see as you move through this chapter that the ability to standardize is easier with some test protocols than with others and with some populations than with others.

As with any process that involves humans, tests have a margin of error. However, audiologists do a number of things to standardize the testing process, to ensure a high degree of confidence that the results are valid and reliable, and to minimize the margin of error. Factors that contribute to the standardization process, including the test environment, the equipment, and the manner in which stimuli are presented, are briefly highlighted here.

One of the most critical factors in obtaining accurate hearing test results is the test environment. Many people who have a hearing test ask if they are going into the "bank vault" or "the chamber," which may be accurate descriptions for their perception of the audiometric sound booth. A sound booth is a room that has been constructed to minimize the ambient (environmental) noise levels to meet the standards of the American National Standards Institute (ANSI) and to ensure that the noise will not interfere with test accuracy. Although they are eerily quiet, it is a myth that these rooms are soundproof, because true soundproofing is not possible.

The listener is separated from the audiologist by a sound-treated wall during testing. The wall usually has a window so that the audiologist and patient have visual access to each other, although the listener should not receive visual cues from the audiologist during testing. The audiologist is able to hear the patient via a talk-back microphone.

Equipment is the next important component in obtaining valid results. A number of pieces of equipment are used to administer the hearing test battery. For example, an audiometer is a piece of equipment that can produce a range of calibrated signals, such as tones or speech. An audiometer is used during most aspects of an audiologic evaluation. Audiometers range in size from portable, such as those that might be used in school screenings, to large diagnostic ones with a full range of options. All audiometers are capable of producing pure tones across the frequency and intensity range for assessing hearing. Computerized audiometers, in addition to producing signals for hearing testing, automatically record and incorporate results into the medical record. These audiometers are also connected directly to equipment that develops prescriptive-fitting information for hearing aids (discussed in more detail in Chapter 4).

Equipment must function in a standardized manner. This means that if an individual has a hearing test in the morning in Ohio and then in the evening in California the results will be the same once the individual's own consistency (called test–retest reliability) is considered, assuming that person's hearing has not changed during the day.

Standard functioning of equipment is verified through calibration. Calibration is the process of matching the characteristics of a piece of equipment to a specific standard. As noted by Wilbur (2002), "checking calibration is necessary to ensure that an audiometer produces a pure tone at a specified level and frequency, that the signal is present only in the transducer [e.g., headphone] to which it is directed, and the signal is free from distortion or unwanted noise interference" (p. 50).

Audiometric equipment is required to meet both equipment manufacturer standards and current ANSI standards (American Academy of Audiology, 2000). Equipment must undergo electroacoustic verification of function at least annually to document calibration. This verification is generally performed by a trained technician, contracted by the audiologist, due to the specialized equipment needed to complete this testing. In addition, most audiologists perform a daily biological calibration or check, where they listen to the auditory stimuli presented through the range of transducers (e.g., all earphones, bone oscillator, and speakers) to verify the function of the equipment prior to testing a patient.

The last aspect of standardization addressed here is how the signal is delivered to the listener's ear, or what type of transducer is used. Most individuals assume that they have to wear big, clunky headphones, again, perhaps because of their experience with hearing screenings. Headphones or earphones with cushions that fit on or around the pinna, also called supra-aural earphones, are still common in hearing testing. It is critical to ensure accurate placement of these earphones so that they are over the opening of the external auditory meatus (see Chapter 2) and not collapsing the ear canals (an artifact that would result in the measure of a hearing loss when none may be present).

Insert earphones, another type of earphone, with disposable foam plugs that fit into the ear canal, are now frequently used in hearing testing. Many patients report that insert earphones are more comfortable than supra-aural earphones. Many audiologists use this type of earphone because it bypasses a few traditional issues in hearing testing, such as collapsed canals and cross-hearing, which is discussed later in this chapter. Both types of earphones are used for air conduction testing.

As noted in Chapter 2, humans hear through both air conduction and bone conduction. Bone conduction bypasses the outer ear and middle ear. The bone-conducted signals stimulate the mechanism of the inner ear by gently vibrating the bones of the skull. Bone conduction testing is performed using a transducer known as a bone oscillator or bone vibrator. This type of transducer is generally placed on the mastoid bone behind the pinna for testing, but it is occasionally placed on the forehead.

In addition to these transducers, the signal may be presented through a speaker in the booth, often referred to by audiologists as *sound field testing*. Speakers are strategically placed in the booth, and the output from the speakers is calibrated based on where the listener will be seated in the booth. Sound field testing is used in a number of situations, including setting up a real-world listening environment within the test booth, verifying hearing aid fitting, and conducting hearing testing with a child who may be reluctant to use earphones (no matter how much the audiologist insists that the "listening hat" is fun to wear).

STEPS IN THE HEARING EVALUATION

Now that you understand the basics of the standardization process, you are ready for the specific steps of a hearing evaluation (which you know is more complicated than a hearing screening). The first step in any comprehensive evaluation is for the audiologist to obtain a systematic case history. Questions in the case history include issues related to otologic (ear) health as well as to general health, concerns regarding hearing and listening issues, family history, and the impact of hearing and listening on functional abilities. Generally, case history information is obtained on a questionnaire completed prior to the evaluation. In addition to a case history questionnaire, audiologists often provide a questionnaire on functional listening behaviors to be completed by the individual, his or her family members, or the classroom teacher. Both sets of information provide insight into the hearing abilities of the patient and may help to direct the test battery.

The audiologist reviews the case history information at the beginning of the evaluation and asks for clarification or additional information as the evaluation begins. This information provides insight into a possible etiology, or cause, of the hearing loss; facilitates understanding of complaints that precipitated the assessment; and directs recommendations and a treatment plan. In addition, a comprehensive case history provides an understanding of patient and family expectations and an opportunity to develop rapport with the patient and his or her family.

Before testing, the audiologist looks in the individual's ear canal. This should happen in conjunction with a careful look at the external ear, including examining for skin tags, pits, growths on the pinna, or asymmetry between the two ears. These conditions may provide clues for a hearing loss, because parts of the outer ear and the inner ear develop simultaneously and from the same type of tissue during fetal development. The audiologist then uses an otoscope, an instrument with a magnifying lens and a light, to visualize the ear canal and eardrum.

Many individuals believe that too much wax in the ear canal is a common cause of hearing loss. This, however, is a relatively rare occurrence. It is important to remember that earwax, or cerumen, is not dirt, but acts to protect and lubricate the ear canal. The old adage that you should "stick nothing in your ear smaller than your elbow" is a good one. Most individuals' ear canals are self-cleaning, and oftentimes mechanical manipulations of the ear canal, such as using a Q-tip in an attempt to clean out the wax, interferes with both the function of the earwax and the normal health of the ear canal.

Examination of the ear also provides insight into the health of the eardrum and, to some degree, the middle ear. If you are curious about what a real eardrum looks like, you are referred to the excellent Web site "Audiology Forum: Video Otoscopy" at www.rcsullivan.com/www/ears.htm or the textbooks of Hawke, Keene, and Alberti (1990) or Pulec (2001) to review photographs of both healthy ear canals and abnormalities of the ear and ear canal.

Pure Tone Audiometry

After the examination, the audiologist tests the person's hearing using pure tone audiometry. This test procedure has been the cornerstone for audiologic evaluations for nearly a century. During pure tone audiometry, the patient is seated in the sound booth. Generally, the patient is positioned to minimize visual cues from the audiologist so that the individual does not know when a tone is presented based on seeing the audiologist's movements.

Tones are presented across a range of frequencies in the octaves between 250 and 8000 Hz, which are thought to be the frequencies most important for understanding speech. The listener is told to respond each time he or she detects the presence of the tone. This response might include a hand raise, a verbal response ("yes, I hear it"), or pressing a response button. Actually, any consistent response will do, including an angry "no" as once stated by a 3-year-old each time a tone was presented!

The intensity of the tone is decreased each time the listener responds until the tone can no longer be heard. Listener responses are bracketed (e.g., the tone is increased and decreased in intensity as the listener responds or does not respond to hearing the tone) until the audiometric threshold is obtained for that frequency. An *audiometric threshold* can be defined as "the intensity at which an individual can just barely hear a sound 50% of the time; all sounds louder than a threshold can be heard, but sounds below a threshold cannot be detected" (Mendel, Danhauer, & Singh, 1999, p. 258).

Once the threshold is obtained at one frequency for one ear, it is recorded on an audiogram, a graph that depicts hearing as a function of frequency (**Figure 3-1**). The threshold for each frequency tested is recorded for each ear individually by air conduction, which is done by using earphones.

The audiogram has been used for reporting hearing test results for nearly 70 years and is another way to standardize the audiometric results (Bunch, 1943). The frequency of the signal in hertz (Hz) is represented on the horizontal axis and is read from low to high frequency. This is similar to facing a piano keyboard and noting that the lower frequency sounds are toward the left and the higher frequency sounds are toward the right. The intensity of the signal in decibels (dB) with a hearing level referent (dB HL) is reported on the vertical axis, which ranges from the less intense sounds at the top of the audiogram to the more intense ones at the bottom.

As with most graphs, note that symbols are used (see the bottom of Figure 3-1). Standardized symbols are recommended by the American Speech-Language-Hearing Association (1990) and are a convention used by the majority of audiologists. The horizontal line at zero, which is bolded on most audiograms, represents what is known as the *audiometric zero*, or the average hearing abilities for young adults. The dB HL, the decibels hearing level noted previously, is a decibel scale that refers to the accepted standards for typical or normal hearing, with 0 dB representing the average normal hearing for each audiometric frequency (Mendell, Danhauer, & Singh, 1999).

Taking a look at an audiogram that represents some familiar sounds (**Figure 3-2**) helps to illustrate the intensity and frequency of a number of common sounds, including speech. This is also a graphic representation of the information presented earlier in Chapter 2 (Table 2-1). If a listener's audiometric information is superimposed on this audiogram of

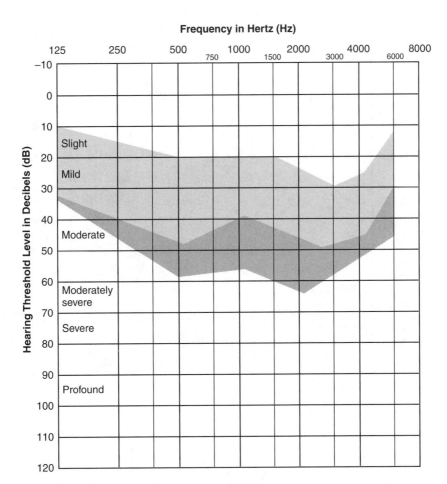

Frequency in Hertz (Hz)

	AIR		BONE		NO RESP.	UNAIDED	AIDED
	NO MASK	MASK	NO MASK	MASK			
RIGHT EAR	O	△	<	[	↙		
LEFT EAR	X	□	>	]	↘		
SOUND FIELD					↓	S	A

LEGEND OF SYMBOLS

Figure 3-1

Standard Audiogram with Audiometric Symbols

Image courtesy of Brad Ingrao, AuD.

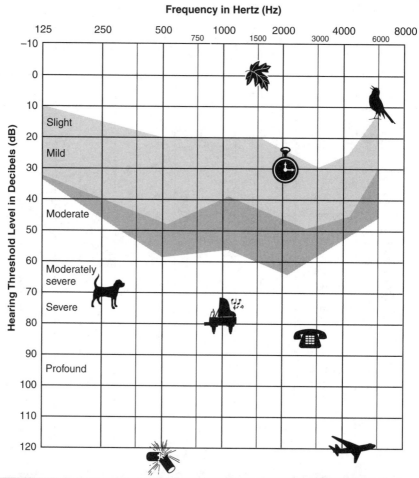

Figure 3-2

Frequency and Intensity of Some Familiar Sounds

Image courtesy of Brad Ingrao, AuD.

familiar sounds, it becomes obvious what types of sounds are audible to the listener and what sounds are likely not to be heard clearly or at all. Some audiologists use this type of familiar sounds audiogram as a counseling tool for the patient and his or her family.

Once all frequencies are tested via air conduction, a similar procedure is used for stimuli presented via bone conduction. Recall that the bone oscillator is placed either behind the pinna on the mastoid or, more rarely, on the forehead, and the thresholds for the octave frequencies of 250–4000 Hz are obtained. Comparing the bone conduction results to the air conduction results helps to address the type of hearing loss, which is highlighted later in this chapter. This is an appropriate time to state that the head does not do a good job of shielding the ears from each other, particularly for bone-conducted stimuli and sometimes for air-conducted stimuli. Again, in the interest of obtaining reliable results, the audiologist has to be sure that if the right ear is being tested that the results are actually those from the right ear.

A rookie mistake is to put the wrong earphone on or in the ear so the right earphone is on the left ear. An audiologic convention is to indicate the right earphone with a red marker and the left earphone with a blue marker, which is also carried over to marking hearing aids to indicate the correct ear. In addition, many audiologists mark the right ear symbols on the audiogram in red and the left ear symbols in blue.

Another way that results can actually not be from the ear that the audiologist thought was being tested is related to the concept of crossover. With crossover, the sound travels from the ear being tested, either across or around the head, and stimulates the ear that is not being tested. This happens nearly all of the time with bone conduction testing and on occasion with air conduction testing, such as when there is a significant difference in hearing between the ears (e.g., 40 dB or greater) or when there is a conductive hearing loss. When this occurs, the audiologist puts noise in the nontest ear, called *masking*, to keep that ear busy so that the responses obtained are truly from the ear being tested.

Note that masked symbols are listed on the symbol key for the audiogram in Figure 3-1. Once you become more comfortable with interpreting audiograms, you will be able to identify when masking was used and perhaps even to understand why it was used (e.g., asymmetric hearing loss).

With all this focus on testing pure tones, you may be asking yourself what many patients ask when they arrive for a hearing test: Why spend so much time focusing on listening to beeps in a quiet room when most people report difficulty hearing speech? As noted in Chapter 1, one way to estimate difficulty in hearing speech is by calculating the pure tone average (PTA), or the average of the thresholds obtained at 500, 1000, and 2000 Hz for an individual unaided ear. The PTA is a quick way to classify degree of hearing loss and helps to estimate hearing difficulty related to speech understanding.

Speech Audiometry

Another aspect of the test battery is speech audiometry, techniques where speech stimuli are presented in a standardized manner in a variety of ways to further assess the auditory system. Many of the same principles used with pure tone audiometry apply to speech audiometry. The idea with speech audiometry is to present the stimuli in a calibrated and standardized manner. Most audiologists accomplish this by using standardized stimuli recorded on a CD or in a sound file on their computer presented through the calibrated audiometer and earphones. Some audiologists use a technique known as monitored live voice (MLV), where the stimulus is spoken by the audiologist and the presentation is calibrated by gauging the V/U meter on the audiometer.

The speech reception or recognition threshold (SRT) has many similarities to pure tone audiometry. Instead of using a tone as the stimulus, *spondees*, or words with equal stress on each syllable (e.g., *baseball, hotdog*), are used. Notice that this is a threshold test; so the audiologist is looking for the least intense level at which the listener can repeat these words 50% of the time. If the listener cannot repeat the words due to speech limitations, modifications can be made, including pointing to pictures of the spondee words.

In some cases, listeners cannot discriminate the words although they are able to discern that speech is being presented. In this case, the audiologist will obtain a speech detection threshold (SDT), or the least intense level at which the listener can identify a speech stimulus is present. The SRT is generally in agreement with the PTA within 5 to 12 dB, with the SDT often better or lower than the PTA (related to the broadband nature of the stimulus, among other factors) (American Speech-Language-Hearing Association Committee on Audiologic Evaluation, 1988).

At this point, your next logical question should be related to why so much time is spent detecting auditory information (e.g., threshold measures) when most people have little need to listen to speech presented at the least intense level that they can just barely hear. This detection information gives the audiologist one part of the puzzle. But, you are right, suprathreshold testing (or perception of auditory information above threshold) is very important to most listeners.

The next type of speech audiometry test that is performed is to obtain a word recognition score (WRS), which you may also see referred to as a *speech recognition score* or as *speech discrimination testing*. WRS is presented at a suprathreshold level, generally a specific level above the SRT, such as 30 or 40 dB SL (sensation level, which can be described as a sound intensity in reference to a threshold for an individual listener's threshold). This is generally both an audible and comfortable listening level for patients—they can both hear the speech and tolerate the level at which it is presented. The stimuli for this test are again standardized, using lists of monosyllable words selected because they are phonemically balanced or phonetically balanced within a list of words. Both of these concepts refer to the frequency at which certain phonemes (speech sounds) occur either in the list or in general American English speech (for more information on phonemes, see Chapter 6).

Audiologists have a range of standardized test materials from which to choose, and lists of either 25 or 50 words are presented per ear. The test is generally presented in an *open set* manner, whereby the audiologist presents the word and the listener is expected to repeat what he or she hears. Some of the word lists use a *closed set* approach, whereby the listener chooses from a predetermined set of words, similar to a multiple-choice test.

A WRS, reported as a percentage, is obtained for each ear. Patients often confuse this percentage score with the percentage of hearing loss, or a calculation based on pure tone results. This type of percentage of hearing loss model is often used in workers' compensation cases for noise-induced hearing loss, but it is irrelevant for addressing communication function in the general practice of audiology. However, the WRS can provide critical information regarding the *fidelity* of the auditory system. Many individuals with a hearing loss report that even when speech is made louder it is not clearer. This is often reflected in word recognition testing. When speech is presented at a higher intensity level, the listener's ability to recognize speech is evaluated. The results of this test help to address issues of clarity or distortion in the auditory system (Wilson & McArdle, 2008). In addition, this information can help to guide prognosis for success with hearing aids.

Your next observation is likely to be that most people do not listen to speech in quiet rooms under headphones. Again, an astute observation. A key concept is that speech understanding in quiet is often a poor predictor for speech understanding in less than optimal listening environments, such as when background noise is present. The hearing and listening abilities of individuals with hearing loss are generally more impacted by a poor signal-to-noise ratio (SNR) than are their peers with typical hearing abilities, as discussed in Chapter 2.

Many individuals with hearing loss note that they can often "get by" in quiet listening situations, but that they have tremendous functional communication difficulties when background noise is present. This is as true for individuals with mild hearing losses as it is for those with more severe degrees of hearing loss. Assessment of *speech-in-noise* (SIN) skills, a type of speech audiometry test, should be part of the test battery to assess functional listening abilities. A number of standardized SIN tests are available and can be presented either through the earphones or in the sound field. It has been proposed that measuring SNR loss is an important domain of auditory functioning (Wilson & McArdle, 2008). This may be particularly important for children in schools where poor SNR abilities inherent in the auditory system can have a negative synergy with a poor classroom SNR (as described in Chapter 2).

SPECIAL CONSIDERATIONS

The test battery discussed to this point focuses on behavioral techniques for listeners who are willing and able participants in the process. However, obtaining valid and reliable audiometric results from a patient who may be less willing to participate presents a set of challenges. Audiologists are resourceful in their desire to obtain accurate test results, so they have developed a number of modifications of the behavioral test battery that can maximize the ability to obtain valid test results from young children. Several of these modifications are briefly discussed in the following paragraphs.

Behavioral testing is based on a stimulus–response paradigm, where a stimulus, such as a tone or word, is presented and a consistent response, such as raising the hand or repeating a word, is desired. With young children, the stimulus–response bond is often not as obvious as it is to more sophisticated listeners or the bond will need to be shaped a bit. One example of this is the visual reinforcement audiometry (VRA) technique used with children approximately 6 to 24 months of age.

During VRA, stimuli are presented either through the sound field or with insert earphones and the child is "rewarded" for localizing, or turning his or her head, toward the stimuli. This reward generally consists of several types of reinforcers, most often the lighting of an animated toy hidden in a smoked Plexiglas box or the starting of video clips projected on a screen in the test booth. This technique can be very effective, provided appropriate conditioning techniques are utilized.

One concern is that if sound field testing is performed ear-specific information is not obtained. In that case, and if the child is either uncooperative with wearing earphones or consistent results are not obtained with earphones, the audiologist must work diligently to continue to reevaluate the child on a regular basis to acquire ear-specific results in a timely manner. Some audiologists reevaluate children every 6 to 12 months based on factors ranging from the perception that parents will not follow up to the fact that insurance will not pay for more frequent testing. The goal should always be to obtain the most comprehensive results in a timely manner, and the audiologist must be proactive in explaining this issue to families, third-party payers, and educators, among others.

Between 24 and 36 months of age, children often understand the stimulus–response technique required for pure tone audiometry but lack the attention and/or motivation to participate in the task. A creative audiologist can engage a child using a technique called conditioned play audiometry (CPA). This technique is similar to standard pure tone audiometry with an important twist—the response is turned into a game. When the child perceives the tone, he or she is asked to complete a specific task, such as putting a peg in a peg board, dropping a block in a bucket, or putting a stacking ring on a stacker. This test modification also involves a careful conditioning phase, but once completed it is generally possible to obtain a complete and reliable audiogram from a toddler or preschooler, often to the surprise of the child's parents.

Modification of speech audiometry techniques, such as pointing to pictures of spondee words or words on a word recognition list, can also be used with young children. Most typically developing children are able to complete the standard audiometric test battery described earlier in this chapter, often with minimal modifications, by the age of 5.

ADDITIONAL TEST CONSIDERATIONS

Note that the types of audiometric testing presented in this chapter focus on behavioral results, or measuring hearing based on behavioral responses presented by the listener. There are many more tests in the test battery than presented in this chapter, many of which are classified as physiologic or electrophysiologic. These test procedures elicit a response from the auditory system with cooperation from the patient; however, a behavior response is not required. Examples of these types of tests are tympanometry, a simple test that provides information about the function of the middle ear system; otoacoustic emissions (OAEs), a test that correlates to outer hair cell function of the inner ear and is used as one of the protocols for newborn hearing screening; and auditory brainstem response testing, in which responses to auditory stimulation are recorded by electrodes attached to the head. An in-depth discussion of these tests is beyond the scope of this text; however, these tests support the cross-check principle and can provide additional information about the type, degree, and configuration of hearing loss.

Review of Types of Hearing Loss

One of the purposes of audiometric testing is to obtain information that contributes to a *differential diagnosis* of hearing loss, which refers to determining the particular site of lesion or etiology for the hearing disorder. As noted in Chapter 2, types of hearing loss generally fall into the categories of conductive, sensorineural, mixed, and auditory processing disorders. Types of loss are again briefly reviewed here in preparation for the discussion of audiogram interpretation.

CONDUCTIVE HEARING LOSSES

Conductive hearing losses are related to disorders of the outer or middle ear. The etiology may include otitis media (middle ear infection), otosclerosis (a degenerative disease that involves bony growth in the footplate of the stapes), or a skull fracture that has resulted in a fracture of the ossicular chain. Conductive hearing loss is often classified as a loss of loudness. Once the intensity of the signal is increased, the individual with the hearing loss has no loss of clarity of the signal. Conductive hearing losses are generally medically treatable. Thus, prompt and accurate identification of this type of hearing loss is critical so that an appropriate referral can be made.

In the unusual case in which the conductive hearing loss cannot be treated medically, individuals generally have tremendous success with hearing aids, providing that there are no medical contraindications for use of amplification. A special type of implantable hearing aid, the bone anchored hearing aid (BAHA), was initially developed for use with this population and is discussed in further detail in Chapter 5.

SENSORINEURAL HEARING LOSSES

Sensorineural hearing losses are related to disorders of the inner ear or the auditory (VIIIth) nerve. The etiology may be related to noise exposure, exposure to drugs that are ototoxic (or damaging to the inner ear), aging of the auditory system, or autoimmune ear disease. Sensorineural hearing losses are often associated with a loss of clarity. Even when the intensity of the speech is increased, the speech signal does not sound clearer to the listener.

Sensorineural hearing losses are generally not medically treatable; however, a wide range of options of nonmedical treatment and management are available. In addition, due to the fact that sensorineural hearing losses often coexist with other types of medical problems, a medical examination by an otologist (physician who specializes in ear disease) is often necessary. Note that a number of red flags require immediate medical referral, including sudden onset of hearing loss; difference between ears; or tinnitus in one ear only.

With recent technological advances, the term *sensorineural* can be broken into its component parts of sensory (cochlear) or neural (VIIIth nerve), which can further contribute to a differential diagnosis of hearing loss. This differentiation can be important in terms of pinpointing the etiology of the hearing loss and directing prognosis such as, for example, diagnosing auditory neuropathy/dys-synchrony (AN/AD).

AN/AD, a recently identified disorder, refers to when cochlear function is normal but that the VIIIth nerve fails to carry electrical signals to the brain in a synchronous manner, resulting in auditory information not being relayed consistently. The identification of AN/AD has been critical in understanding why some children with mild-to-moderate hearing losses, identified by audiometry, have had such poor word recognition and poor functional use of residual hearing. AN/AD has considerable variation among individuals and can fluctuate significantly within an individual.

In the past, individuals with AN/AD were lumped into the group of people with sensorineural hearing losses, although they generally had much more difficulty with communication than would be anticipated by their audiograms. Many of these children rejected hearing aid use and were often unsuccessful in achieving educational goals. Having the ability to differentiate between cochlear and retrocochlear hearing loss, in this case, helps to direct rehabilitation efforts. The progress of patients with AN/AD is often slow and, generally, they do not demonstrate much benefit from hearing aids, but are successful with cued speech/language and speechreading methods, which are discussed in Chapters 7 and 8, respectively.

One of the most common causes of sensorineural hearing loss is genetic, either as a component of a genetic syndrome or as a nonsyndromic sensorineural hearing loss (NSSHL). Many people believe that genetic hearing losses are always congenital. However, recent research on the genetic mechanisms of hearing loss indicates that the onset can occur at any time in an individual's life (Steel, 1998).

Every child with sensorineural hearing loss should have a genetic evaluation to help determine the etiology of the hearing loss, the prognosis for treatment, and the direction for management. Contrary to urban legend, the purpose of a genetic evaluation is not to eradicate Deaf culture. Some hearing losses are part of genetic syndromes that can involve multiple medical conditions. Therefore, the results of a genetic evaluation can positively contribute to a d/Deaf or hard-of-hearing individual's health and well-being.

MIXED HEARING LOSS

A mixed hearing loss is a combination of both conductive and sensorineural hearing loss. This may happen as the result of a genetic condition or as a combination of etiologies, such as a child with a sensorineural hearing loss who then develops a middle ear infection. As with conductive hearing losses, identification of a mixed hearing loss is critical, because medical intervention may be able to resolve the conductive component. This is important in terms of being able to provide improved hearing, which is a crucial factor for many listeners. Recall from Chapter 2 that decibels are on a logarithmic scale. If a listener can recover even a few decibels of hearing, it can contribute to improved perception of speech.

AUDITORY PROCESSING DISORDERS

Moving into the central auditory system, we might encounter instances of auditory processing disorders (APD). APD is referred to by a number of names, including central auditory processing disorder (CAPD). Auditory processing disorders refer to

> …difficulties in the processing of auditory information in the central nervous system (CNS) as demonstrated by poor performance in one or more of the following skills: sound localization and lateralization; auditory discrimination; auditory pattern recognition; temporal aspects of audition, including temporal integration, temporal discrimination (e.g., temporal gap detection), temporal ordering, and temporal masking; auditory performance in competing acoustic signals (including dichotic listening); and auditory performance with degraded acoustic signals. (American Speech-Language-Hearing Association, 2005, p. 2)

Most auditory processing disorders occur in individuals with normal peripheral hearing acuity, otherwise reported as normal results on an audiogram. In addition, these disorders are not thought to be a result of higher-order global deficits such as autism, mental retardation, or attention deficit disorder. Based on the definition presented, it is easy to understand why the category of auditory processing disorders can be confusing.

Another way to address this is to consider auditory processing disorders as a breakdown in auditory abilities resulting in diminished learning (e.g., comprehension) through hearing, even when peripheral hearing acuity is normal. This fact is critical, because many individuals with auditory processing disorders report hearing difficulties similar to those with peripheral hearing loss (e.g., cannot hear well in the presence of background noise, difficulty discriminating between similarly sounding words, etc.). Often, patients with auditory processing disorders report subtle, yet significant, issues, particularly in less than optimal listening environments.

A test battery approach is recommended to assess auditory processing skills, using techniques that tax the auditory system; however, the discussion of specific tests and their interpretation is beyond the scope of this text. It is critical to understand that both children and adults who report subtle listening issues can benefit from further testing, particularly if the information gained may assist them educationally or vocationally.

Auditory processing disorders can result from genetic factors; pathologies of the central auditory nervous system, such as multiple sclerosis; or injuries, such as a traumatic brain injury. Although auditory processing disorders, as described here, focus on individuals with normal peripheral hearing acuity, differences in listeners with sensorineural hearing losses may also be explained by auditory processing deficits, as has been discussed in addressing individual variations in older adults.

A brief list and descriptions of commonly occurring hearing disorders are presented in **Table 3-1.**

Table 3–1

Overview of Commonly Occurring Hearing Disorders

Type of Hearing Loss	Disorder	Description
Conductive	Otitis media with effusion (OME)	This disorder is an infection or inflammation of the middle ear, often in conjunction with an upper respiratory infection. Otitis media can occur in any person of any age; however, it is most common in young children under the age of 9, with more than 75% of children experiencing one episode of otitis media by their first birthday (NIDCD, 2009).
	Otosclerosis	This is an abnormal bony growth on the footplate of the stapes (one of the bones of the middle ear). The bone becomes fixated so the stapes cannot move freely. This bony growth and fixation adds mass to the system, requiring more energy to stimulate the middle ear. This results in a loss of energy transfer, which translates into a conductive hearing loss. The cause of otosclerosis is unknown. It is most common in Caucasian women of childbearing age, and the hearing loss is often noted during or soon after pregnancy, suggesting a possible hormonal component (NIDCD, 2009). Otosclerosis also tends to occur in families, suggesting a possible hereditary and/or genetic cause. As noted in Chapter 3, many conductive hearing losses can be addressed medically. A common treatment for otosclerosis is stapedectomy, a surgical procedure in which the immobile stapes is removed and replaced with a prosthetic one. This allows the middle ear bones to move, thus restoring or improving hearing (American Academy of Otolaryngology-Head and Neck Surgery, 2009). In some cases, people with otosclerosis are fit with hearing aids.

| Sensorineural | Noise induced hearing loss (NIHL) | Exposure to levels of noise that can damage the inner ear can result in a permanent sensorineural hearing loss. This type of loss is particularly prevalent in individuals who have occupational (e.g., industrial machinery) or recreational (e.g., firearms) exposure to levels of noise that can damage hearing. These levels of noise are based on the type (e.g., continuous, impact) and the decibel level of the noise over time. The loss can occur from a one-time exposure or repeated exposures over an extended period of time. If individuals are exposed to an 85 dB noise source for 8 hours a day, they are at risk for developing a hearing loss. For every 3 dB above 85 dB, the permissible noise exposure time before possible damage to hearing is cut in half. For example, if a listener is exposed to an 88 dB sound, the maximum exposure should be 4 hours (Dangerous Decibels, 2009). There is significant concern regarding NIHL in children and teens due to extended exposure to music under headphones or the soundtrack of video games. NIHL can be prevented, using the model suggested by Dangerous Decibels (2009): turn the noise down, walk away from the noise source, and use appropriate hearing protection. NIHL is a significant public health issue, and education is a key to prevention. |

(continues)

Table 3-1

Overview of Commonly Occurring Hearing Disorders (continued)

Type of Hearing Loss	Disorder	Description
	Infections	Both bacterial and viral infections can result in sensorineural hearing loss. For example, bacterial meningitis is described as one of the most common causes of acquired severe to profound sensorineural hearing loss in children (Burton, 2009). Other types of infections, such as cytomegalovirus (CMV), measles, and mumps can also result in a hearing loss. One of the critical features for these types of diseases is to try to prevent them through public health immunization programs for children.
Central	Traumatic brain injury	Head injuries, even those that are described as *mild*, can produce damage to the central auditory nervous system that results in an auditory processing disorder. This can be an injury such as a blast injury related to military service, post concussive syndrome related to being hit in the head or being involved in a motor vehicle accident (MVA), or a sports injury. Many of these individuals have normal hearing acuity on a pure tone audiogram. Individuals who have incurred this type of injury may experience tinnitus (e.g., ringing or sound in the ear) and vestibular (or balance) disorders in addition to auditory processing issues (Myers, Wilmington, Gallun, Henry, & Fausti, 2009). Types of difficulties include a poorer ability to listen in noisy environments, to localize auditory information, or to discriminate between similar sounds than would be anticipated for someone with a normal audiogram.

Audiogram Interpretation

We hope that you are not worn down by the preceding discussions of hearing tests and different types of hearing losses! The remainder of this chapter is devoted to interpreting audiometric results, most specifically those obtained from the audiogram. As noted previously, interpreting the audiogram yields some important information: the type of hearing loss (e.g., conductive, sensorineural, or mixed), the degree of hearing loss (e.g., mild, moderate, profound), and the configuration of hearing loss (e.g., flat, sloping in the high frequencies). All of this information provides insight into the diagnosis of hearing and auditory disorders and has a critical role in directing the treatment and management of hearing loss.

Recall that the audiogram is a graphic representation of the hearing test results, reported as air conduction and bone conduction thresholds obtained for each ear individually. The type of hearing loss is determined by comparing the air conduction and bone conduction results at each frequency. Hearing thresholds of 25 dB HL or better (meaning a lower number) for an adult or 15 dB HL or better for a child are consistent with normal peripheral hearing acuity (see Chapter 1). This assumes that the results of the air conduction and bone conduction thresholds are in agreement, or interweaving, and do not differ by more than 10 dB HL.

Figure 3-3 illustrates normal audiometric results. Results are plotted for the right ear. When the gap between the air conduction and bone conduction results is greater than 10 dB at an individual frequency and the bone conduction results fall above 25 dB HL, the results are consistent with a conductive hearing loss. This is typically reported as an air–bone gap, which is illustrated on the audiogram in **Figure 3-4**.

When the air conduction and bone conduction results are interweaving (within 10 dB of each other) and both fall below (or are a higher number than) 25 dB HL for adults or 15 dB HL for children, the results are consistent with a sensorineural hearing loss. This is illustrated on the audiogram in **Figure 3-5**.

When both air conduction and bone conduction scores fall outside the range of normal hearing acuity but there is a gap of greater than 10 dB between them, the results are consistent with a mixed hearing loss. This is depicted on the audiogram in **Figure 3-6**. Again, you should notice the air–bone gap; however, all the results are shifted below the range of normal hearing acuity.

The degree of hearing loss refers to the range that the results fall into on the audiogram. This range was presented in Table 1-1 in Chapter 1, which described the degree of hearing loss based on pure tone audiometry. Audiologists look at each frequency and describe each type within the range. This is depicted in **Figure 3-7**. Although there are some slight variations in labels for degree of hearing loss, most audiologists use this method.

Configuration refers to the shape or pattern of the audiogram, or how the results of the audiogram change as a function of the frequency. Mendel, Danhauer, and Singh (1999) note that the three main configurations are *sloping*, *rising*, and *flat*. The shape of the audiogram is important for both diagnostic and rehabilitation purposes. Many sensorineural hearing losses are thought to have a sloping configuration in which hearing is better in the lower frequencies and poorer in the higher frequencies.

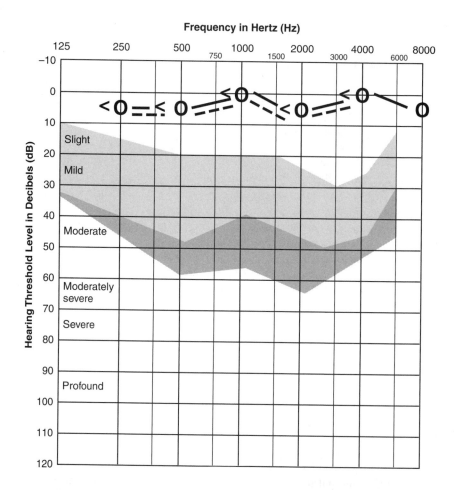

Frequency in Hertz (Hz)

LEGEND OF SYMBOLS

	AIR		BONE		NO RESP.	UNAIDED	AIDED
	NO MASK	MASK	NO MASK	MASK			
RIGHT EAR	O	△	<	[	↙		
LEFT EAR	X	□	>	]	↘		
SOUND FIELD					↓	S	A

Figure 3-3

Normal Hearing Acuity for the Right Ear

Image courtesy of Brad Ingrao, AuD.

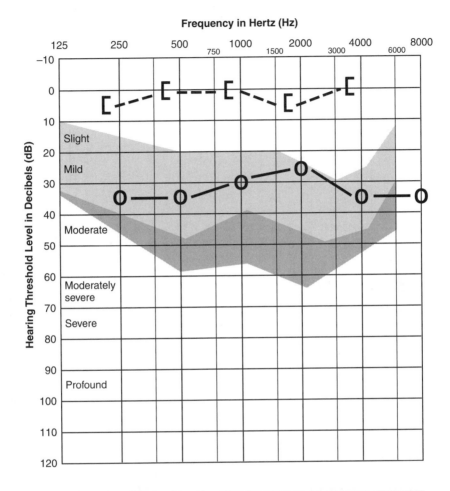

Figure 3-4

Conductive Hearing Loss

Image courtesy of Brad Ingrao, AuD.

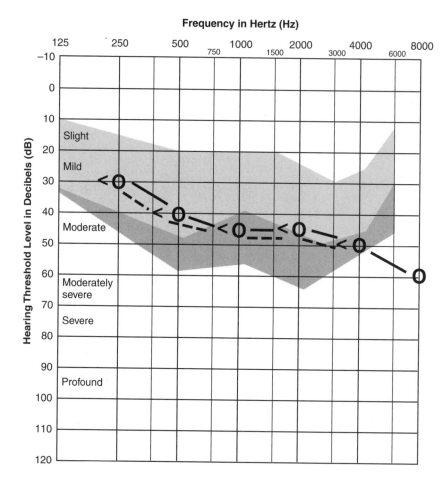

Figure 3-5

Sensorineural Hearing Loss

Image courtesy of Brad Ingrao, AuD.

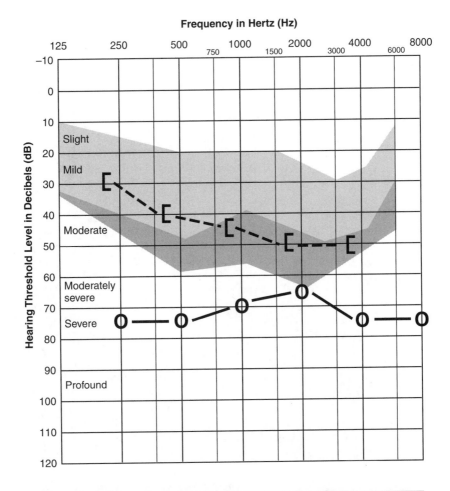

LEGEND OF SYMBOLS							
	AIR		BONE		NO RESP.	UNAIDED	AIDED
	NO MASK	MASK	NO MASK	MASK			
RIGHT EAR	O	Δ	<	[	↙		
LEFT EAR	X	□	>	]	↘		
SOUND FIELD					↓	S	A

Figure 3-6
Mixed Hearing Loss

Image courtesy of Brad Ingrao, AuD.

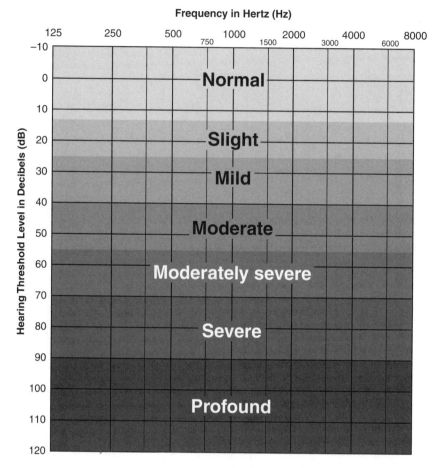

Figure 3-7
Degrees of Hearing Loss
Image courtesy of Brad Ingrao, AuD.

If you think back to the audiogram representing familiar sounds (Figure 3-2), you should have an idea of what this may mean functionally. Many individuals with the type of hearing loss shown in Figure 3-2 indicate that they miss certain sounds, such as high-frequency consonant sounds (e.g., /s/ or /f/) because their hearing is most impaired in the frequencies where these sounds are located (see discussion of phonemes in Chapter 6). Vowel sounds carry the power of the speech signal, but consonant sounds actually carry the meaning. With a sloping type of audiogram, listeners often report that although they know that someone is talking, they cannot make out the words. They hear the power of the vowels, but they cannot differentiate between the consonants.

Becoming familiar with the audiogram assists you in understanding the type, degree, and configuration of the hearing loss, but, more important, with additional practice you can learn how this information is likely to impact individuals in their daily listening situations. How might these results impact speech and language development (see also Chapter 6)? If a child has a severe sensorineural hearing loss at 4000 Hz, it is unlikely that he or she will be able to effectively produce certain speech sounds without appropriate amplification and remediation. Because perception and production of a speech sound are considered to mirror each other, the information about a listener's ability to detect sound provides insight into potential speech, language, and literacy issues (see Chapters 6 and 7).

Summary of Major Points

The profession of audiology uses an evidence-based practice model to shape clinical decisions. Evidence-based practice uses a combination of the audiologist's clinical experience and expertise and current research findings. However, the ability to obtain consistent results, particularly from a challenging patient, entails the art and science of audiology. The bottom line is that listening to the patient and establishing a rapport are as important as the science behind the testing.

Now that you have completed this chapter, we hope that all or most of your questions that you had at the beginning have been answered. If not, you might want to dialogue with your instructor or read some of the references listed at the end of the chapter. Specifically, we hope that you understand the process of hearing testing and how the results of the audiologic test battery contribute to the diagnosis and treatment of hearing loss.

The overall intent of this chapter was to provide a brief introduction to the construct of audiologic evaluation. The *Key Concepts* were as follows:

- Hearing screening

- Hearing evaluation

- Causes of hearing loss

- Interpreting results of a hearing evaluation

With respect to hearing screening, it was stated that

- A hearing screening is not the same as a hearing evaluation. The purpose of a hearing screening is to identify those in the general population who have, or who are likely to have, a hearing loss.

- Recently, hearing screening programs have been applied to newborn infants as part of universal newborn hearing screening (UNHS) programs.

■ Although hearing screening programs provide a foundation for identification of hearing loss, they have many limitations.

With respect to hearing evaluation, we remarked that

■ Hearing, or audiologic, evaluation is made up of a battery of tests. This battery is designed to quantify hearing and listening skills.

■ Most audiologists have incorporated the cross-check principle into audiologic evaluations.

■ One of the cornerstones of an audiologic evaluation is the ability to standardize the process.

■ Any comprehensive evaluation of hearing involves several steps.

■ Pure tone and speech audiometry are essential in an audiologic evaluation.

In the section on the causes of hearing loss

■ One of the purposes of audiometric testing is to obtain information that contributes to a differential diagnosis of hearing loss, which refers to determining the particular site of lesion or etiology for the hearing disorder.

■ Conductive hearing losses are related to disorders of the outer or middle ear. The etiology may be related to many causes, including otitis media (middle ear infection), otosclerosis (a degenerative disease that involves bony growth in the footplate of the stapes), or a skull fracture that has resulted in a fracture of the ossicular chain.

■ Sensorineural hearing losses are related to disorders of the inner ear or the VIIIth nerve. The etiology may be related to noise exposure, ototoxic drugs (i.e., drugs damaging to the inner ear), aging of the auditory system, or autoimmune ear disease.

■ Mixed hearing losses are a combination of both conductive and sensorineural hearing loss. This may happen as the result of a genetic condition or as a combination of etiologies, such as a child with a sensorineural hearing loss who develops a middle ear infection.

■ Auditory processing disorders (APD) are referred to by a number of names, including central auditory processing disorders (CAPD).

In the section on audiogram interpretation

■ The audiogram provides some important information: the type of hearing loss (e.g., conductive, sensorineural, or mixed), the degree of hearing loss (e.g., mild, moderate, profound), and the configuration of hearing loss (e.g., flat, sloping in the high frequencies).

■ The audiogram is a graphic representation of the hearing test results, reported as air conduction and bone conduction thresholds obtained for each ear individually. The type of hearing loss is determined by comparing the air conduction and bone conduction results at each frequency.

■ When the gap between the air conduction and bone conduction results is greater than 10 dB at an individual frequency and the bone conduction results fall above 25 dB HL, the results are consistent with a conductive hearing loss.

■ When the air conduction and bone conduction results are interweaving (within 10 dB of each other) and both fall below (or are a higher number than) 25 dB HL for adults or 15 dB HL for children, the results are consistent with a sensorineural hearing loss.

■ When both air conduction and bone conduction scores fall outside the range of normal hearing acuity but there is a gap of greater than 10 dB between them, the results are consistent with a mixed hearing loss.

Now that you understand the basics of the anatomy and physiology of the ear and the essentials of a hearing evaluation, you are ready to learn about amplification and other assistive technologies. We begin with hearing aids in Chapter 4.

Chapter Questions

Note: Some answers to the questions can be found in the chapter; however, others have a variety of possible responses based on the students' backgrounds and experiences.

1. What is the function of a hearing screening? At what age should one have a screening?

2. What are the limitations of a hearing screening?

3. What are the major components of an audiologic evaluation? What are the major steps?

4. Briefly explain the cross-check principle.

5. List and briefly describe the factors that contribute to the standardization of the audiologic evaluation.

6. What is a hearing threshold?

7. How is hearing represented on an audiogram? Be sure to include the representation of hearing by the left ear and the right ear.

8. Briefly describe crossover. How does the audiologist address this issue?

9. What is speech audiometry? How is it similar to or different from pure tone audiometry?

10. If you were designing your own hearing test battery, what types of tests might you include?

11. List and provide examples of the various types of hearing losses. Relate the losses to the results on an audiogram.

12. What information does an audiogram provide?

13. If you had an opportunity to converse with the authors, what burning questions would you ask them? Share and discuss these questions with your instructor and classmates.

Challenge Questions

Note: *Complete answers are not in the text. Additional research/reading is required. In some cases, reading further or elsewhere in the text might provide some information to guide a response to a particular question.*

1. This chapter mentions that the standard for normal hearing for children is different from that for adults. What are some reasons for this difference? Do you think this might be related to the development of speech and language? Why or why not?

2. UNHS is available in most states in the United States. What are some limitations of UNHS? Are these limitations similar to those stated for hearing screenings in general? Is UNHS critical for early intervention (e.g., see Chapter 9)? Why or why not?

3. Do the results of an audiogram lead to the recommendation of a hearing aid? Cochlear implant? Why or why not? [Note: Additional information may be gleaned from either Chapter 4 or Chapter 5.]

Suggested Activities

1. The major focus of this chapter was on hearing tests, audiograms, and hearing losses. We recommend a visit to your local speech, language, and hearing clinic (typically, there is one at a university). With adequate permission, it should be instructive to observe the testing battery for each of the following individuals:

   ■ A child younger than 2 years of age

   ■ A child between 2 and 5 years of age

   ■ A child between 5 and 10 years of age

   ■ A teenager

   ■ An adult

   Report your experiences and observations to your instructor or to the rest of your class.

2. Ask the audiologist to show you (under appropriate conditions; i.e., not violating privacy laws) audiograms depicting the following:

   ■ Hearing losses from slight to profound (i.e., according to PTAs)

   ■ A range of hearing loss types, from conductive to sensorineural

   If possible, ask the audiologist to test your hearing. Report your experiences and observations to your instructor or to the rest of your class.

References

American Academy of Audiology. (2000). Audiology clinical practice algorithms and statements. *Audiology Today* (Special Issue), 32–49.

American Academy of Audiology. (2004). Audiology: Scope of practice. *Audiology Today, 16*(3), 44–45.

American Academy of Otolaryngology-Head and Neck Surgery. (2009). *Fact sheet: What you should know about otosclerosis.* Available online: http://www.entnet.org/HealthInformation/ otosclerosis.cfm. Accessed November 30, 2009.

American Speech-Language-Hearing Association. (1990). Guidelines for audiometric symbols. *ASHA, 32*(Suppl), 25–30.

American Speech-Language-Hearing Association. (1997). *Guidelines for audiologic screening.* Rockville, MD: ASHA.

American Speech-Language-Hearing Association. (2005). *(Central) auditory processing disorders—The role of the audiologist.* Available online: www.asha.org/policy. Accessed December 12, 2008.

American Speech-Language-Hearing Association Committee on Audiologic Evaluation. (1988). Guidelines for determining threshold level for speech. *ASHA, 30,* 85–89.

Audiology Forum. Video otoscopy. Available online: www.rcsullivan.com/www/ears.htm. Accessed August 22, 2009.

Bunch, C. (1943). *Clinical audiometry.* St. Louis, MO: CV Mosby.

Burton, M. (2009). Acquired sensorineural hearing loss. In J. Graham & D. Baguley (Eds.), *Ballantyne's Deafness* (7th ed., pp. 101–114). London: Wiley.

Centers for Disease Control and Prevention. (2008). NHANES III: National Health and Nutrition Examination Survey. Available online: www.cdc.gov/nchs/products/elec_prods/subject/nhanes3 .htm. Accessed December 5, 2008.

Crandall, C., & Smaldino, J. (2002). Room acoustics and auditory rehabilitation technology. In J. Katz (Ed.), *Handbook of clinical audiology* (5th ed., pp. 607–630). Philadelphia: Lippincott Williams & Wilkins.

Dangerous Decibels. (2009). *Information center: Hearing loss.* Available online: http://www.dangerous decibels.org/hearingloss.cfm. Accessed November 30, 2009.

Hawke, M., Keene, M., & Albert, P. W. (1990). *Clinical otoscopy: an introduction to ear diseases.* New York: Churchill Livingstone.

Jerger, J., & Hayes, D. (1976). The cross-check principle in pediatric audiometry. *Archives of Otolaryngology, 102*(5), 614–620.

Kochkin, S. (2005). MarkeTrak VII: Hearing loss population tops 31 million people. *Hearing Review, 12*(7), 16–29.

Kochkin, S., Luxford, W., Northern, J., Mason, P., & Tharpe, A. (2007). MarkeTrak VII: Are 1 million dependents with hearing loss in America being left behind? *Hearing Review, 14*(10), 10–36.

Martin, F. N., & Clark, J. G. (2009). *Introduction to audiology* (10th ed.). Boston: Pearson.

Mendel, L. L., Danhauer, J. L., & Singh, S. (1999). *Singular's illustrated dictionary of audiology*. San Diego, CA: Singular.

Myers, P. J., Wilmington, D. J., Gallun, F. J., Henry, J. A., & Fausti, S. A. (2009). Hearing impairment and traumatic brain injury among soldiers: Special considerations for the audiologist. *Seminars in Hearing, 30*(1), 5–27.

NIDCD. (2009). National Institute on Deafness and Other Communication Disorders. Available online: http://www.nidcd.nih.gov/health/hearing/otitism.htm#what. Accessed November 28, 2009.

Niskar, A. S., Kieszak, S. M., Holmes, A. E., Esteban, E., Rubin, C., & Brody, D. J. (2001). Estimated prevalence of noise-induced hearing threshold shifts among children 6 to 19 years of age: The third national health and nutrition examination survey, 1988–1994, United States. *Pediatrics, 10*(1), 40–43.

Paul, P. (2009). *Language and deafness* (4th ed.). Sudbury, MA: Jones & Bartlett.

Petrak, M. (2000). Integrating physiologic technologies for hearing evaluation in infants and small children: An overview. Available online: www.audiologyonline.com/articles/article_detail.asp?article_id=217. Accessed December 4, 2008.

Pulec, J. L. (2001). *Atlas of otoscopy*. San Diego, CA: Singular/Thomson Learning.

Steel, K. P. (1998). A new era in the genetics of deafness. *The New England Journal of Medicine, 339*(21), 1545–1547.

Wilbur, L. (2002). Calibration: Pure tone, speech, and noise signals. In J. Katz (Ed.), *Handbook of clinical audiology* (5th ed., pp. 607–630). Philadelphia: Lippincott Williams & Wilkins.

Wilson, R., & McArdle, R. (2008). Change is in the air—in more ways than one. *The Hearing Journal, 61*(10), 10–15.

Wolfe, J., & Rogers-Scholl, J. (2008). Better *sooner* rather than later: So says the JCIH. *The Hearing Journal, 61*(10), 54.

Further Readings

Bess, F., & Humes, L. (2008). *Audiology: The fundamentals*. Philadelphia: Lippincott Williams & Wilkins.

Hepfner, S. (1997). *The audiogram workbook*. New York: Georg Thieme Verlag.

Madell, J., & Flexer, C. A. (2008). *Pediatric audiology: Diagnosis, technology, and management*. New York: Thieme.

Stach, B. (1998) *Clinical audiology: An introduction*. San Diego, CA: Singular.

HEARING AIDS AND OTHER ASSISTIVE TECHNOLOGY

There is little doubt that the single most important invention to help the hearing-handicapped child is the electronic hearing aid. There is an old adage ". . . as we hear, so we shall speak," and it is this very close relationship between hearing, speech, and language that is important to the deaf child. Several electronic gadgets have been invented to help the deaf child, including voice pitch indicators, speech timing equipment, vowel indicators, voice/non-voice meters, speech spectrum displays, visible speech machines, etc. None of these inventions, however, is more fundamental to the deaf child's education and ability to learn speech than a properly fitted hearing aid.

—Northern & Downs (1984, p. 269)

Key Concepts

After completing this chapter, readers should have a basic understanding of:

- Brief history of hearing aids
- Components and styles of hearing aids
- Regulations and standards
- Considerations in fitting of hearing aids
- Assistive technology options
- Future trends

This chapter covers the basics of hearing aids, starting with a brief history and ending with developments that are on the horizon. Components common to all styles of hearing aids are discussed. Current styles of hearing aids are reviewed, and we compare and contrast each in terms of benefits and limitations. Features available in hearing aids that enhance hearing and listening are also highlighted. In addition, we provide the critical steps of the fitting process. Finally, an introduction to assistive technology is presented. Either in addition to or in place of hearing aids, assistive listening devices are sometimes the best solution for hearing needs.

The passage that introduces this chapter, from the classic text by Northern and Downs, is a snapshot of the historic perspective on hearing aids. It was published over 25 years ago; however, in many ways it is as relevant today as it was then (if we ignore a few of the dated words and phrases). This passage provides a glimpse of how the constantly changing technology of hearing aids contributes to the quality of life for individuals with hearing loss. In the years since the passage first appeared, the increase in both technological and non-technological options has been astounding.

Our message here should not be interpreted to mean that hearing aids are the only option for individuals with hearing loss. Nevertheless, hearing aid technology is now flexible enough to accommodate a wide range of hearing loss, from a very small device designed to give a boost of amplification to address early hearing loss in Baby Boomers to hearing aids powerful enough to provide awareness of environmental sounds to those individuals who are d/Deaf or hard of hearing.

You might be thinking that the topic of hearing aids and assistive technology is somewhat dry. We shall do our best to make it interesting, albeit we cannot promise to make it as colorful as some of the current earmolds! We do think you will obtain a basic understanding and appreciation of amplification and assistive listening devices.

Consider the words of Staab (2002): "The function of a hearing aid is to amplify sounds to a degree and manner that will enable a person with a hearing impairment to use his or her remaining hearing in an effective manner" (p. 631). In short, hearing aids are devices designed to *aid* the ability to hear. They are not, as some individuals might think, bionic ears or cures for a hearing loss.

A few individuals who are fit with hearing aids report being disappointed with the result, to the point of saying that hearing aids do not work. Their expectation is that the hearing aid will restore their hearing to normal, meaning that they will be able to hear like a person without a hearing loss. This is a common fallacy (and the same is the case for individuals with cochlear implants, as discussed later in Chapter 5). Even though current hearing aids are amazing computers that process sound and deliver it efficiently to the ear, they cannot restore hearing to normal levels. The limitations do not lie in the hearing aid, but rather with the individual's auditory system, which impacts how sound is processed. The hearing aid is only as good as the user's realistic expectations, and the hearing aid is only a device that supports hearing.

Along this line of thinking, it is important to establish that one of the goals of using amplification is "...to ensure that sounds are audible across the widest possible frequency range at a comfortable level" (Dillon, Ching, & Golding, 2008, p. 168). Although the hearing aid provides information to the ear, the actual use of this information occurs at the level of the brain of the listener. Listeners should be able to "use their heads," so to speak, to understand the message.

Whether a person is involved in a conversation in a noisy restaurant, reacting to a siren of a passing ambulance, or listening to a favorite TV show, all of these environments require that accurate and clear information be provided by the hearing aid. This fact drives many of the decisions made in the selection of hearing aids, from the specific style to whether to use one or two hearing aids (always surprising to us; because people have two ears, we would expect that they would understand that each ear would need a hearing aid).

For professionals such as teachers, educational interpreters, and speech-language pathologists, knowing the basics of how a hearing aid works and how to troubleshoot (e.g., check for problems, provide basic maintenance like changing a battery, etc.) problems are important. In our view, troubleshooting is a critical skill for teachers and speech-language pathologists, given the breakdowns that are bound to occur during a typical school day, especially with young children. We have provided a few brief guidelines with respect to troubleshooting; however, readers are encouraged to seek hands-on experience if they will be working with students, patients, or consumers who use hearing aids.

We hope that the introduction to this chapter has stimulated you to think about a few questions related to hearing aids and the *Key Concepts* listed at the beginning of the chapter. These questions might include:

■ How do hearing aids work?

■ What do hearing aids look like?

■ What are the benefits and limitations of hearing aids?

■ Why would an individual need two hearing aids?

■ How is an individual fitted with hearing aids?

■ What are assistive listening devices?

■ What does the future look like?

These questions, and we hope many more, are addressed throughout this chapter and set the stage for Chapter 5 on cochlear implants.

Brief History of Hearing Aids

Believe it or not, hearing aids have been around since humans have had the ability to hear. Early "hearing aids" of animal horns or shells placed close to the ear were used to collect sound and direct it to the ear canal. We venture to guess that you have used one of the simplest hearing aids available—cupping your hand behind your ear. The cupping of the hand behind the ear has been estimated to provide about 14 dB of amplification (also referred to as *gain*) in the 1500 Hz range, an area where someone with a hearing loss may need a bit of a boost (deBoer, 1984).

Prior to the discovery of electricity, nonelectric hearing aids were available. These included ear trumpets, conversation tubes, and ear inserts—all of which funnel sounds toward the ear canal. Early versions of mechanical hearing aids were so large that they had to be supported by a table, not particularly convenient or cosmetically appealing for the user!

The earliest electric hearing aids appeared at the beginning of the twentieth century (Berger, 1984; Lybarger & Lybarger, 2000). These hearing aids used a carbon microphone, which was originally used in a telephone. The early hearing aids, although small enough to be worn, were only useful to individuals with mild-to-moderate hearing loss (see Chapter 1 on degrees of hearing impairment). One of the greatest limitations was that these devices sounded noisy and scratchy. Consequently, carbon microphone hearing aids had limited popularity among individuals with hearing loss.

Vacuum tubes were developed in the early 1900s and integrated into hearing aids in the early 1920s (Berger, 1984; Lybarger & Lybarger, 2000). The vacuum tubes were relatively small, making it possible to produce a hearing aid that could fit into the pocket of a shirt. However, these hearing aids required a relatively large battery pack. Miniaturization resulted in vacuum tube aids becoming smaller in the 1940s, with the battery placed directly into the hearing aid rather than in a separate pack. Vacuum tube hearing aids were used into the 1950s when transistors were introduced.

The invention of the transistor at Bell Labs in 1948 revolutionized many aspects of American life, causing huge improvements in televisions, radios, telephones, and hearing aids (Berger, 1984; Lybarger & Lybarger, 2000). Hearing aids were the first product to use the transistor (http://www.hearingaidmuseum.com/). Transistors allowed for continued miniaturization, resulting in progressively smaller and more powerful hearing aids during the 1950s and 1960s. In fact, these hearing aids had sufficient amplification for individuals with severe and profound hearing losses. Only two styles of hearing aids were available until the late 1950s: (1) body aids, which were about the same size as current handheld calculators, and (2) eyeglass hearing aids, which were built into and fit in the temples of eyeglasses.

Historically, hearing aids used analog processing of sound, suggesting that their main ability was merely to amplify sounds (Levitt, 2007). Processing with analog technology was often reflected by comments made by people with hearing loss: "I can hear the sound but I can't understand what is being said." This statement is generally noted in less than optimal environments, such as when background noise is present.

Pascoe (1991) described analog hearing aids as having technology similar to the grooves of a phonograph record to resemble the sound. Many of you might be too young to remember the phonograph, which was a sound-reproducing machine that played records made from vinyl. In this case, the songs were pressed into soundtracks embedded in the vinyl. Although the phonograph was used for decades as a device for listening to music, the quality of the sound it was able to reproduce was limited. The combination of the needle that played the record and the recording on the vinyl itself resulted in a poor quality, with popping and background noise often audible in the recording.

It should be easy to see why analog hearing aids are no longer a popular choice (or actually an available choice, because very few manufacturers continue to produce them). Just as the phonograph and vinyl records have been replaced by digital music players and digital media storage, the analog hearing aid has been replaced by the digital hearing aid. Nearly 90% of the hearing aids sold in the United States in 2006 were digital hearing aids (Kirkwood, 2006).

Now, a few comments about this fascinating technology. Basically, digital hearing aid technology, similar to the process used by other digital devices, converts sound waves into binary information. A digital hearing aid changes an electrical signal by an analog-to-digital (A/D) converter. This converter separates the signal into a series of separate bits, or basic units of information. These bits represent the characteristics of the sound input, including frequency, intensity, and timing aspects.

When the signal is digitized, more advanced processing can happen quickly and nearly automatically. The signal is changed back to an analog signal, because our ear is not able to understand the binary code. At this point, it is converted by a digital-to-analog (D/A) converter (Sandlin, 2001). The in-depth details of digital signal processing are beyond the scope of this chapter.

The foundation for digital hearing aids was developed during World War II (Levitt, 2007). Researchers at Bell Labs used a digital computer to simulate a high-frequency gain hearing aid for individuals with hearing loss (Levitt, 2006). The first wearable digital hearing aids were introduced in the mid-1980s (prototype digital hearing aids prior to this time were transported in a wagon, a significant limitation for the potential user!). Ricketts (2009) noted that most hearing aid manufacturers are currently moving toward their third or fourth generation of digital hearing aids.

The development of digital hearing aid technology has been the most significant advance in the field since the introduction of electric hearing aids. To paraphrase the classic Oldsmobile slogan, "It's not your father's hearing aid." In essence, digital hearing aids are able to accommodate listener needs not addressed by previous generations of hearing aids (Sandlin, 2001). For example, current digital hearing aids are able to handle issues that have frustrated individuals with hearing loss for years, including minimizing acoustic feedback, or the whistle that is sometimes heard from a hearing aid when sound escapes and is reamplified. In addition, digital hearing aids can increase audibility of sounds that are of interest to the listener (such as speech) while reducing competing noise (such as background conversations). Digital hearing aids also provide for connectivity with devices such as telephones or computers through wireless Bluetooth transmission (Levitt, 2007; Ricketts, 2009). Marriage (2009) indicated that although digital hearing aids cannot overcome distortions present in the cochlea, advances have created compensation for limitations in previous hearing aids.

You can learn more about the history of hearing aids by visiting either the Hugh Hetherington On-line Hearing Aid Museum (www.hearingaidmuseum.com) or the Kenneth Berger Hearing Aid Museum and Archives (http://ehhs.kent.edu/spa/museum.cfm). You can also visit the Berger Museum located at Kent State University in Kent, Ohio.

Hearing Aid Components

All hearing aids, regardless of the style or processing, are made up of three basic components: microphone, amplifier, and receiver (Sweetow, 2007; Tye-Murray, 2009). The two general types of microphones are directional, picking up sounds coming from the front of the hearing aid, and omnidirectional, picking up sounds from all directions (Tye-Murray, 2009). Directional microphones help the listener hear an individual speaker in a noisy environment. In contrast, omnidirectional microphones help the listener to be connected in that environment. Many digital hearing aids incorporate automatic directional microphones, which help the listener to understand speech in the presence of background noise while adapting to a number of listening situations.

In essence, the microphone picks up acoustic energy in the environment, such as speech or environmental noise, and converts it to an electrical signal. The electrical signal generated by the microphone is then routed through an amplifier. The amplifier provides relative amplification based on the hearing loss and a prescription for gain, which is discussed later in this chapter. Once the signal is amplified, it is directed to the receiver of the hearing aid, where it is converted back to an acoustic signal and delivered to the listener's ear canal.

A hearing aid may also be considered a signal processor that alters a signal input to improve its audibility for the wearer. The term *audibility* refers to being able to hear and understand speech. Audibility of the speech signal is important to the hearing aid wearer because greater audibility translates into improved speech intelligibility, which addresses the goal of most people who wear hearing aids—being able to understand speech (Souza, 2009). However, the trade-off is that this increased audibility must be provided to the wearer without distorting the sound quality or having the incoming signal at a level that is perceived as uncomfortably loud for the listener (Gudmundsen, 1997).

An Aside on Hearing Aid Batteries

Regardless of the style of hearing aid, its power source is a battery, described by Preves and Curran (2000) as "the unsung heroes in hearing aids" (p. 38). In general, the smaller the hearing aid, the smaller the power source, which also limits the battery's life. The vast majority of hearing aids are powered by button cell batteries designed specifically for hearing aids. These batteries have come a long way since hearing aids were powered by a large battery pack carried in the hand or strapped to the leg of the hearing aid wearer (Bloom, 2003).

Battery life is a frequent topic of discussion among hearing aid wearers. They state, often with indignation, that their watch battery only needs to be changed once a year but that their hearing aid battery needs to be changed weekly. In addition, another frequent comment is that hearing aid batteries cost too much, although they are generally around one dollar per cell. When one is spending $6000 or more on two hearing aids, the cost of batteries may seem irrelevant, similar to an analogy of purchasing a high-performance luxury car then stressing about the cost of the premium gasoline needed to run it.

Currently, virtually all hearing aid batteries are zinc air. Battery life is measured in hours, not days. Therefore, a person who wears hearing aids for 20 hours a day is likely to experience shorter battery life than the more casual hearing aid wearer (as long as that person remembers to turn the hearing aid off when not wearing it). When a hearing aid wearer inquires about the length of time a battery will last, the answer is always "it depends."

In general, digital hearing aids require more "juice" than analog hearing aids. This can be a transition for a person who switches to a digital hearing aid. A trade-off, however, is that digital hearing aids provide a low-battery warning, either in the form of a tone or a voice alerting the user that it is time to change the battery.

The concept of hearing aids powered by rechargeable batteries has been and continues to be explored. However, at this time, neither rechargeable nor extended life batteries have become a reality. This is due, in part, to the energy required to supply the hearing aid (Bloom, 2003). Solar-powered hearing aids and rechargeable nickel–metal hydrate batteries may both hold promise for the future.

Styles of Hearing Aids

Hearing aids come in a variety of styles but can be placed into two general categories: behind-the-ear styles and custom products that fit into the ear canal. Behind-the-ear hearing aids, also referred to as BTEs, are standard in size. The components fit into a small case worn behind the pinna (see ear structures in Chapter 2). The customized portion of the BTE—the earmold—is the part that attaches it into the ear canal. Custom products come in a variety of sizes—in-the-ear (ITE), in-the-canal (ITC), or completely-in-the-canal (CIC)—but all are similar in that the components fit into a custom shell fabricated from a mold of the individual's ear. BTEs have been available since the 1950s, whereas the custom products have been widely available since the late 1970s for the larger styles and the late 1980s for the CICs.

Each style has benefits and limitations. Much of the focus is often on the perceived cosmetic benefits of the style of hearing aid. BTEs are often perceived as less cosmetically appealing than custom hearing aids. However, style requires a broader understanding of a listener's needs than cosmetics alone. Hearing loss, listening demands, potential for growth of the ear, among many other factors, must be considered. For example, a physician who uses hearing aids with a stethoscope may find that the acoustics and physical location of the CIC hearing aids really meet her needs. A teenager involved in sports may prefer a BTE style. Custom products tend to be a bit less durable than BTEs, and if a soft earmold is forced into the ear canal during physical contact it is less likely to break and cut the ear canal than the hard case generally used with custom products. A brief review of each style of hearing aid is provided in the ensuing paragraphs.

BEHIND-THE-EAR HEARING AIDS

In the early 1960s, continued miniaturization of components resulted in hearing aids that could be worn behind the ear. Not surprisingly, this style of hearing aid is referred to as a behind-the-ear style of hearing aid, or BTE (see **Figure 4-1**).

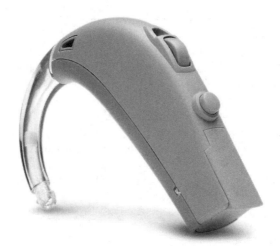

Figure 4-1
Behind-the-Ear Hearing Aid
Photo courtesy of Oticon, Inc.

BTE hearing aids provide significant benefits in terms of power and features. Although BTEs are appropriate for anyone with a hearing loss, they are also the most appropriate choice for more severe degrees of hearing loss or for listeners with more complex hearing needs. For example, BTEs are the most appropriate choice for children, because these aids can be adjusted to address changing listening demands and can accommodate growing ears by remaking the earmold. Directional microphones, one method for improving signal-to-noise ratio, are easily built into these hearing aids, addressing the problem of noise so common for individuals with sensorineural hearing loss. BTEs are powered by batteries, generally larger than those used in custom products, which may be easier to handle for individuals with vision issues or restricted dexterity.

BTEs have options, such as direct auditory input (DAI), that allow them to be connected to external audio sources, such as MP3 players, and provide a high-quality audio signal. Because BTEs are the style of hearing aid that has been around the longest, they are often perceived as less technologically advanced. However, technological advances are often included in BTEs first, due to the ability to build new components into the larger case.

Over the years, BTEs have become smaller and available in a range of colors and patterns, which appeal to wearers who want to express their own personal flair. As an audiologist at Ohio State, the second author occasionally receives requests for hearing aids cased in scarlet and grey, the Ohio State University colors. She recently fit a young man with Down syndrome with green and yellow hearing aids, as a tribute to his favorite company, John Deere. The popularity of this style of hearing aid has continued since its inception and has been reinvented many times over the past four decades. It continues to be the most popular style of hearing aid today, accounting for 56% of all hearing aid sales in 2008, in part due to the recent introduction of the open-fit or slim-tube BTEs (Kirkwood, 2008).

Earmolds for BTEs

As noted previously, the BTE style of hearing aid requires some type of method to hold the hearing aid in the ear. The two options at this point are an earmold (see **Figure 4-2**), which is custom made and fabricated from an impression made of the wearer's ear, or a standard dome used as part of the newer generation of open-fit BTEs connected by a slim tube (see **Figure 4-3**).

A well-fit earmold continues to be a critical factor in the success of a BTE hearing aid. As stated by Valente and colleagues (Valente, Valente, Potts, & Lybarger, 2000):

> Earmolds are designed to seal the ear canal, correctly couple the hearing aid to the ear from an acoustical viewpoint, retain the hearing aid on the pinna, be comfortable for an extended period of time, modify the acoustic signal produced by the hearing aid, be able to be easily handled by the patient, and be cosmetically appealing. (p. 71)

To make an earmold that meets the expectations presented by Valente et al. (2000), an excellent impression of the ear canal is required. Most audiologists use silicone material that is injected into the ear canal with a syringe. The impression takes about 10 minutes to set and harden. When removed from the ear canal, the audiologist should have an accurate impression of the ear, which is then sent to an earmold laboratory.

A major issue for the hearing aid wearer is to ensure that the fit is good. This allows the wearer to adjust the hearing aid to the volume level needed for audibility without having

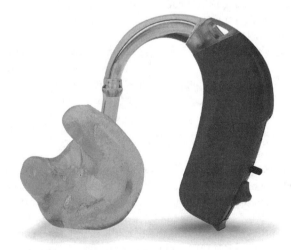

Figure 4-2
Behind-the-Ear Hearing Aid Attached to a Standard Earmold
Photo courtesy of Oticon, Inc.

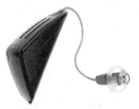

Figure 4-3
**Behind-the-Ear Hearing Aid Attached to Slim-Tube Fitting with a
Dome Style of Open Mold**
Photo courtesy of Oticon, Inc.

feedback. An ill-fitting earmold can be uncomfortable to wear and can result in a sore in
the ear canal. Clearly, if an earmold is uncomfortable the hearing aid is not likely to be
worn. The chance of having an ill-fitting earmold is minimized if the audiologist makes a
good impression of the ear canal (often easier said than done in a squirming toddler) and
dialogues with the hearing aid user about the perception of the fit of the earmold.

Just as there is a range of styles of hearing aids, there is also a range of styles of earmolds.
In addition, earmold materials range from lucite, which is a rigid material, to silicone,
which is soft and adheres to the shape of the ear canal in response to the wearer's body
heat. The selection of a particular style and material is based on a number of factors, including acoustic parameters, degree of hearing loss, allergies to certain components, or desire
for a specific material or a specific color or pattern (and there are interesting and appealing colors and patterns!).

A few earmold laboratories and hearing aid manufacturers are moving away from the
use of silicone impressions to the use of a 3D laser scan of the ear, with dimensions of the
individual ear developed by computer software. From this scan, a custom earmold or hearing aid shell is designed; this process is thought to result in a more accurate, better quality
impression than those created from the more traditional methods.

IN-THE-EAR AND IN-THE-CANAL HEARING AIDS

In-the-ear hearing aids, or ITEs (see **Figure 4-4**), and in-the-canal hearing aids, or ITCs
(see **Figure 4-5**), are both custom-made hearing aids in which all of the components are
housed in a case or shell made from an impression of the wearer's ear.

These hearing aids are considered to be self-contained. The case fits into the ear canal,
with the primary difference being that the ITE fills more of the concha, or the C-shaped
area, of the ear canal than the ITC. A number of wearers view these hearing aids as more
convenient than having a hearing aid with an earmold. Custom hearing aids may be easier to insert into the ear for some individuals (Upfold, May, & Battaglia, 1990). In addition, the sound quality for both the ITC and ITE is reported to be more natural because

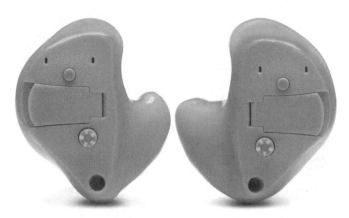

Figure 4-4
In-the-Ear Hearing Aid
Photo courtesy of Oticon, Inc.

the microphone of the hearing aid is in the ear canal rather than behind the pinna, as is the case with BTEs.

Although current ITEs can accommodate nearly any degree of hearing loss, ITCs tend to be more appropriate for no greater than moderate-to-severe hearing losses, due to their limited ability to provide sufficient gain and the possibility of acoustic feedback. These styles of hearing aids tend to be somewhat less durable than BTEs in terms of moisture and wax entering the receiver, which is housed directly in the hearing aid and close to the ear canal.

Individuals who wear one of these styles of hearing aids need to be fastidious about keeping the part of the aid worn in the ear clear of wax, either by using a wax loop (a tool

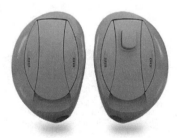

Figure 4-5
In-the-Canal Hearing Aid
Photo courtesy of Oticon, Inc.

that looks like a mini paperclip) or by changing the wax guards, which are designed to limit the amount of wax entering the hearing aid. ITEs are also more limited with respect to their use in conjunction with assistive technology, discussed later in this chapter. However, with ever-evolving wireless connectivity, this situation is likely to change in the next few years.

COMPLETELY-IN-THE-CANAL HEARING AIDS

Completely-in-the-canal, or CIC (see **Figure 4-6**), hearing aids are custom hearing aids in which all components fit into the ear canal only. These aids do not extend into the concha. Initially designed to address primarily high-frequency hearing loss, their main benefits were considered to be cosmetic and in reducing the occlusion effect, or the perception that the ear feels plugged, as reported by many wearers, particularly those with high-frequency hearing loss.

The CIC style addresses many issues that kept individuals from being previously successful with hearing aids, including the reduction of wind noise (important for sports or working outside) and the ability to use the hearing aids comfortably without feedback on the telephone or with a stethoscope. Because the components of this hearing aid are closer to the eardrum, less electronic gain is required compared to other styles, which also reduces the risk of acoustic feedback (Tye-Murray, 2009). These hearing aids also provide increased gain (or amplification) in the high frequencies, improving audibility for those with normal hearing in the lower frequencies and having a hearing loss in the higher frequencies—a common type of hearing loss that was difficult to fit with a hearing aid before the introduction of the CIC.

CICs are best for individuals with a mild-to-moderate hearing loss, although there are some exceptions to this guideline, primarily based on the physical size and shape of the ear canal. Physical limitations of the ear canal make this style of hearing aid an inappropriate choice as often as degree of hearing loss does. Because the CIC hearing aid fits into the ear canal, it has a removal cord built into the case (which has been trimmed off more than once by a well-meaning hairstylist).

The small size of the CIC renders it the least flexible in terms of options. It can be argued that the small size of the hearing aid itself and of the battery that powers it makes

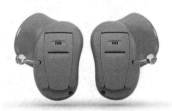

Figure 4-6
Completely-in-the-Canal Hearing Aid
Photo courtesy of Oticon, Inc.

it a less than optimal choice for those with visual or dexterity issues (as has been attested to by the number of these aids that have been mistaken for a nut of some type, popped in the mouth, and chewed by the wearer—usually salvaged before swallowed, but usually not before the case is damaged by the teeth). The CIC is the most temperamental style of hearing aid because it is most sensitive to moisture and cerumen. Some wearers have changed to a different style of hearing aid due to the number of repairs needed by the CIC, even though the sound quality of the hearing aid was good. A disadvantage of all custom hearing aids is that the wearer is without a hearing aid if the aid needs to be repaired; in contrast, it is not unusual for an audiologist to be able to provide a hearing aid on loan while a BTE is being repaired.

Are Two Ears Better Than One? Binaural Hearing Aids

A question frequently asked by individuals who are considering hearing aids is if they really need two hearing aids. For some, this appears to be a perception that they are being oversold; that is, they only really "need" one hearing aid but are sold two by an unethical audiologist only wanting to make money. Others state that wearing one hearing aid is "bad enough," but that wearing two would be unacceptable from a cosmetic perspective or with regard to their self-perception. The question of one hearing aid versus two hearing aids (also known as monaural versus binaural amplification) can be answered based on evidence from years of research, along with the listener's communication demands and needs.

Simply stated, two hearing aids are better than one, assuming that both ears have a hearing loss. This is based on what is known as the *binaural (two ear) advantage*. If listeners have a hearing loss in one ear only, they are still candidates for a hearing aid; however, if someone tries to fit them with two hearing aids in this case, it is likely that that person is only looking to make money!

Ross (2006) pointed out that, in the "early days" of hearing aids, the decision to amplify only one ear was based on the fact that hearing aids were big and bulky, and most listeners were able to tolerate only one hearing aid. In general, the ear with the poorer hearing ability was the one fit with the hearing aid. In the past 30 years, the strength of the evidence supports the use of binaural hearing aids. Ross (2006) stressed that there is "...an overwhelming preponderance of evidence that supports the notion that for most hearing-impaired, two ears are better than one" (p. 36). Pascoe (1991) suggested that hearing aids should be sold in pairs similar to eyeglasses.

The benefits of having two ears (i.e., binaural hearing) have been well documented. Localizing the sound source, which is important for listening in noise and in providing direction of the sound (which is important for safety), is one of the most basic benefits of binaural hearing. Another benefit is binaural summation; that is, having the sum of information received at the two ears is greater than its parts. Improved speech understanding in noise, also known as *binaural squelch*, is yet another binaural benefit. The central auditory system can compare the input from the two ears and "squelch" the noise to some extent. Wearing a hearing aid in both ears minimizes the auditory deprivation inherent in not amplifying a hearing loss. Most important, hearing with two ears improves the quality of sound perceived by the listener (Pascoe, 1998; Ross, 2006). In short, two ears are better than one.

A classic study by Silman and his colleagues (Silman, Gelfand, & Silverman, 1984) provided additional insight into the importance of binaural hearing/binaural amplification. People with bilaterally sensorineural hearing loss who use a hearing aid only on one ear demonstrate what has been termed as *late-onset auditory deprivation*. This is categorized by statistically poorer word-understanding abilities (which have decreased over previous results) in the unaided ear. This type of change is related to auditory deprivation of the central auditory nervous system (CANS). The "use it or lose it" conclusion of this line of research provides additional evidence for the importance of binaural hearing aids.

Current hearing aid technology allows for the synchronization of two hearing aids through a wireless connection, which enhances the adaptive abilities of the two aids. As noted by Marriage (2009), this binaural synchronization is an innovation that truly enhances the ability to use the two ears together to maximize the binaural benefit, just as the auditory system is designed to do. Hearing aid wearers using this type of synchronization are better able to track sound sources for localization purposes. In addition, improved sound clarity has been noted (Marriage, 2009).

Hearing Aid Regulations and Standards

Now that we have resolved the debate on one versus two hearing aids, let us proceed to regulations and standards. The sale, dispensing, and fitting of hearing aids are regulated by the federal government, specifically by the Food and Drug Administration (FDA). This regulation is designed to protect consumer safety and to ensure efficacy of products (Food and Drug Administration, 2009).

One example of a regulation is the role of the physician. A physician does not have to approve or supervise the fit of a hearing aid; however, if an individual chooses to not see a physician prior to obtaining the hearing aid, he or she must sign a *Physician Waiver*. Medical clearance is needed for certain types of situations, such as when the individual is younger than age 18 or presents a "red flag" condition, such as asymmetric hearing loss, conductive hearing loss, or drainage from the ear canal. In these cases, an examination by a physician, preferably an otolaryngologist (also referred to as ear, nose, and throat physician, or ENT) is required. Note that medical clearance does not provide permission for the fitting of a hearing aid; it only verifies that there is no medical reason why the individual cannot use a hearing aid. It also confirms that the hearing loss cannot be medically or surgically treated.

One of the main reasons for federal and state regulation of hearing aids is the perception that consumers believe they are going to be "ripped off" when they purchase a hearing aid. This perception is fueled by the bait-and-switch advertising seen in newspapers ("buy one get one free") or on TV infomercials. You have probably seen one of these fine "bionic rechargeable hearing aids" advertised for only $14.95. The old adage of "if it's too good to be true, it is" applies to hearing aids. In any case, the individual with a hearing loss should enter into a relationship with an audiologist who seeks to understand communication needs and addresses how to support the listener's goals. The hearing aid should not be viewed as a purchase, but as an investment, which will need maintenance and care.

With respect to standards, hearing aid manufacturers use an approach to defining terms and for outlining performance parameters. This standard, known as American National Standards Institute (ANSI) S3.22, has been the defining document for hearing instrument performance since 1976 (Frye, 2005). This is a way to ensure that the hearing aid is working in the manner that the manufacturer indicates that it should. It is also one way to verify selection of the hearing aid, which is discussed later.

The ANSI standard encompasses a significant number of parameters, including those frequently used in describing hearing aid function, such as gain, MPO, and distortion. *Gain* is defined as how much a quiet sound is amplified. *Maximum power output*, or MPO, addresses how a more intense sound drives the hearing aid (Frye, 2005). Another parameter considered in hearing aid function is *distortion*, which translates into the sound quality of the hearing aid. Obviously, low levels of distortion in a hearing aid are critical, because this helps to ensure that the speech signal is clear.

These are important terms for calibrating the hearing aid against the standard, but they can also be used to ensure that the hearing aid is working for the wearer. If the hearing aid has too little gain, users will not hear what they want or need to hear. If the MPO is too high, minimally the hearing aid will be uncomfortable; but, more important, the sound may be so intense that it can damage the wearer's hearing.

Hearing Aid Fitting

The selection and fitting of hearing aids should be viewed as part of a process and not merely as part of the sale of a product. The foundation of all hearing aid fittings begins with a comprehensive evaluation of hearing, including assessing the listener's ability to understand speech in quiet and in the presence of noise, as mentioned in Chapter 3. Several factors have to be considered, including the listener's needs and expectations, etiology of the hearing loss, and language skills. With respect to a child, the parents' expectations, the school's acoustical environment, and the type of school program are additional factors that must be considered. Other factors, including physical issues (e.g., manual dexterity) and financial considerations, also come into play.

Individuals with hearing loss often ask the question, "What hearing aid is best for me?" This question is often related to a specific manufacturer or style of hearing aid, sometimes augmented by information from what has been a success (or failure) for friends or family members. The answers to this question are as unique as the individuals themselves. It is the audiologist's responsibility to learn as much as he or she can about the listener, including his or her lifestyle and communication needs, to assist in selecting the best hearing solutions. For example, if an individual perspires heavily or expects to use hearing aids while playing sports, selecting a hearing aid that is moisture resistant may be the best choice. This choice will limit the decision; in this case, the logical choice is the BTE, and a small number of hearing aids are actually moisture resistant.

In general, the fitting of a hearing aid requires a two-step process: verification and validation. After these steps, it is important to consider the issues of orientation and acclimatization. Taken together, all of these concepts contribute to a successful fitting.

VERIFICATION

Verification of the hearing aid requires the use of techniques to ensure that the hearing aid meets specified goals (Kruger & Kruger, 1994). The specified goals are often based on a prescriptive method for fitting the hearing aid. Just as a prescription medication addresses a patient's specific issue or concerns, a prescriptive method for hearing aid fitting ensures that the amount of amplification prescribed in the hearing aid addresses the listener's specific communication issues.

There are two distinct approaches of prescriptive methods. One approach strives to maximize comfort for the listener, based on the recognition that one aspect of sensorineural hearing loss is abnormal perception of loudness. These methods are generally based on the hearing thresholds obtained during the audiologic evaluation (Bagatto et al., 2005). The second approach seeks to maximize audibility for the listener and is based on hearing measures above the listener's threshold (Bagatto et al., 2005).

An example of a prescriptive method based on comfort would be the National Acoustic Lab-NL1 (NAL-NL1). An example based on audibility is the Desired Sensation Level (DSL). Each method has its own strengths and provides a goal or target to guide the hearing aid fitting. The most important aspect of verification is not the actual prescription that is selected, but the fact that the audiologist actually spends time verifying the hearing aid fit to ensure that the aid does what it is anticipated to do in terms of amplification.

Audiologists select and order hearing aids from the manufacturer of their choice, based on a number of parameters. When the hearing aids are delivered to the audiologist, most perform a conformity check as one step in the hearing aid verification process. This step, also known as electroacoustic analysis (EAA), ensures that the hearing aid is working appropriately and meeting the ANSI standards discussed earlier.

The next step is to adjust the hearing aid for the wearer's specific hearing loss. Current digital hearing aids are programmed with computer software through a wireless interface, a process known as *programming* the hearing aid. As noted by Ross (2007), this programming requires incorporating specific amplification goals, known as *targets*. These targets can be modified based on the particular individual's ear canal size and shape.

Digital hearing aids can be adjusted for nearly unlimited changes. The audiologist can shape the signal being heard by the listener, add multiple programs for specific situations, and customize features, such as adding a low-battery alert signal. The hearing aid wearer is able to change programs either by pushing a button on the hearing aid or by using a remote device (which may resemble a small MP3 player remote or even be part of a wristwatch).

Some features are automatic, meaning that the hearing aid is "smart"; it can make decisions based on the listening environment. Consider the example provided earlier of an adaptive directional microphone, whereby the listening environment directs the type of microphone response. Another advantage of digital hearing aids is that they can sometimes be upgraded when the manufacturer makes changes, often as easily as a software upgrade can be installed on a laptop computer.

Once the hearing aid is programmed for the listener, other types of verification methods may be applied, including what is described as *real ear*, or probe microphone, measures. For example, the output of the hearing aid can be measured by placing the aid in a small coupler, presenting a signal as an input, and measuring the intensity of the output. This measurement is made in a 2-cc coupler, designed to simulate the dimensions of the average adult ear (Ross, 2007). Obviously, most ears differ from this average simulated ear. In the case of this real ear verification, the fit of the hearing aid is verified objectively, but in the listener's own ear, by placing a small microphone into the ear canal close to the eardrum. Measurements are made, using a variety of signals, in both unaided and aided situations.

VALIDATION

The second major step of the hearing aid fitting process is validation. *Validation* is the functional assessment of the hearing aid; that is, does the hearing aid work the way the user needs it to work in the real world? If the hearing aid and its programs have been verified, but the hearing aid user cannot hear well, it is unlikely that the fitting will be successful.

A number of factors can be considered in validation, including: (1) the wearer's satisfaction with the hearing aid; (2) the actual use time, which is recorded in the digital hearing aid and can be verified by the audiologist; (3) the impact that fitting of the hearing aid has had on significant others; and (4) improvement in overall quality of life (Cox, 2003). Questionnaires or inventories are often used as part of the validation process. Some are self-assessment instruments, such as the *Satisfaction with Amplification in Daily Life* (SADL) (Cox & Alexander, 1999). Others address observations of the listener's ability to hear in a specific situation (e.g., classroom, etc.), such as the *Listening Inventory for Education* (LIFE) (Anderson & Smaldino, 1998).

Audiologists may also use speech understanding in noise as a measure of validation. Two examples of tests that are used for this purpose are the *Quick Speech in Noise* (QSIN; Killion, Niquette, Gudmundsen, Revit, & Banerjee, 2004) and the *Hearing in Noise Test* (HINT; Nillson, Soli, & Sullivan, 1994). Both of these tests simulate real-world situations of listening in noise that can be set up in the audiologic booth.

In addition to audiologists, validation of hearing aid fitting may be performed in real-world environments by individuals who interact with the listener, including parents, speech-language pathologists, and educators. There are a number of tools and techniques that can be utilized to ensure that hearing aid fitting is set effectively and is working on a daily basis. Similar techniques can be applied to validating the setting of a cochlear implant processor (Chapter 5). The *Ling 6 Sound Test* is one prominent example of such a validation procedure and is discussed in Chapter 8.

ORIENTATION AND ACCLIMATIZATION

One of the most important steps in the fitting process is that of hearing aid orientation. The hearing aid user and his or her family members must understand how to use and maintain the new hearing aids. This orientation includes discussing how to insert the hearing aid into the ear, how to change the batteries, how to keep the hearing aid clean and in good working order, how to troubleshoot potential problems, and how to use the hearing aid with other devices (e.g., using the t-coil for telephone use or enabling Bluetooth to use a cell phone or computer). This is also an important time to discuss realistic expectations and the limitations of amplification. In most cases, this is also the time to answer questions and help listeners get started with their hearing aids.

Most hearing aids are dispensed with what is referred to as a *trial or adjustment period*, allowing the individual to use the hearing aids in various situations; that is, "to kick the tires," so to speak. A typical trial period is often 30 days, and the listener has the opportunity to use the hearing aid in actual situations. The audiologist can make adjustments to the programs based on feedback from the individual. This trial period may be complimentary or at a minimal cost, so the individual can see the benefits of the hearing aid without the investment of purchasing it outright.

The trial period acknowledges acclimatization, an important step in the fitting process. *Acclimatization* refers to changes in speech understanding that happen over the time of the initial fitting of the hearing aid, usually thought to be most noted in the first 30 to 90 days of being fit (Mueller & Powers, 2001). This is a process of adjustment and accommodation on the part of the individual with a hearing loss. Many individuals wait to be fit with a hearing aid long after they recognize that they have a hearing loss. A significant number of individuals wait 15 years or more (Kochkin, 2009).

With respect to "waiting," we should mention *auditory plasticity*, or the brain's ability to change, which is related to what has been described as *auditory deprivation* (Billings & Tremblay, 2007). This type of deprivation impacts the brain's ability to code auditory information, including the frequency, intensity, and timing aspects of the signal. In essence, a hearing loss not only impacts the ear's ability to hear, but also the brain's ability to perceive sound. Billings and Tremblay (2007) report that "...the typical person being evaluated by an audiologist for hearing aids or a cochlear implant has an auditory system that has likely undergone significant deprivation-related physiological changes...." (p. 5).

In essence, introducing sound to an auditory system that has been deprived of sound is likely to alter the way in which sounds are perceived and represented by the ear. New research is focused on how hearing aids might interact with the auditory system to change auditory plasticity. When first fit with a hearing aid, most individuals need a period of adjustment or acclimatization to sound perception.

Ultimately, the success of a fitting is defined by the individual who is able to use the aids effectively and efficiently to enhance his or her communication. As noted previously, many individuals with hearing loss initially expect that hearing aids will *cure* their hearing loss. Once it is established that hearing aids do not cure hearing loss, most listeners are able to establish reasonable goals for the hearing aid fitting. Despite popular myths, most individuals with hearing aids adjust well and enjoy the benefits of improved communication. In addition, it is not unusual for spouses or other family members to provide unsolicited testimonials about how much the hearing aid has changed their lives.

Once individuals are fit and the aids are adjusted, they will need to know about the care and maintenance of the hearing aids. In the cases of children or older adults, it is possible that someone other than the user will be responsible for the care of the hearing aids and for troubleshooting issues that may arise. A basic troubleshooting guide is provided in Table 4-1.

Table 4-1

A Practical Guide for Understanding Hearing Aids

Before Getting Started

It is important to have basic information to understand hearing aid function. Knowing the manufacturer, the model, and serial number can be helpful and can provide additional information in the future, such as guiding the types of assistive technology that may be recommended (e.g., FM system). Having a copy of the user manual provided with the hearing aid can also provide some useful information. Many hearing aid manufacturers now have instructional manuals online.

Tools and Hearing Aid Kit

A number of tools are useful in checking and maintaining hearing aids. These tools can be purchased through a local audiologist, online from a site such as *HARC Mercantile* (http://harc.com), or as part of a hearing aid care kit from a manufacturer (e.g., the Otikids program through Oticon; more information at http://www.oticonchildren.com). Tools in a care kit may include the following:

- Hearing aid battery tester

- Stethoset or listening earmold to listen through the hearing aid

- Wax loop: A small tool bent like a 1/2 paperclip for cleaning debris from earmold or hearing aid receiver

- Brush: Small brush for cleaning debris from opening of earmold or hearing aid receiver

- Air blower for earmold: Forces air though tubing of earmold

- A small cleaning cloth or sanitized *audio wipes,* specially designed disinfecting towelettes

(*continues*)

Table 4-1	*A Practical Guide for Understanding Hearing Aids (continued)*

Checking and Changing the Battery

Most current hearing aids have a low battery indicator, either a tone or a voice indicator that states that the battery is "low." A quick check can be accomplished by turning the hearing aid to the "on" position (usually by closing the battery door, which is the on/off switch for most hearing aids) and cupping the hearing aid in your hand. If you hear "feedback" (a whistling sound), the hearing aid is working. If no feedback is heard, the battery should be changed.

It is critical to know the correct size of the hearing aid battery. The battery has a positive (+) sign on the flat (silver colored) side of the battery. This + should be matched with the + in the battery compartment of the hearing aid. The battery is always placed in the battery compartment (and not directly into the case of the hearing aid), and the battery door should close with little resistance when the battery is inserted correctly.

When the hearing aid is not in use, the battery compartment should be open. This turns the aid off and extends the life of the battery. The battery contacts should be kept clean. If the contacts become corroded (which may be observed by discoloration), they should be cleaned with cotton swabs dipped in isopropyl alcohol or with a clean pencil eraser. If this is a frequent problem, an aerosol spray of contact restorer may be used. Moisture in the hearing aid can contribute to an issue with corrosion.

Moisture

Although some hearing aids are now moisture resistant, hearing aids are not designed to be immersed in water. Humid climates result in malfunction of hearing aids due to moisture exposure. In addition, hearing aids may be a victim of perspiration when worn in activities such as sports.

Efforts should be made to keep hearing aids dry. In some cases, moisture droplets may be observed in the tubing of the earmold. In other cases, a filter in an earhook (the plastic piece that attaches the body of the behind-the-ear hearing aid to the earmold) is distended, blocking sound from reaching the ear.

Tools to keep the hearing aid dry include a hearing aid desiccant or dehumidifier kit, generally consisting of silica beads or gel, or the *Dry and Store*, a storage kit designed to remove moisture and to sanitize the hearing aid (http://www.dryandstore.com/). In cases of chronic moisture buildup, an air blower can be used to clear the earmold tubing and sweat bands on BTE hearing aids.

Table 4-1	*A Practical Guide for Understanding Hearing Aids (continued)*

Storing the Hearing Aids

When hearing aids are not being worn (which should be only when the wearer is sleeping), they should be safely stored for protection. If a desiccant kit is used, this is a logical place to store the hearing aids. The storage boxes that come with hearing aids are also a good storage option. If children will be removing their hearing aids during the school day, an option for safe storage should be developed. It is critical that hearing aids be stored away from pets, as dogs in particular seem to be attracted to the smell of earwax and end up chewing and destroying the hearing aid.

Listening Check of Hearing Aids

Most adult listeners are able to address whether their hearing aids are working well. However, in children or older adults, a change in their behavior is often the primary indicator that the aid is not working effectively. A validation process, such as the Ling Test outlined in Chapter 8, may be of benefit for a check. In addition, you can listen through a hearing aid stethoset or listening earmold to better perceive the amplification in the way that the wearer experiences the hearing aid.

Basic Troubleshooting

If a hearing aid is not working or seems to be working less than optimally, there are some things that can be easily checked and often easily addressed.

The Hearing Aid Is Dead

- Change the battery

- Check tubing of earmold for occlusion with wax or debris (separate the earmold from the hearing aid and see if the aid works without the earmold attached)

- Clean the receiver of the hearing aid or the sound bore (opening) to earmold with wax loop or brush

- Make sure hearing aid is in the "on" position and that the program is appropriate (e.g., not in a "mute" program)

(continues)

Table 4-1	**A Practical Guide for Understanding Hearing Aids (continued)**

The Hearing Aid Sounds Weak

- Battery may be weak; change the battery
- Check tubing in earmold or receiver in custom products for wax or debris
- Make sure that the earmold is securely attached to the hearing aid
- Make sure the earmold is positioned appropriately in the hearing aid
- For open fit, change dome
- Store in desiccant or drying device to remove potential sources of moisture

The Hearing Aid Is Whistling (Feedback)

- Check that the hearing aid is correctly positioned in the ear
- Check earmold or receiver for earwax
- Check ear canal for occlusion with earwax
- Check fit of earmold or hearing aid case
- Check earmold tubing to determine if cracked or loose and needs to be replaced

Assistive Technology

Despite the high quality of digital technology, hearing aids cannot optimize communication for all listening situations. Think of the variety and complexity of listening situations you find yourself in on a daily basis—listening on the telephone, both landline and cellular; listening in a large lecture hall; listening as the passenger from the backseat of the car; listening to music through an MP3 player; having a conversation in a noisy restaurant; hearing effectively while playing a pick-up game of basketball, just to name a few. Each of these situations involves a unique listening environment in terms of the acoustic environment, the signal-to-noise ratio, and the technology interface. These are the same variety of situations that present challenges for individuals with hearing loss. It is also important to acknowledge that even the best hearing aid cannot overcome hearing issues that result from damage to the cochlea, based on the demands of dynamic listening situations.

Compton-Conley (2009) remarked that all listeners, regardless of hearing abilities, share four communication demands:

1. Face-to-face communication with other people

2. Enjoyment of electronic media (radio, stereo system, television, the soundtrack at the movies, etc.)

3. Telephone communication

4. Awareness of environmental sounds and situations (doorbell, fire alarm, pager, etc.)

Although hearing aids may be beneficial in all of these situations, other types of technology may address these situations more effectively or efficiently. These other types of technology are often referred to as ALDs, or assistive listening devices. This type of technology may also be known as HAT, or hearing assistance technology. They have been referred to as being like "binoculars for the ears" (Compton-Conley, 2009).

As noted by Compton-Conley (2009), there are two categories of these devices: auditory and nonauditory. The topic of ALDs for people with hearing loss is an important one, but an in-depth description of the available options is beyond the scope of this chapter. However, we want to provide you with a brief overview of some options that are available to individuals with hearing loss. We shall proceed from classrooms to telephones to television and, finally, to the use of alerting devices.

Devices to address face-to-face communication are designed to overcome issues of poor room acoustics, such as distance from the speaker, reverberation in the room, and background noise. Most of these devices use a remote microphone or a microphone placed near the speaker or attached directly to the sound source, such as an MP3 player or DVD player. These microphones can be wireless and use a receiver added to a hearing aid, as in a frequency modulated system (FM system) (see **Figures 4-7**, **4-8**, and **4-9**), or they can be wired directly to the hearing aid. Both types of microphones capture the sound from the source, whether it is a person speaking or a DVD player, and allow the listener to access a clean, clear sound (Compton-Conley, 2009; Tye-Murray, 2009). The use of remote microphone technology has frequently been described as having "whatever the person is listening to being about 6 inches away from his or her ear." FM systems have been used in schools for many years.

You may have been in a classroom lecture in which the speaker's words are represented by visual information (i.e., printed words), such as real-time closed captioning or Communication Access Real Time Translation (CART). The CART system operator uses a machine similar to those used by court reporters that is fed to a computer from where it is displayed on a computer monitor, for a small group, or onto a screen, such as in the classroom or lecture hall setting. This type of captioning can provide great information to individuals with all degrees of hearing loss as long as they are able to read.

Being able to use the telephone is an important aspect of communication, from catching up with a friend who lives out of town to reporting an emergency. Telephones are generally difficult to accommodate because they tend to be higher-frequency filters, which both changes the tone of the speaker's voice (which is why your friends may sound differ-

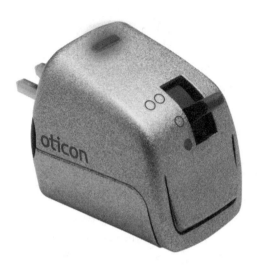

Figure 4-7
FM Receiver That Attaches to a Hearing Aid

Photo courtesy of Oticon, Inc.

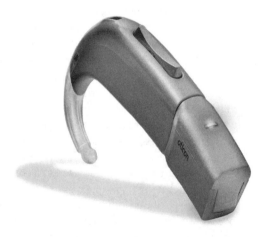

Figure 4-8
FM Receiver Attached to a Hearing Aid

Photo courtesy of Oticon, Inc.

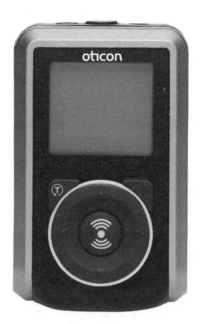

Figure 4-9
FM Transmitter, Worn by the Person Speaking, to Transmit His or Her Voice Directly to the Listener's Ear (Receiver)
Photo courtesy of Oticon, Inc.

ent on the phone than in person) to transposing information to a range that is difficult for the individual with a hearing loss to perceive. Many hearing aids have a telecoil, or *t-coil*, option, which picks up and sends the electromagnetic information from the telephone directly into the hearing aid. In the past, these t-coils were activated with a switch; however, current digital hearing aids often have an automatic t-coil that is activated when the phone is close to the hearing aid. Amplified telephones and telephone amplifiers are also available and may be an option.

If an individual is unable to hear over the telephone, options such as Voice Carry Over (VCO), also known as *read and talk*, are available (Compton-Conley, 2009). VCOs are used in conjunction with telephone relay services, so the speaker is able to talk to the operator who translates what is said to the individual with a hearing loss, who then views the message in print on an LCD screen.

One of the complaints that family members of individuals with hearing loss often express is related to the volume of the television; that is, the TV is often louder for family members with typical hearing. Obviously, most television shows are currently closed captioned. However, other options are available, such as the use of an infrared television listening device. An infrared transmitter is placed near the speaker on the television, and the listener wears a small infrared receiver as headphones. The listener can adjust the personal receiver to a volume level that he or she is able to hear while family members are able to listen to the volume at the level they prefer. This type of device has contributed to domestic tranquility in many households.

The last category of ALDs to be addressed is alerting devices. These alerting devices may include those for safety, such as with a fire alarm, to awakening with an alarm clock. These devices often incorporate tactile information, such as vibration, or visual information, such as a flashing light, as part of alerting the user. An alarm clock may include a vibrating device that shakes the bed when it is time to wake up. Lights may flash when the phone or the doorbell rings.

There are as many specialized listening situations as there are individuals with hearing loss. Medical professionals with hearing loss may use an amplified stethoscope, some with visual displays. Listening in places such as churches and movie theaters may provide a special challenge, which is met with many options, such as infrared systems and rear-projection closed captioning. For an overview of many types of devices that are available, the reader is referred to HARC Mercantile (www.harcmercantile.com).

The Future

Based on the speed of changes in technology, we can only speculate on the transformations ahead in hearing aids and assistive technologies for individuals with hearing loss. Clearly, the sky should be considered the limit. With the ability to load more music of digital quality on smaller and smaller devices, such as a mini-MP3 player, many scholars have speculated that future hearing aids will be built into devices such as the iPod (Yanz, 2006). Hearing aid and cell phone manufacturers have both been exploring options to build hearing aids directly into cell phones for a number of years.

Even though we do not have a crystal ball, a couple of things are evident about the future of hearing aids and assistive technology devices. The developments and changes in technology that drive new hearing aids make it likely that some of the information included in this chapter will be outdated by the time this book is published. Although the fundamentals are likely to remain the same, providing a foundation for you to understand important aspects of hearing aids, rapid technological changes are inevitable.

It is also anticipated that the discoveries designed to address enhancing communication for individuals with hearing loss will benefit all listeners, regardless of hearing status. An example of this type of technological advance can be viewed in the development of closed captioning for television. Originally designed to allow an individual with hearing loss to appreciate and understand programs on television, it is likely that you have also benefited from closed captioning when you are watching your favorite sporting event in a bar or restaurant setting.

It is likely also that hearing aids that address performance in listening situations will be manufactured, but with an eye toward other types of concerns expressed by individuals with hearing loss, such as cosmetics and extended battery life. One product currently available that incorporates a future perspective is manufactured by Lyric Hearing. This product is described as "the world's only 100% invisible hearing device that is worn 24/7 and delivers a natural sound" (Lyric Hearing, 2009, n.p.). Currently available only to adults, it is placed deep in the ear canal by the audiologist. The hearing aid utilizes a proprietary battery that lasts for up to 120 days.

The Lyric hearing aid offers a number of benefits. It is reported to provide an excellent, natural sound quality that is available to the listener 24 hours a day. The wearer has a personal hearing situation available "on demand" so that he or she is able, for example, to hear a standard alarm clock without having to "turn on" his or her ears by putting in the hearing aid. The current restrictions for the Lyric are that it is only available for individuals with mild-to-moderate hearing loss and that its fit may be limited based on size and shape of the person's ear canal. The cost and relatively small number of audiology practices currently dispensing the Lyric product may also be seen as a limitation. However, Lyric is likely to set the stage for many more technological advances that address cosmetics and extended wear.

Sweetow and Henderson-Sabes (2004) state that recent discoveries in neuroscience suggest that training may enhance listening skills and even build changes into the auditory system for an individual with a hearing loss. An excellent example of a program that incorporates these neuroscience discoveries is *Listening and Communication Enhancement* (LACE), a self-paced computer program described as "physical therapy for the ears." LACE helps to develop listening skills for situations where the individual with a hearing loss has difficulty. The program uses an adaptive approach and can be completed in about 30 minutes a day over the period of a month (Sweetow & Henderson-Sabes, 2004).

Data on the LACE program demonstrate both reduced returns of hearing aids by wearers and improved satisfaction with hearing aids for LACE users when compared to those who do not participate in this type of program (Martin, 2007). As suggested by Edwards (2009), it is likely that there will be a proliferation in these types of "brain games" as part of the aural rehabilitation process associated with obtaining a hearing aid.

To conclude the chapter, we offer a quote from Josephine Timberlake, a former editor of *Volta Review*, a publication of the Alexander Graham Bell Association devoted to education of children and adolescents who are d/Deaf or hard of hearing:

> If you have been hesitating about buying a hearing aid, don't wait, get it now. The manufacturers have already done a superb job. There is no doubt that the majority of hard of hearing people can be helped very much indeed by one of the instruments available today. The longer you put off using an instrument, the harder it will be for you to learn to enjoy it. Make the plunge, learn to manage the kind you select, compare notes with other users. And then, when the wonderful improvements we hear about actually materialize, you will appreciate them much more than if you prolong the waiting. (Timberlake, as cited in Pascoe, 1998, p. 135)

Although this quote sounds as if it was written about current and future hearing aid technology, it was actually in an article published in the *Volta Review* in 1945. Timberlake's enthusiasm for hearing aids perhaps would be even more true today than for the state-of-the-art hearing aids she was referring to in the post-World War II era. She also acknowledged that adjustment to the hearing aid requires acclimatization, aural rehabilitation, and support from family members, friends, and fellow hearing aid users. And, of course, the benefits will outweigh the challenges.

Summary of Major Points

Now that you have completed this chapter on hearing aids, we hope that you have found a few answers to your questions that you developed at the beginning of the chapter. If your questions did not get answered, then we encourage you to do additional reading and/or to dialogue with your instructor.

The overall intent of this chapter was to provide some information on the *Key Concepts*, as follows:

- Brief history of hearing aids
- Components and styles of hearing aids
- Regulations and standards
- Considerations in fitting of hearing aids
- Assistive technology options
- Future trends

With regard to the history of hearing aids

- Early hearing aids involved animal horns or shells placed close to the ear to collect sound and direct it to the ear canal.

- Prior to the discovery of electricity, nonelectric hearing aids were available. These included ear trumpets, conversation tubes, and ear inserts—all of which funnel sounds toward the ear canal.

- The earliest electric hearing aids appeared at the beginning of the twentieth century. These hearing aids used a carbon microphone, which was originally used in a telephone. Although small enough to be worn, these hearing aids were only useful for individuals with mild-to-moderate hearing loss.

- Transistors allowed for miniaturization, resulting in progressively smaller and more powerful hearing aids during the 1950s and 1960s. These hearing aids had sufficient amplification for individuals with severe and profound hearing losses.

- The development of digital hearing aid technology has been the most significant advance in the field since the initial introduction of electric hearing aids. Digital hearing aids provide for connectivity with devices such as telephones or computers through wireless Bluetooth transmission.

With respect to the components and styles of hearing aids

- All hearing aids, regardless of the style or processing type, are made up of three basic components: microphone, amplifier, and receiver.

- The two general types of microphones are directional, picking up sounds coming from the front of the hearing aid, and omnidirectional, picking up sounds from all directions.

- The amplifier provides relative amplification based on the hearing loss and a prescription for gain.

- Once the signal is amplified, it is directed to the hearing aid's receiver, where it is converted back to an acoustic signal and delivered to the listener's ear canal.

- Hearing aids are powered by batteries.

- Hearing aids come in a variety of styles that fall into two general categories: behind-the-ear hearing aids and custom products that generally fit into the ear canal.

- Each style of hearing aids provides benefits and limitations.

- Just as there is a range of styles of hearing aids, there is also a range of styles of earmolds.

- Simply stated, two hearing aids are better than one, assuming that both ears have a hearing loss.

With respect to regulations and standards

- The sale, dispensing, and fitting of hearing aids are regulated by the federal government, specifically by the Food and Drug Administration (FDA).

- This regulation is designed to protect consumer safety and to ensure efficacy of products.

- With respect to standards, hearing aid manufacturers use an approach to defining terms and outlining performance parameters.

With regards to the fitting of hearing aids

- All hearing aid fittings begin with a comprehensive evaluation of hearing, including assessing the listener's speech understanding ability in quiet and in the presence of noise.

- The fitting of a hearing aid requires several steps: verification, validation, orientation, and acclimatization.

- Verification of the hearing aid requires the use of methods to ensure that the hearing aid meets specified goals.

- Validation is a functional assessment of the hearing aid; that is, does the hearing aid work the way the user needs it to work in the real world?

- One of the most important steps in the fitting process is that of hearing aid orientation. The hearing aid user and his or her family members must understand how to use and maintain the new hearing aid.

- Acclimatization refers to changes in speech understanding that happen over the time of the initial fitting of the hearing aids, usually thought to be most noted in the first 30 to 90 days of being fit. This is a process of adjustment and accommodation on the part of the individual with a hearing loss.

With respect to assistive technology options

- There are two categories of assistive technology devices: auditory and nonauditory.

- Different types of assistive technologies may address particular situations more effectively or efficiently.

- The use of assistive technology options ranges from classrooms to telephones to television and to the use of alerting devices.

With respect to future trends

- Scholars have speculated that future hearing aids will be built into devices such as the iPod. Hearing aid and cell phone manufacturers have both been exploring options to build hearing aids directly into cell phones for a number of years.

- Hearing aids that address performance in listening situations will be manufactured, but with an eye toward other types of concerns, such as cosmetics and extended battery life.

- There will be a proliferation in "brain games" as part of the aural rehabilitation process associated with obtaining a hearing aid.

Chapter Questions

Note: Some answers to the questions can be found in the chapter; however, others have a variety of possible responses based on the students' backgrounds and experiences.

1. Consider the following statement: Hearing aids do not cure the hearing loss; that is, with a hearing aid, an individual does not gain normal or typical hearing ability. Is this statement accurate? Why or why not?

2. Describe the history of the development of the hearing aid. Start with the earliest "hearing aids" to the advent of digital hearing aids. State three to five major points of this history.

3. The development of digital hearing aid technology has been the most significant advance in the field since the initial introduction of electric hearing aids. Why is this the case?

4. List and describe the three major components of a hearing aid (excluding the battery!).

5. Describe the two major categories of styles of hearing aids. What are the advantages and limitations of each category?

6. What are earmolds? Discuss two to three major points from the section on earmolds.

7. Why are two hearing aids better than one, if two hearing aids are necessary?

8. List at least three major points from the section "Hearing Aid Regulations and Standards."

9. What are the major steps in the fitting of hearing aids?

10. List and briefly describe the various types of assistive technologies mentioned in this chapter.

11. If you had an opportunity to converse with the authors, what burning questions would you ask them? Share and discuss these questions with your instructor and classmates.

Challenge Questions

Note: *Complete answers are not in the text. Additional research/reading is required. In some cases, reading further or elsewhere in the text might provide some information to guide a response to a particular question.*

1. Do you think that digital hearing aids are as effective as cochlear implants? Why or why not? You might want to read and study Chapter 5 to obtain additional information.

2. Do you think that advances in technology such as digital hearing aids will eradicate Deaf culture? Why or why not? Should deaf children (younger than 18 years old) of hearing parents have the opportunity to benefit from such technology? Why or why not? Who should make this decision? [Note: We asked this previously and will ask this question again after you read Chapter 5!]

3. Will we ever reach the stage where a specific technology—be it digital hearing aid or something more advanced—would make an individual with a hearing loss exactly like an individual with typical or normal hearing (i.e., with respect to hearing ability)? Why or why not?

Suggested Activities

1. Visit the local speech and hearing center or clinic in your community or at your university. Ask personnel to show you the following:

   ■ Various kinds of individual hearing aids, from BTEs to ITEs and so on

   ■ How to make a wax impression of the ear

■ Examples of other assistive devices

■ Computers or programs to adjust settings on a digital hearing aid

Compare your findings on the above activities with the information discussed in this chapter. Are there similarities? Differences?

2. Visit your local school district. Ask the relevant personnel about the number of children in d/Deaf or hard of hearing programs who wear digital or analog hearing aids. Ask about the kinds of amplification systems used in the classrooms.

■ Visit a few of these classrooms. Observe the types of hearing aids that children wear. Report on the use of the amplification systems.

■ Interview one or two students who wear a digital hearing aid (at the upper elementary or middle school would be best). How do these students feel about their aids? Benefits? Disadvantages?

Compare your findings on the above activities with the information discussed in this chapter. Are there similarities? Differences?

References

Anderson, K. L., & Smaldino, J. (1998). *Listening inventory for education (L.I.F.E.)*. Tampa, FL: Educational Audiology Association.

Bagatto, M., Moodie, S., Scollie, S., Seewald, R., Moodie, S., Pumford, J., & Liu, K. P. R. (2005). Clinical protocols for hearing instrument fitting in the desired sensation level method. *Trends in Amplification, 9*(4), 199–226.

Berger, K. W. (1984). *The hearing aid, it's operation, and development* (3rd ed.). Livonia, MI: National Hearing Aid Society.

Billings, C. J., & Tremblay, K. L. (2007). "Hearing aids and the brain": What's the connection? *The ASHA Leader, 12*(7), 5, 23.

Bloom, S. (2003). Today's hearing aid batteries pack more power into tinier packages. *The Hearing Journal, 56*(7), 17–24.

Compton-Conley, C. (2009). Hearing solutions: Assistive listening devices. Available online: www.betterhearing.org/hearing_solutions/listeningDevicesDetail.cfm. Accessed January 17, 2009.

Cox, R. M. (2003). Assessment of subjective outcome of hearing aid fitting: Getting the client's point of view. *International Journal of Audiology, 42*, S90–S96.

Cox, R. M., & Alexander, G. C. (1999). Measuring satisfaction with amplification in daily life. The SADL scale. *Ear and Hearing, 20*(4), 306–320.

deBoer, B. (1984). Performance of hearing aids from the pre-electronic ear. *Audiologic Acoustics, 23,* 34–55.

Dillon, H., Ching, T., & Golding, M. (2008). Hearing aids for infants and children. In J. R. Madell & C. Flexer (Eds.), *Pediatric audiology: Diagnosis, technology, and management* (pp. 168–182). New York: Thieme.

Edwards, B. (2009, July 12). Innovation science: Brain games. Message posted to http://brentblog.typepad.com/brentblog/2006/05/brain_games.html.

Food and Drug Administration. (2009). Device regulation and guidance. Available online: www.fda.gov/downloads/MedicalDevices/DeviceRegulationandGuidance/GuidanceDocuments/ucm127091.pdf. Accessed July 30, 2008.

Frye, G. J. (2005). Understanding the ANSI standard as a tool for assessing hearing instrument functionality. *Hearing Review, 12*(5), 22–27, 79.

Gudmundsen, G. I. (1997). Physical options. In H. Tobin (Ed.), *Practical hearing aid selection and fitting* (pp. 1–16). Washington, D.C.: Department of Veterans Affairs.

Killion, M. C., Niquette P. A., Gudmundsen, G. I., Revit, L. J., & Banerjee, S. (2004). Development of a quick speech-in-noise test for measuring signal-to-noise ratio loss in normal-hearing and hearing-impaired listeners. *Journal of the Acoustical Society of America, 115*(4, Part 1), 2395–2405.

Kirkwood, D. H. (2006). Survey probes the economic realities of the dispensing business. *Hearing Journal, 59*(3), 19–32.

Kirkwood, D. H. (2008). Economic turmoil threatens to reverse recent growth in the hearing aid market. *Hearing Journal, 61*(12), 9–12.

Kochkin, S. (2009). Hearing solutions: The impact of treated hearing loss on quality of life. Available online: www.betterhearing.org/hearing_solutions/qualityOfLifeDetail.cfm. Accessed November 5, 2009.

Kruger, B., & Kruger, F. M. (1994). Future trends in hearing aid fitting strategies: With a view towards 2020. In M. Valente (Ed.), *Strategies for selecting and verifying hearing aid fittings* (pp. 300–342). New York: Thieme.

Levitt, H. (2006). Digital hearing aids: From wheelbarrows to ear inserts. Paper presented at the 4th ASA/ASJ Joint Meeting, Honolulu, HI; November 20, 2006.

Levitt, H. (2007). A historical perspective on digital hearing aids: How digital technology has changed modern hearing aids. *Trends in Amplification, 11*(1), 7–24.

Lybarger, S. F., & Lybarger, E. H. (2000). A historical overview. In R. S. Sandlin (Ed.), *Hearing aid amplification: Technical and clinical considerations* (pp. 1–35). San Diego, CA: Singular.

Lyric Hearing. Available online: www.lyrichearing.com. Accessed July 1, 2009.

Marriage, J. (2009). New developments in hearing aids for children and adults. *ENTNews, 18*(2), 71–72.

Martin, M. (2007). Software-based auditory training programs found to reduce hearing aid return rate. *The Hearing Journal, 60*, 8.

Mueller, H. G., & Powers, T. (2001). Consideration of auditory acclimatization in the prescriptive fitting of hearing aids. *Seminars in Hearing, 22*(2), 103–124.

Nillson, M., Soli, S., & Sullivan, J. (1994). Development of the hearing-in-noise test for the measurement of speech reception thresholds in quiet and noise. *Journal of the Acoustical Society of America, 95*(2), 1085–1099.

Northern, J. L., & Downs, M. (1984). *Hearing in children* (3rd ed.). Baltimore, MD: Williams and Wilkins.

Pascoe, D. P. (1991). *Hearing aids: Who needs them?* St. Louis, MO: Big Bend Books.

Pascoe, D. P. (1998). Hearing aids: Selection considerations. In H. G. Mueller & J. W. Hall (Eds.), *Audiologists' desk reference, Volume 2* (pp. 113–158). San Diego, CA: Singular.

Preves, D. A., & Curran, J. R. (2000). Hearing aid instrumentation and procedures for electroacoustic testing. In M. Valente, H. Hosford-Dunn, & R. J. Roeser (Eds.), *Audiologic treatment* (pp. 1–58). New York: Thieme.

Ricketts, T. (2009). Digital hearing aids: Current "state of the art." Available online: www.asha.org/public/hearing/treatment/digital_aid.htm. Accessed June 30, 2009.

Ross, M. (2006). Are binaural hearing aids better? *Hearing Loss, 27*(2), 32–37.

Ross, M. (2007). Evaluating the performance of a hearing aid in the real-ear. *Hearing Loss, 28*(5), 28–32.

Sandlin, R. E. (2001). Digital hearing aids: Hype, hoax, or hope. *Audiology OnLine.* Available online: www.audiologyonline.com/articles/article_detail.asp?article_id=293. Accessed June 30, 2009.

Silman, S., Gelfand, S. A., & Silverman, C. A. (1984). Late-onset auditory deprivation: Effects of monaural vs. binaural hearing aids. *Journal of the Acoustical Society of America, 76*(5), 1357–1362.

Souza, P. (2009). Severe hearing loss: Recommendations for fitting amplification. *Audiology OnLine.* Available online: www.audiologyonline.com/articles/article_detail.asp?article_id=2181. Accessed June 20, 2009.

Staab, W. J. (2002). Characteristics and use of hearing aids. In J. Katz (Ed.), *Handbook of clinical audiology* (5th ed., pp. 631–686). Baltimore, MD: Lippincott Williams & Wilkins.

Sweetow, R. W. (2007). Hearing aid technology. In R. Carmen (Ed.), *The consumer handbook on hearing loss and hearing aids: A bridge to healing* (2nd ed., pp. 104–124). Sedona, AZ: Auricle Ink Publishers.

Sweetow, R. W., & Henderson-Sabes, J. (2004). The case for LACE: Listening and communication enhancement training. *The Hearing Journal, 57*(3), 32–38.

Tye-Murray, N. (2009). *Foundations of aural rehabilitation: Children, adults, and their family members* (3rd ed.). Clifton Park, NY: Delmar/Cengage Learning.

Upfold, L., May, A., & Battaglia, J. (1990). Hearing aid manipulation skills in an elderly population: A comparison of ITE, BTE, and ITC aids. *British Journal of Audiology, 24*(5), 311–318.

Valente, M., Valente, M., Potts, L. G., & Lybarger, E. H. (2000). Earhooks, tubing, earmolds, and shells. In M. Valente, H. Hosford-Dunn, & R. J. Roeser (Eds.), *Audiology Treatment* (pp. 59–104). New York: Thieme.

Yanz, J. L. (2006). The future of wireless devices in hearing care: A technology that promises to transform the hearing industry. *The Hearing Review 13*(1), 18–20, 93.

Further Readings

Burkey, J. (2007) *Overcoming hearing aid fears: The road to better hearing.* Piscataway, NJ: Rutgers University Press.

Carmen, R. (Ed.). (2009). *The consumer handbook on hearing loss and hearing aids: A bridge to healing.* Sedona, AZ: Auricle Ink Publishers.

Dillion, H. (2001). *Hearing aids.* New York: Thieme.

Hearing Loss Association of America. (2009). *The consumer's guide to hearing aids.* Bethesda, MD: HLAA.

Schaub, A. (2008). *Digital hearing aids.* New York: Thieme.

COCHLEAR IMPLANTS

*Hearing with a cochlear implant, I realized . . . was going to be like a stone skipping across the surface of a lake. I would have to learn to glide over the soundstream, not always fully in contact with it but getting the general meaning. I would have to learn to backfill the important information in my mind. I would have to give up the expectation that it would truly feel like hearing, and learn to use the implant as a tool that would enable me to do something that resembled hearing. It would not **be** hearing. It would just be **equivalent** to hearing.*

—Chorost (2005, p. 79)

Key Concepts

After completing this chapter, readers should have a basic understanding of:

- History and nature of cochlear implants
- Candidacy requirements and considerations
- Benefits and limitations of cochlear implants
- Other types of implantable hearing devices
- Cochlear implants and the Deaf culture
- Future trends

The chapter opening quote reflects Michael Chorost's experience with a cochlear implant (CI), as documented in his book *Rebuilt* (Chorost, 2005). Chorost makes the analogy that receiving a cochlear implant is similar to becoming a *cyborg*, or a cybernetic organism, a term reportedly coined in 1960 to describe a human being whose body has been taken over, in whole or in part, by electromechanical devices. This idea feeds the perception of cochlear implants by much of the general population—that it is a "bionic ear" (similar to what was stated about digital hearing aids in the previous chapter). In fact, Chorost (2005) compares the experience of receiving a cochlear implant to the experience of Steve Austin, the main character of the 1970s classic TV show *The Six Million Dollar Man*. Austin was a test pilot who was given bionic limbs and organs following an accident, essentially being "rebuilt."

Wilson and Dorman (2008) portray cochlear implants as "...among the great success stories of modern medicine" (p. 695). Clark (2009) goes as far as describing the multi-channel cochlear implant, the current type of implant device, as "the first clinically successful sensory interface between the world and human consciousness" (p. 3). Note that more than 120,000 people worldwide have received cochlear implants, and the devices are regarded as the most successful neural prosthesis available (Pfingst, 2008; Zeng, 2009).

The other side of this story has been presented as a controversy, because some believe that the goal of cochlear implants is to "eradicate" deafness, threatening to eradicate Deaf culture at the same time. The truth about cochlear implants is that they are somewhere between a technological miracle and a cultural threat. In any case, the value and importance of cochlear implants often depend on one's perspective or schema.

The purpose of this chapter is to provide an overview of the history, nature, and current status of cochlear implants, including a brief discussion of the controversies and conflicts with Deaf culture. You will notice many parallels between the topics in this chapter and those discussed in Chapter 4 on hearing aids (such as benefits and troubleshooting guidelines). Although cochlear implants were initially designed to address issues faced by individuals with severe-to-profound hearing loss, the lessons learned from their use have advanced understanding in all areas of hearing loss, from speech and language development in children to understanding the development of the central auditory nervous system.

A subtle aside in this chapter is what to call individuals who have received cochlear implants. In Chapter 4, the authors were careful to utilize terminology that described the person using the hearing aid, and we settled on *hearing aid wearer* or *hearing aid user*. In the cochlear implant literature, individuals with hearing loss who are fit with a cochlear implant are most often referred to as *patients*. This might seem like "antics with semantic," because the difference between a *wearer* and a *patient* seems insignificant or awfully thin. We shall use *patient* interchangeably with other terms (e.g., *individual, listener*) in this chapter, and we hope our readers put the use of these terms in perspective.

Nevertheless, it is important to recognize that the term *patient* denotes a *medical model* approach to hearing loss—that hearing loss may be perceived as a *disease* to be cured. The use of this term, *patient*, ties into the discussion on the tension between cochlear implants and Deaf culture discussed later, and frames one of the major points of this discussion for some scholars in the cochlear implant debate: Does having a profound hearing loss make one a patient with a disease that should be cured or an individual who is part of a culture? You might remember this as the debate between clinical (i.e., medical) and cultural perspectives of deafness, as mentioned in Chapter 1 (for further details, see Paul, 2009).

As you read this chapter, you should think of questions that might be or should be answered. Your questions should be related to the *Key Concepts*. Here are a few to get you started:

- What is significant about the history of cochlear implants?
- What is the nature of cochlear implants?
- Who is or can become a candidate for the implants?
- Is one implant as good as two implants or fittings?
- What other implantable devices are available?
- What is the tension between Deaf culture and implantation?
- What are the research findings on the effects of cochlear implants?
- What does the future hold?

We are sure that you have other questions; however, we hope that we will answer or address most of them by the time you finish the chapter.

History of Cochlear Implants

Although cochlear implants are considered a modern development, the concept of electrical stimulation of the auditory system has been explored for more than 200 years. Alessandro Volta, an Italian scientist credited for the invention of the battery, was interested in electrical stimulation resulting in evoking sensation of the auditory system (Zeng, 2004). Volta conducted these stimulating experiments on himself around 1800, and his perception of placing the end of a 50-volt battery in each ear is recounted by Zeng (2004):

> ...at the moment when the circuit was completed, I received a shock in the head, and some moments after I began to hear a sound, or rather noise in the ears, which I cannot well define: It was kind of a crackling with shocks, as if paste or tenacious matter had been boiling.... This disagreeable sensation, which I believe might be dangerous because of the shock in the brain, prevented me from repeating this experiment.... (p. 2)

Although these "shocking" results indicated the potential for electrical stimulation of the auditory system, they did not bode well for its practical use for hearing.

Research continued in this area in the intervening years; however, it was not until the 1950s when electrical stimulation of the auditory nerve resulted in the perception of hearing in two deaf patients in France (Djourno & Eyries, 1957). Although the research of the 1950s was promising, researchers were discouraged when listeners reported that speech delivered by this electrical stimulation to the auditory nerve was unintelligible (Loizou, 1998). This initial line of research ignited additional studies in providing hearing by electrical stimulation for deaf individuals, particularly in experiments by House and his colleagues, which became the foundation for the future of the cochlear implant (House, 1974; House & Urban, 1973).

The first commercially available cochlear implant was the 3M House implant, introduced in 1972. This implant used a single-channel electrode and was approved for use in the United States by the Food and Drug Administration (FDA) in 1984. As you will note from information provided in this chapter, the single-channel electrode was a beginning; albeit, it did a poor job of replicating the speech signal to the inner ear. At the time, the main benefit of this single-channel cochlear implant was as an aid to lipreading (Bilger, 1983).

Devices using a multiple-channel electrode were introduced in 1984 with the Symbion device, a six-channel electrode, developed at the University of Utah (Niparko & Wilson, 2000; Zeng, 2004). Since that time, maximizing information from the use of both electrode types, the depth of insertion of the electrode into the cochlea, and processing strategies have been the focus in cochlear implantation up to the current multichannel implants. Current electrodes have 22 to 24 channels available and are generally capable of delivering information to significantly fewer channels than those available. Research suggests that high levels of speech understanding can be obtained for adults with five to eight independent channels of input, whereas children may benefit from input from additional channels (Loizou, Dorman, & Tu, 1999).

The Nature of Cochlear Implants

Now that we have provided a little history about cochlear implants, let us discuss the basic nature of this type of device. Zeng (2004) described cochlear implants as "... the only medical intervention that can restore partial hearing to a totally deafened person via electrical stimulation of the residual auditory nerve" (p. 1). This description provides a good foundation for understanding the cochlear implant. It is a medical intervention relying on electrical stimulation that is designed for individuals with severe-to-profound degrees of hearing loss. Cochlear implants were designed with the knowledge and understanding that not all individuals with a significant hearing loss can benefit from hearing aids.

To understand the basics of how a cochlear implant works, it is important to consider how the cochlea codes sound. The basilar membrane, a flexible membrane within the cochlea in the inner ear, is displaced, or moved, by cochlear fluid. This process is associated with mechanical stimulation of the inner ear from the sound reaching the outer ear (see Chapter 2 for details on anatomy and physiology). As described by Loizou (1998), these displacements contain information about the frequency, which is perceived by the listener as pitch of the signal. The displacements of the basilar membrane bend the hair cells attached to the membrane. This bending of hair cells results in the electrochemical substances being released that cause neurons to fire and transmit information about the auditory signal to the brain (Loizou, 1998).

In the case of a severe-to-profound sensorineural hearing loss, the hair cells attached to the basilar membrane are damaged and cannot translate sound to neural impulses, and this is considered a hallmark of hearing loss. Loizou (1998) describes this simply by explaining that sound information is able to travel through the outer, middle, and inner ear, but never makes it to the brain due to the broken link of the damaged hair cells. Essentially, the sound reaches a dead end. One of the concerns is that the auditory neurons close to the damaged hair cells also deteriorate due to a lack of stimulation. In the case of an individual with a profound hearing loss, a significant number of hair cells and auditory neurons are damaged. The fact that most profound sensorineural hearing losses are related to damage to the hair cells is one of the foundations of the development of the cochlear implant.

Another consideration in this hearing process is the tonotopic organization of the basilar membrane of the cochlea (mentioned in Chapter 2). *Tonotopic organization* refers to the representation of frequencies on specific areas of the basilar membrane. You could think of this as similar to the organization of a piano keyboard. High-frequency information is coded at the basal end of the cochlea where low-frequency information is coded at the apex.

With this background on the cochlea, we can proceed to the operation of the cochlear implant. The electrode of the cochlear implant also has a tonotopic organization that simulates that of the basilar membrane. In contrast to hearing aids, which are designed to amplify sounds that are detected through a damaged portion of the ear (see Chapter 4), cochlear implants bypass the damaged hair cells and stimulate the auditory nerve directly. Auditory signals are generated from the auditory nerve to the brain, which recognizes the signal as sound. Tye-Murray (2009) describes the cochlear implant as the device that "replaces the hair-cell transducer system by stimulating the auditory nerve directly, bypassing the damaged or missing hair cells" (p. 111). However, as noted by the National Institutes on Deafness and Communication Disorders (NIDCD, 2007), hearing through a cochlear implant is perceived differently from typical hearing, and it takes time and practice to learn/relearn the interpretations of sounds.

The three major manufacturers of cochlear implants are Advanced Bionics, Cochlear Americas, and MED-EL. Although there are some significant differences between processing strategies or electrode stimulation philosophies with individual manufacturers, all CI devices have the same components. The cochlear implant itself has both internal and external components. The internal components include an internal receiver and an electrode array. An internal receiver (**Figure 5-1**) is surgically placed in the mastoid bone of the skull, and an electrode array (**Figure 5-2**) is surgically inserted into the cochlea. The electrode array has the same tonotopic organization as the cochlea. This electrode divides sounds into frequency bands, and then stimulates the area of the basilar membrane of the cochlea that corresponds to the sounds being received. The only visible evidence of the internal placement of a cochlear implant is a small scar behind the ear from the surgical incision.

External components of the cochlear implant include the processor, microphone, and transmitter. Wilson and Dorman (2008) note that the most critical components of the cochlear implant are the microphone and the speech processor. The role of the microphone is to pick up sounds in the environment. The role of the speech processor is to transform the information from the microphone input to a set of stimuli that can be transmitted to the electrode array in the cochlea.

In the past, the microphone and speech processor were worn on the body, consisting of a large processor the size of early MP3 players and often worn on the chest. Current

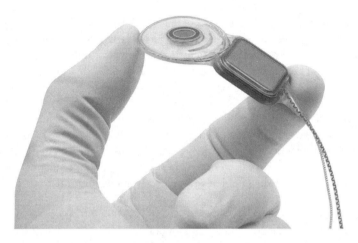

Figure 5-1
Internal Receiver of the Cochlear Implant
Photo courtesy of Cochlear Americas.

cochlear implant processors are at ear level, similar in size to larger behind-the-ear hearing aids (see **Figure 5-3**; see also BTEs in Chapter 4).

When thinking of the external components of a cochlear implant, it is important to dispel the myth that the cochlear implant is invisible. The external components of a cochlear implant are visible, similar in size to a hearing aid, which is a significant improvement over the early devices that were worn on the body, from both an acoustic and cos-

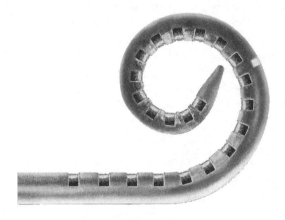

Figure 5-2
Electrode Array
Photo courtesy of Cochlear Americas.

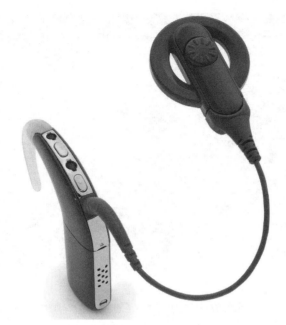

Figure 5-3
External Processor of the Cochlear Implant
Photo courtesy of Cochlear Americas.

metic perspective. The adult in **Figure 5-4** is shown wearing the external processor of the cochlear implant.

How do the external components of the cochlear implant communicate with the internal components? The transcutaneous, or through the skin, link between the internal and external devices is magnetic. The advantage to this type of link is that the skin is closed over the components that are implanted, which is convenient and minimizes the risk of infection (Wilson, 2004). At present, all available cochlear implant devices use this type of transcutaneous link for coupling the external components to the internal components. Therefore all implant users have a magnet implanted in their mastoid area (i.e., in the bone behind the ear) in order for the external processor to communicate with the internal electrode.

An important aspect of the external processor is the strategy used to encode the auditory signal. Similar to the programming of hearing aids, the implant's processor must be programmed for the individual's needs and should be based on the development of his or her listening experience. This processing strategy refers to how speech and other sounds are represented. These are based on models that try to mimic our understanding of how the auditory system functions.

Processing strategies may take into account aspects such as how frequency is coded, how noise is filtered, and the nonlinear nature of the auditory system. One common approach

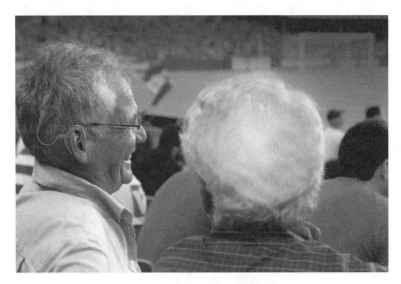

Figure 5-4
Adult Wearing a Cochlear Implant
Photo courtesy of Cochlear Americas.

used is for the processor to analyze the spectral peaks of the auditory information. If you are around a CI user or interact with the CI team, it is likely that you will become familiar with the names of some of these strategies: advanced combination encoder (ACE), spectral peak (SPEAK), HiResolution (HiRes), and continuous interleaved sampling (CIS) (Wilson & Dorman, 2008).

Cochlear Implant Candidacy and Considerations

Now we have arrived at one of the most controversial—albeit most important—issues with cochlear implant; that is, candidacy. One of the keys to success with cochlear implants is that candidates for the surgery and the rehabilitation process are, or should be, carefully selected. Decisions for candidacy are influenced by a number of factors, including audiometric criteria; developmental, social, communication, and occupational considerations; and reasonable expectations. As with hearing aids, the FDA oversees the production and distribution of cochlear implants within their products and medical procedures division in the Medical Devices unit (FDA, 2009).

According to the FDA (2009), a significant number of considerations impact potential success with a cochlear implant, including the following issues that should be taken into account for an individual patient or wearer:

- The length of time that the patient has been deaf; individuals who have been deaf for a short time do better than those who have been deaf a long time.

- The age at onset of the deafness; that is, whether patients were deaf before they could speak.

- The rate at which individuals can learn; the quicker the better.

- The quality and dedication of the learning support structure.

- The health and structure of the individual's cochlea; in particular, the number of nerve (spiral ganglion) cells that exist in the cochlea.

- Implanting variables, such as the depth and type of implanted electrode and the signal-processing technique.

- Intelligence and communicativeness of the patient.

These considerations again highlight the significant number of factors, many of which require patient commitment, for the implant to be successful.

When cochlear implants were first approved by the FDA, the criteria were strict, including limiting the surgery to adults only. As stated by Kreuger and her colleagues (Kreuger, Joseph, & Rost, 2008), candidacy criteria for cochlear implantation in the United States have progressively expanded, based on advances in technology, speech-coding strategies (see Chapter 7), and surgical techniques that have resulted in significant improvements in auditory-only hearing abilities in cochlear implant recipients.

The FDA criteria differ for adults and children and may differ based on the actual device being implanted. In addition, candidacy criteria may vary somewhat from implant center to implant center. As noted by Tye-Murray (2009), one of the key candidacy requirements for cochlear implant in either a child or adult is a permanent severe or profound sensorineural hearing loss as well as good general health. General FDA criteria for cochlear implantation in an adult (age 18 and older) include bilateral severe-to-profound sensorineural hearing loss (>70 dB HL; see Chapter 1) and receiving limited benefit from appropriately fitted hearing aids, which may be defined as a score of 50% or less on a test requiring open-set recognition of sentences, such as the *Hearing in Noise Test* (HINT), presented in a quiet environment.

Considerations for children are somewhat more restricted than for adults. Anatomically and physiologically, the cochlea is adult-like at birth, so implantation is feasible from a physical perspective. However, a number of other considerations must be addressed. Pediatric implant candidates, those aged 12 months to 17 years, must have a bilateral, profound sensorineural hearing loss. In addition, these children must demonstrate minimal or no benefit from appropriately fitted hearing aids.

In children younger than age 4, lack of benefit may be determined by use of a validation measure, such as tracking auditory developmental milestones by using the *Infant-Toddler Meaningful Identification Scale* (IT-MAIS). In addition, verification of poor word recognition abilities, as documented by performance of less than 20% correct on an open-set word recognition test such as the *Lexical Neighborhood Test* (LNT), may also be a criterion. Lack of hearing aid benefit in an older child would be verified by specific audiometric test results, such as poor performance on an open-set word recognition test or an open-set sentence test. *Open-set identification* refers to a test in which the possible response is not determined from a predetermined, or closed, set of responses, but rather has unlimited response possibilities.

The FDA criteria indicate that cochlear implants are appropriate for children 12 months and older; however, several sites have included children younger than 12 months in investigational studies. Research suggests that implants are safe for children between 7 and 12 months. The benefits of early implantation have been discussed in the literature; one of the most compelling outcomes is that early implantation has the greatest likelihood of the child developing spoken language skills that are commensurate with aged-matched hearing peers (Hammes, Novak, Rotz, Willis, Edmondson, & Thomas, 2002; James & Papsin, 2004; see also, Chapter 9). A further discussion of the research on cochlear implants is presented later in this chapter.

Cochlear implant surgery and follow-up is generally covered by most third-party private insurers, as well as Medicaid and Medicare. Insurers may have more stringent candidacy requirements than those of an individual implant center. A common concern is the low reimbursement rates for cochlear implant services. There is a perception that fewer centers are now providing implants than in the past due to escalating costs of newer technology in the face of poor insurance reimbursement.

TEAM APPROACH

Many of the concepts highlighted in Chapter 4 in terms of partnership in fitting an amplification device are also applicable in the cochlear implant process. Receiving a cochlear implant is part of a process that begins with identification of the hearing loss and ends with ongoing adjusting or tweaking of the processing strategy to maximize speech understanding. The implant surgery itself, in the hands of a skilled otolaryngologist and with a healthy patient, is a relatively minor step in the process for most patients.

The likelihood of a successful outcome with a cochlear implant is maximized when the implant is done as part of a team approach, which may include an audiologist, speech-language pathologist, otolaryngologist, psychologist, social worker, educator, and the patient and his or her family.

This team will collect appropriate data, which follow the person who has received the implant over time. This approach requires a significant commitment by all members of the team to follow a protocol and for the patient to participate in aural habilitation/rehabilitation so that the implanted individual's brain learns how to make use of the sound being delivered and to use that sound to stimulate hearing. Obtaining a cochlear implant, if done well, is labor intensive, entailing many visits to the implant center, much speech-language therapy, and an ongoing commitment for the patient to learn to use this auditory information.

The second author recently encountered a young woman who had opted to undergo cochlear implant surgery. She had attended an educational program and a college for d/Deaf and hard of hearing students and had primarily used American Sign Language

(ASL) to communicate. When the woman started dating a man with a hearing loss, who communicated primarily via spoken English, she decided to obtain a cochlear implant.

This woman shared that her results were "disappointing." She indicated that she used her processer as "an expensive magnet on her fridge" (recall that the external processor is connected to the internal components by a magnet). When asked to explain her disappointment, she stated that she thought that after she had this surgery she would wake up and be able to hear—and, frankly, it was just too much work to learn to use this new auditory information. The woman added that she thought that this "miracle ear" would "make her hear" and that she really did not understand that she would have to do so much in the process.

This sad story underlies the fact that the common misperception, mentioned previously, is that the cochlear implant is a miracle cure for deafness—the bionic ear as stated in the introduction to this chapter. The reality is that success with a cochlear implant is hard work on the part of all individuals involved. It also requires honest communication among all team members, and an assurance that once the surgery is completed the resources for success will be available, including speech-language therapy, educational support, and perhaps a hearing aid for the nonimplanted ear, as is discussed later.

Communicating reasonable expectations and outcomes with the implant may be one of the most important roles of the team. It is also important to remember that if a person interested in pursuing an implant attends a seminar at a hospital or looks on YouTube for the experiences of others, the implant users featured are often the "superstars." So, it should be highlighted, as they say on infomercials, that "these results may not be representative as individual results may vary."

BENEFITS AND LIMITATIONS OF COCHLEAR IMPLANTS

Here is another story that ties into the benefits and limitations of cochlear implants. The second author was recently at a meeting at which a woman who had received bilateral cochlear implants was the keynote speaker. This woman had lost her hearing as an adult as the result of an autoimmune inner ear disease. Her hearing loss progressed over a period of about 8 years, resulting in a severe-to-profound hearing loss. She received minimal benefit from hearing aids. Her initial cochlear implant surgery was about 8 years ago, with an implant to her other ear about 2 years ago.

This woman described the cochlear implant as a "technological marvel." She listed all the things that she was now able to hear that she could not with hearing aids: a pen writing on paper, traffic noise, her own chewing. She noted that in addition to improved speech understanding, the cochlear implant connected her to the world. The woman also stated that learning to listen with a cochlear implant, even for someone who had years of experience as a hearing person, was a challenge. It required dedication and work, but it was worth it.

This woman's story is echoed by the vast majority of individuals who have chosen to pursue a cochlear implant. The outcomes of individuals who have received implants have been carefully studied for more than 30 years. Ongoing changes in technology and implant candidacy suggest that the story of the cochlear implant is still in the process of being written. However, despite controversy, current research highlights benefits based on carefully collected outcome data, much of which are longitudinal.

Within 6 months of implantation of a multichannel monaural cochlear implantation in adults, significant increases in speech understanding and in health utility are noted (Palmer, Niparko, Wyatt, Rothman, & de Lissovoy, 1999). Numerous studies have demonstrated considerable quality-of-life benefits for adults with severe-to-profound hearing impairment who use either hearing aids or cochlear implants over no amplification; however, these results are more significant for CI users (Cohen, Labadie, Dietrich, & Haynes, 2004).

One of the important questions has been related to differences in adult individuals who are prelingually versus postlingually deafened. Conventional wisdom has been that individuals who are postlingually deafened are strong candidates for a cochlear implant; however, it has been suspected that those who are prelingually deafened will receive no benefit from a cochlear implant. Recent research dispels this myth and indicates that significant improvements in speech understanding, speech production, and quality of life are noted among prelingually deafened adults who pursue cochlear implantation (Klop, Briaire, Stiggelbout, & Frijns, 2009).

Outcomes for cochlear implants in children have also been well studied; albeit, there is still considerable controversy. The landscape for cochlear implantation outcomes in children continues to shift due to earlier identification of hearing loss, universal newborn hearing loss screenings, and changes in candidacy criteria that have provided CIs to children at younger ages. It is clear that cochlear implants have provided improved access to auditory information for d/Deaf or hard of hearing children when the research is well designed.

Hirsh (1966) predicted that improved auditory skills would play a role in accelerated speech and language development for children who have profound hearing losses. Research has certainly supported this prediction. Geers (2004) reported that, when compared to children with profound hearing loss who use hearing aids, children with cochlear implants demonstrate improved speech perception abilities, improved oral communication abilities, closer approximation of language skills to hearing peers, increased use of speech in children in total communication programs, and acceleration of acquiring reading skills.

Again, the cochlear implant is not a miracle cure; however, several research outcomes are roughly similar to those for children with no hearing loss. Note, however, that recent research indicates that some children who have cochlear implants continue to demonstrate lags in a few areas of language development compared to their hearing peers (Geers, Moog, Biedenstein, Brenner, & Hayes, 2009). Nevertheless, this research suggests that outcomes are significantly better for children who receive a cochlear implant at an earlier age and that the results help to direct the future of aural habilitation programs. It is obvious that many factors go into decision making related to cochlear implantation in children, including the fact that hearing aid technology for children with severe-to-profound hearing loss also continues to improve, which may continue to challenge these outcomes.

Years of research indicates that cochlear implants have had a significant positive impact on the quality of life for children with profound hearing loss at what appears to be a net economic savings to society due to reduced educational costs (Cheng, Rubin, Powe, Mellon, Francis, & Niparko, 2000). Furthermore, children with cochlear implants may derive additional benefits that have, to date, been limited to adults. For example, good music recognition abilities and music enjoyment have recently been reported in children who use cochlear implants, which has not generally been found to be the case for adults with cochlear implants (Trehub, Vongpaisal, & Nakata, 2009). For an additional perspective on the effects of cochlear implants on the educational and literacy levels of d/Deaf and hard of hearing children, readers are referred to the work of Paul (2009, e.g., Chapter 4). There is also a brief discussion of this research on speech and language development in the next chapter (Chapter 6).

Other than philosophical issues related to cochlear implantation, the limitations or negative outcomes with cochlear implants have been reported to be minimal. The surgery itself has been found to be very safe in healthy individuals. As noted earlier in the chapter, establishing appropriate expectations for outcomes is a critical factor in the individual's success or failure with the cochlear implant. A potential negative outcome that has been documented in the literature is that of nonuse: a person is implanted then opts not to use the implant—recall the refrigerator magnet example mentioned earlier.

There are several reasons for nonuse, including the age at the time of implant, the educational setting, lack of family support, failed psychological adjustment, or an inability to adapt to the signal (Raine, Summerfield, Strachan, Martin, & Totten, 2008). Although a very small percentage of patients who are implanted (e.g., less than 5%) exhibit nonuse, this issue highlights the importance of carefully selecting candidates for implant surgery. If the patient opts not to use the cochlear implant once it is implanted, the cost of the surgery and rehabilitation is incurred without the benefit of the device being received.

Special consideration should be given to nonuse of cochlear implants in the pediatric population. As with the vast majority of decisions made in children's lives, informed consent is not given by the patient prior to the decision to pursue an implant. Currently, children are being implanted at younger ages when informed consent is not feasible. In older children, although not required, the notion of informed consent must be seriously considered. As noted by Archbold, Nikolopoulos, and Lloyd-Richmond (2009), although the cochlear implant electrode is surgically implanted, the decision to use the external processor can be made later by older children. In a study following pediatric cochlear implant users over a 7-year period, Archbold et al. (2009) reported that 83% of children were full-time users and 17% of children were part-time users. Educational placement was one of the major factors between full-time and part-time users.

Nonuse in children appears to be related to a number of complex factors resulting in intermittent use over time. Another issue in nonuse is the child's objection to the implant prior to the surgery. Archbold et al. (2009) indicated that none of the children who participated in their study became total nonusers if they were implanted prior to age 5 years. In addition, they suggest that the "likelihood of nonuse is minimised by careful preparation and decision making before implantation and by careful long-term follow-up afterwards" (p. 38).

Finally, we think it is important to provide a few basic guidelines related to troubleshooting, similar to what was presented in Chapter 4 on hearing aids. These guidelines are discussed in **Table 5-1**.

Table 5-1

A Practical Guide for Understanding Cochlear Implants

Before Getting Started

Similar to our guidelines for hearing aids, it is important to have basic information. Knowing the manufacturer, model, and serial number is critical. In addition, knowing the recommended program for each listening environment or the appropriate program for specific situations (e.g., coupling an FM device to the CI) is important. Currently, most CI processors are ear level (BTE); however, it is possible that one may encounter an older body worn processor. CI manufacturers provide manuals and troubleshooting guides for specific products online.

Tools

A number of tools are useful in checking and maintaining cochlear implants. These tools can be obtained from the implant center. The tools in a "care kit" may include the following:

- Battery tester

- Supply of batteries

- Monitor headphones: Specific to each processor, these headphones are plugged into the processor to provide you the opportunity to know that sound is being transmitted (however, this does not allow you to make any judgment about the quality of the sound). In some cases, there is an automatic "shut off" when using the monitor headphones to minimize battery drain.

- Lapel microphone

- Depending on your comfort level and the support options provided to the implant user, additional components are available, such as earhooks, extra cords, and microphone.

Table 5-1	*A Practical Guide for Understanding Cochlear Implants (continued)*

Checking and Changing the Battery

Cochlear implant processors may have either disposable or rechargeable battery packs. Cochlear implant batteries are offered by some of the battery manufacturers, which are generally labeled *power 675 batteries*, to accommodate the additional power demands of the cochlear implant. When the need to change batteries is identified, all batteries in the battery holder should be changed. Proper insertion of the batteries is required; consult the user or troubleshooting manual for specific guidance.

Electrostatic Discharge (ESD)

Electrostatic discharge is familiar to anyone who lives in a dry climate in the winter. It is the built-up electric discharge or a *shock*, resulting in your hair standing on end when you remove your hat in the winter, or when you rub your feet on the carpet and touch another person or object. The concern is that these minor shocks may damage the cochlear implant processor. Current CI processors incorporate features to protect against electrostatic damage. Although the risk of ESD exposure is minimal, you should use common sense in handling the processor. Prior to touching the processor, you should touch a conductive surface, such as metal, before handling the external processor (Hedley-Williams, Sladen, & Tharpe, 2003). In addition, antistatic mats may be used with computer equipment in the classroom, and antistatic computer monitor covers should be considered for the person with a cochlear implant.

Moisture

As with hearing aids, the external processor of a cochlear implant is sensitive to exposure to moisture. Efforts should be made to keep the CI processor dry. The *Dry and Store*, a storage kit designed to remove moisture and to sanitize the CI components (http://www.dryandstore.com/), can be useful in storing and protecting the processor.

(continues)

Table 5-1	**A Practical Guide for Understanding Cochlear Implants (continued)**

Basic Troubleshooting

In most cases, it is more difficult to accurately listen to a CI processor than to a hearing aid. A daily listening check, using something like the Ling Sound Test (see Chapter 8), is critical. Error codes can be displayed on the LCD of the CI processor. Consulting the user manual or troubleshooting guide for the processor can direct troubleshooting and resolve the issue. Some general basic troubleshooting tips are offered here.

The Listener Reports a Buzzing/Distorted Sound from the Processor

- Check for sources of electromagnetic interference, such as cell phone towers, battery chargers, and security systems

- Try moving away from the potential source of the interference

- If buzzing persists, turn off processor and contact the audiologist

The Processor Is Not Working or Is Intermittent

- Change batteries or recharge battery pack

- Check microphone for debris

- Check cords for cracks or needs for replacement

BIMODAL AMPLIFICATION AND BILATERAL COCHLEAR IMPLANTS

Because we are on the topic of benefits of cochlear implants, we now turn our attention to bimodal amplification and bilateral implants. In Chapter 4, we debated the issue of one hearing aid versus two. In a similar vein, are two ears better than one with regard to cochlear implants? The answer is essentially "yes."

Historically, cochlear implants have been fit monaurally, or to only one ear. Many factors must be considered when determining which ear to fit for unilateral implantation. In some cases, cochlear implant users were discouraged from using a hearing aid in the opposite ear, and in other cases the implant user tried to maximize residual hearing in the non-implanted ear. Recently, bimodal (hearing aid in one ear and cochlear implant in the other ear) or bilateral cochlear implants (implant in each cochlea) have been the source of considerable research interest. Based on research results, bimodal fitting or bilateral implantation is becoming the standard in the cochlear implantation process.

As noted by Ching and her colleagues (Ching, van Wanrooy, & Dillion, 2007), bilateral implantation and bimodal fitting both address improving binaural hearing and avoiding auditory deprivation in the nonimplanted ear (see similar discussion in Chapter 4). Essentially, either bimodal amplification or bilateral cochlear implantation demonstrates significant benefits over cochlear implant alone or hearing aid alone. Both adults and children demonstrated significant improvements in sentence understanding in noise with bimodal amplification when compared to cochlear implant alone or hearing aid alone (Luntz, Shpak, & Weiss, 2005). Localization abilities, important for directionality and for being able to listen effectively in noisy environments, have also shown improvement for many listeners with bimodal amplification over the cochlear implant or hearing aid alone (Ching, Incerti, & Hill, 2004). Bilateral cochlear implantation has been shown to address some of the complaints of current CI users, such as difficulty hearing in less than optimal listening environments in localizing the direction of sound, because it has often been perceived as coming from directly at the ear or inside the head (Litovsky, Johnstone, & Godar, 2006).

Most current research suggests that, in addition to localization and listening in noise, speech perception in quiet environments is significantly improved with bilateral cochlear implants than with monaural implants (Eapen & Buchman, 2009). These advances have provided more natural hearing abilities for those with severe-to-profound hearing loss that contribute to both communication ability and quality of life. These advances also set the stage for improved processing strategies designed to maximize binaural benefits.

Other Types of Implantable Hearing Devices

In this section, we proceed to other types of implantable hearing devices. These implantable hearing devices are typically for individuals who cannot benefit from typical traditional hearing aids, discussed in Chapter 4.

BONE ANCHORED HEARING AID (BAHA)

The bone anchored hearing aid, or BAHA, is an implantable hearing aid designed to address conductive hearing loss, mixed hearing loss, or single-sided deafness (SSD). It has been approved for use in the United States since 1996. Individuals who have chronic conductive or mixed hearing loss may not benefit from hearing aids for a number of reasons. Some individuals with conductive hearing losses may have constant drainage from the ear that prohibits healthy or comfortable placement of a hearing aid or earmold in the ear canal. In a few cases, individuals have an absent ear canal, also known as aural atresia, which excludes the use of hearing aids that require placement in an ear canal.

The BAHA uses the concept of bone conduction, or how sound is delivered to the inner ear by vibration of the bones in the skull. Recall from previous chapters (e.g., Chapters 2 and 3) that this is a method for testing hearing. Bone conduction oscillators have been used in hearing aids in the past; however, they have not been popular due to cosmetics (these aids require a headband) and poor sound quality. The BAHA system bypasses the middle ear system and delivers the sound signal directly to the inner ear. A titanium abutment, or screw, is surgically implanted in the bone of the skull behind the ear.

Similar to a cochlear implant, an external sound processor is used that is attached to the abutment. The processor can be seen in the photograph of the child in **Figure 5-5**. The processor allows for the sound to be picked up and delivered directly to the inner ear.

The BAHA can be safely implanted in both children and adults. BAHA users have been found to have significantly better speech understanding ability than with traditional bone conduction hearing aids and also improved ability to hear in the presence of background noise (Snik et al., 2004; Yuen, Bodmer, Smilsky, Nedzelski, & Chen, 2009). Just as with hearing aids, the BAHA is designed with consideration to how listeners live their lives, including an adapter to connect an MP3 player or cell phone directly to the processor.

AUDITORY BRAINSTEM IMPLANT (ABI)

A relatively obscure type of implantable hearing device is the auditory brainstem implant (ABI). This device, with the electrode array implanted directly into the brainstem, is designed to address neural pathologies of the auditory system, such as those that occur in neurofibromatosis type 2 (NF2). Individuals with this type of hearing loss generally have no residual hearing ability and demonstrate no ability to make use of auditory information, often relying primarily on speechreading.

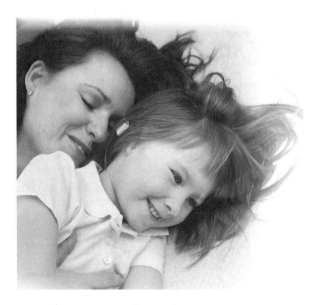

Figure 5-5
Child Wearing a Bone Anchored Hearing Aid (BAHA)
Photo courtesy of Cochlear Americas.

The first ABI surgery was performed in 1979 (Maini, Cohen, Hollow, & Briggs, 2009). Analogous to the fact that the cochlear implant replaces a damaged portion of the auditory system, the ABI bypasses the damaged auditory nerve and is implanted directly into the brainstem. Research suggests that those who receive an ABI demonstrate a significant improvement in speech perception over speechreading alone, although nearly 20% of all individuals implanted note no benefit from the device (Maini et al., 2009). Many patients experience mild nonauditory effects, such as tingling or vibration, at the onset of sound. Overall, the ABI can increase the patient's quality of life significantly (Matthies et al., 2000).

Deaf Culture and Cochlear Implants

Any chapter on the topic of cochlear implants would be incomplete without considering the perceived impact of this technology on Deaf culture. The positive outcomes outlined in this chapter may be interpreted or perceived in a number of ways, depending on the viewpoint being considered. As mentioned in Chapter 1, this is also construed as a debate between clinical proponents of deafness and those who espouse the cultural view (see also, Paul, 2009). We do not think that this is an *either/or* situation. There are benefits to both viewpoints—albeit, this text focuses primarily on the clinical perspective.

Lane (1992) indicted "the hearing establishment" as part of a movement against Deaf culture, and identified the technology of cochlear implantation as a "linchpin" in this movement. He described the motivation for cochlear implantation as financial and profoundly political; that is, done in the name of benevolence toward people with hearing loss, with the desire for the hearing to dominate the Deaf. Lane also resurrected the term, *audism*, which refers to the concept that individuals who hear or who behave as hearing are somewhat superior to those who do not hear. Audism is viewed as a form of discrimination against individuals who are d/Deaf. This term was initially introduced in a doctoral dissertation by Tom Humphries at the University of Cincinnati in 1977 (Harrington, 2009).

The early years of cochlear implantation were certainly a tumultuous time with regard to opinions on cochlear implants and the role implants play, if any, in relation to the status of Deaf culture. Individuals who are either direct (have a hearing loss) or indirect (no hearing loss) members of Deaf culture often vilified the technology and characterized the otologists performing the surgery as butchers. Conversely, the individuals involved in cochlear implant teams were often zealous, and perhaps sometimes overzealous, with respect to their enthusiasm for this new technology.

Since the early days, it is our perception that the great divide between those who support cochlear implants and those who believe that this technology is a form of audism has narrowed significantly. As we mentioned previously, research has demonstrated both the limitations and benefits of cochlear implants. Although we do not have research data to provide adequate statistics, both authors of this text know of individuals who are members of the Deaf culture who have had cochlear implants. Obviously, there has been somewhat of an attitudinal shift from an earlier period where such decisions would have resulted in ostracism by other members of the Deaf culture.

This narrowing of the divide can also be seen in the position statement on cochlear implantation from the National Association of the Deaf (NAD), described on its Web site as "the nation's premier civil rights organization of, by and for deaf and hard of hearing individuals in the United States of America" (National Association of the Deaf, 2009, n.p.). An online debate regarding positions on cochlear implants was hosted as part of the Public Broadcasting System (PBS) introduction of the televised documentary *Sound and Fury* (2006), which focused on the conflict surrounding cochlear implantation.

Nancy Bloch, the executive director of NAD, has noted that the organization has taken no position on cochlear implantation in adults because it is viewed as an individual choice (PBS, 2006). Initially, the NAD opposed cochlear implantation in children; however, it revised this viewpoint in the NAD Position Statement on Cochlear Implants (2000). In this statement, the NAD discusses technological changes of the past 30 years and how these have improved the quality of life for individuals who are deaf and hard of hearing. The statement focuses primarily on children with hearing loss and the respect for choices made by parents. The NAD statement addresses cochlear implants in the following manner:

> Cochlear implants are not appropriate for all deaf and hard of hearing children and adults. Cochlear implantation is a technology that represents a tool to be used in some forms of communication, and not a cure for deafness. Cochlear implants provide sensitive hearing, but do not, by themselves, impart the ability to understand spoken language through listening alone. In addition, they do not guarantee the development of cognition or reduce the benefit of emphasis on parallel visual language and literacy development. (National Association for the Deaf, 2000, n.p.)

The NAD statement also provides strong action recommendations, including the following:

- Training in issues related to Deaf culture in medical schools

- Early assessment of advanced digital hearing aid technology prior to a cochlear implant decision

- Involvement of professionals in deafness on cochlear implant teams

- A long-term commitment from families for habilitation following implantation

- Fair and equitable insurance coverage for hearing aids and associated services

- Ongoing research, and supporting communication and educational development in a dynamic and interactive visual environment that supports both American Sign Language and English

The struggle between a wellness (or natural) perspective of deafness and the desire to address deafness with cochlear implantation was the focus of the 2001 Academy Award-nominated documentary *Sound and Fury*. The film follows one family's decision-making process regarding cochlear implantation for their two deaf children. It addresses the underlying questions of the potential impact of this surgery on the person's sense of identity in the Deaf culture. This documentary, and its follow-up, *Sound and Fury: Six Years Later*, renders a fascinating perspective on this topic, and like any good film, suspense and surprises. These documentaries are must sees for anyone interested in this topic.

We anticipate that there will be research to document the change in attitudes toward cochlear implantation and, perhaps, toward any form of hearing amplification device. Realistically, we do not expect the divide, mentioned previously, to be completely eliminated. That is human nature. Nevertheless, we hope that there will be a more balanced, comprehensive approach by professionals and medical personnel that would enable the affected individuals and/or their families to render an informed decision. We think it is imprudent to attempt to roll back or ignore the benefits of technology.

Future Trends

Now it is time for us to get out our crystal ball again (which is still fuzzy, at the moment) and offer some predictions for future trends. We believe that improvements in current cochlear implant technology will address function, including changing current components, software, and processing strategies. For example, researchers at the University of Texas are working on microphones that can improve spatial cues and coordinate binaural input between ears. This should result in improved speech recognition abilities in less than optimal environments (The University of Texas at Dallas News Center, 2009).

Future changes in cochlear implants are also likely to address the size of the device and cosmetics. It is anticipated that a completely implantable cochlear implant (CICI) will be available, with no visible external components (Tye-Murray, 2009). In addition, hybrid, or short-electrode, devices using electroacoustic stimulation (EAS) have been in clinical trials and are designed for individuals with more low-frequency hearing abilities than current cochlear implant candidates (Gifford, Dorman, Spahr, Bacon, Skarzynski, & Lorens, 2008).

It is also possible that candidacy requirements will continue to change as "off-label" uses of cochlear implants are explored. A recent example is the use of cochlear implants as treatment for tinnitus, or ringing in the ears, in patients with unilateral hearing loss. This research has demonstrated significant reduction of tinnitus over the postoperative condition, an important outcome for individuals with intractable constant tinnitus that compromises quality of life (Van de Heyning, Vermeire, Diebl, Nopp, Anderson, & De Ridder, 2008). Although it is not likely that the cochlear implant will become a major treatment for tinnitus, in general, these types of findings might contribute to both understanding of the mechanisms and treatment options for those with tinnitus, a debilitating chronic condition for more than 50 million Americans.

If "what's past is prologue," then future technology should continue to provide benefits for individuals with hearing loss, accompanied by controversy and debate. Cochlear implants have been a strong foundation for a clinical standard of care that can apply to other areas for individuals with hearing loss. In addition, cochlear implants have offered a strong basis for the application of systematic and effective aural habilitation/rehabilitation. The area of cochlear implantation has also yielded evidence-based research that has supported changes in implant candidacy and has convinced both proponents and opponents of the technology of its benefits, at least for some individuals with severe-to-profound hearing losses.

With respect to the education of children who are d/Deaf or hard of hearing, we sympathize with the passage below by Nevins and Chute (1996), prophetic perhaps, which appeared about 15 years ago:

> The impact of the cochlear implant on the field of deaf education is only beginning. Early trends seem to indicate the potential for earlier mainstream placement, which has a concomitant impact on the field of regular education and society at large. True mainstreaming, in the sense of full participation in the mainstream of school and society, can only be accomplished if proper assessment and follow-up are components of the process. (p. 201)

In essence, we need to continue to conduct relatively unbiased, research documentation of the effects of cochlear implants on children, adolescents, and adults. The end result should be a better understanding of why and for whom this technology produces the greatest benefits, as noted by Paul (2009; see also the brief discussion in Chapter 6 of this text).

Summary of Major Points

Our goal in this chapter was to provide an overview of the history, nature, and status of cochlear implants. In addition, we discussed briefly the past and current tensions between the issue of cochlear implantations and the Deaf culture. We also retrieved our "crystal ball" and attempted to predict future trends. We hope that we were able to answer or partially answer most of your questions that you created at the beginning of the chapter. If not, we encourage you to read some of the references cited and/or to dialogue with your instructor and classmates.

The overall intent of this chapter was to provide a brief introduction to *Key Concepts*, as follows:

- Basic history and nature of cochlear implants
- Candidacy requirements and considerations
- Benefits and limitations of cochlear implants
- Other types of implantable hearing devices
- Cochlear implants and the Deaf culture
- Future trends

With respect to the basic history and nature of cochlear implants

- The first commercially available cochlear implant was the 3M House implant, introduced in 1972. This implant used a single channel electrode. Devices using a multiple-channel electrode were introduced in 1984, with the Symbion device, a six-channel electrode.

■ Maximizing information from use of both electrode types, depth of insertion of the electrode in the cochlea, and processing strategies have been the focus in cochlear implantation up to the current multichannel implants.

■ To understand the basics of how a cochlear implant works, it is important to consider how the cochlea codes sound.

■ The cochlear implant has both internal and external components. The internal components are an internal receiver, surgically placed in the mastoid bone of the skull, and an electrode array, surgically inserted into the cochlea. External components of the cochlear implant include the processor, microphone, and transmitter.

In the section on candidacy requirements and considerations

■ One of the keys to success with cochlear implants is that candidates for the surgery and the rehabilitation process are carefully selected.

■ Decisions for candidacy are influenced by a number of factors, including audiometric criteria; developmental, social, communication, and occupational considerations; and reasonable expectations.

■ A significant number of considerations impact potential success with a cochlear implant.

■ The FDA criteria differ for adults and children and may differ based on the specific device being implanted.

■ Many of the concepts highlighted in Chapter 4 in terms of partnership in fitting an amplification device are also applicable in the cochlear implant process.

Considering the benefits and limitations of cochlear implants, including bilateral amplification

■ Recently, bimodal (hearing aid in one ear and cochlear implant in the other ear) or bilateral (implant in each cochlea) cochlear implants have been the source of considerable research interest. Based on research results, bimodal fitting or bilateral implantation is becoming the standard in the cochlear implantation process.

■ Essentially, either bimodal amplification or bilateral cochlear implantation demonstrates significant benefits over cochlear implant alone or hearing aid alone.

■ Outcomes for cochlear implants in children have also been well studied; albeit, there is still considerable controversy.

■ Hirsh (1966) predicted that improved auditory skills would play a role in accelerated speech and language development for children who have profound hearing losses. Research has certainly supported this prediction.

■ Other than philosophical issues related to cochlear implantation, the limitations or negative outcomes with cochlear implants have been reported to be minimal.

In discussing other types of implantable hearing devices

■ The bone anchored hearing aid, or BAHA, is an implantable hearing aid designed to address conductive hearing loss, mixed hearing loss, or single-sided deafness (SSD).

■ The BAHA uses the concept of bone conduction, or how sound is delivered to the inner ear by vibration of the bones in the skull.

■ A relatively obscure type of implantable hearing device is the auditory brainstem implant (ABI). This device, with the electrode array implanted directly into the brainstem, is designed to address neural pathologies of the auditory system, such as those that occur in neurofibromatosis type 2 (NF2).

■ Analogous to the fact that the cochlear implant replaces a damaged portion of the auditory system, the ABI bypasses the damaged auditory nerve and is implanted directly into the brainstem.

In the section on cochlear implants and the Deaf culture

■ The early years of cochlear implantation were certainly a tumultuous time related to opinions on cochlear implants and the role implants play, if any, in relation to the status of Deaf culture.

■ Since the early days, it is our perception that the great divide between those who support cochlear implants and those who believe that this technology is a form of audism has narrowed significantly.

■ This narrowing of the divide can also be seen in the position statement on cochlear implantation from the National Association of the Deaf (NAD).

With respect to future trends

■ Improvements in current cochlear implant technology are likely to address function, including changing current components, software, and processing strategies.

■ Future changes in cochlear implants are also likely to address the size of the device and cosmetics.

■ It is also possible that candidacy requirements will continue to change as "off-label" uses of cochlear implants are explored.

■ If "what's past is prologue," then future technology will continue to provide benefits for individuals with hearing loss, accompanied by controversy and debate.

Chapter Questions

Note: *Some answers to the questions can be found in the chapter; however, others have a variety of possible responses based on students' backgrounds and experiences.*

1. Consider the following statement: The cochlear implant is erroneously viewed as a miracle that "cures hearing loss." Is this correct? Why or why not?

2. List three major developments in the history of cochlear implantation.

3. How does a cochlear implant work? [Note: Relate this discussion to the operation of the cochlea.]

4. What are the internal and external components of a cochlear implant?

5. What impacts a successful implantation process? [Note: Consider the FDA's considerations.]

6. Are the candidacy criteria for children different from those for adults? Explain.

7. Describe what is meant by a "team approach" to cochlear implantation.

8. What are the benefits of bimodal amplification or bilateral cochlear implantation? Is this the same as for bilateral digital hearing aids from Chapter 4?

9. What are a few research findings on the benefits of cochlear implants for children and adults?

10. Briefly discuss the other types of implantable hearing devices.

11. What evidence suggests that the concept of audism might be on the decline?

12. What does the future hold (so far!) for cochlear implantations and other devices?

13. If you had an opportunity to converse with the authors, what burning questions would you ask them? Share and discuss these questions with your instructor and classmates.

Challenge Questions

Note: *Complete answers are not in the text. Additional research/reading is required. In some cases, reading further or elsewhere in the text might provide some information to guide a response to a particular question.*

1. What are your views on cochlear implants? Can you support your views with theoretical or research data, or both? Did the information in this chapter influence your views?

2. Is there a positive linear relationship between cochlear implants and reading achievement? Why or why not? Is there a problem with determining "linear relationships," for example, a linear relationship between digital hearing aids and achievement, between "any X" and reading achievement, and so on? Why or why not?

3. We asked this question in Chapter 4 on digital hearing aids; we think it is interesting to include it here for cochlear implants. Do you think that advances in technology such as cochlear implants and other implantable hearing devices will eradicate the Deaf culture? How has your answer evolved from Chapter 4 to now? How do you feel about the decision-making process now?

Suggested Activities

1. Find out the percentage of students who have had cochlear implants in the local schools. Do any of the children have two cochlear implants? How about a hearing aid in one ear and a cochlear implant in the other? Observe the performance of a few of these children (any age level) in selected classrooms. What do you notice about their use of speech and language (in English)? Share your findings with your instructor and with other students in your class.

2. Visit your local speech and hearing center or clinic in the community or at your university. Ask personnel to show you the following:

   ■ Examples of cochlear implants.

   ■ Examples of other implantable hearing devices.

   ■ Is it possible to use a computer to program or adjust settings for a cochlear implant similar to that of a digital hearing aid?

   Share your findings with your instructor and with other students in your class.

3. Interview one or two students who wear a cochlear implant (at the upper elementary or middle school would be best). How do these students feel about their implants? Benefits? Disadvantages? Share your findings with your instructor and with other students in your class.

References

Archbold, S. M., Nikolopoulos, T. P., & Lloyd-Richmond, H. (2009). Long-term use of cochlear implant systems in paediatric recipients and factors contributing to non-use. *Cochlear Implants International, 10*(1), 25–40.

Bilger, R. C. (1983). Auditory results with single channel implants. *Annals of the New York Academy of Science, 405,* 337–342.

Cheng, A. K., Rubin, H. R., Powe, N. R., Mellon, N. K., Francis, H. W., & Niparko, J. K. (2000). Cost-utility analysis of the cochlear implant in children. *Journal of the American Medical Association, 284*(7), 850–856.

Ching, T., Incerti, P., & Hill, M. (2004). Binaural benefits for adults who use hearing aids with cochlear implants in the opposite ear. *Ear and Hearing, 25*(1), 9–21.

Ching, T. Y. C., van Wanrooy, E., & Dillion, H. (2007). Binaural-bimodal fitting or bilateral implantation for managing severe to profound deafness: A review. *Trends in Amplification, 11*(3), 162–191.

Chorost, M. (2005). *Rebuilt: How becoming part computer made me more human.* Boston: Houghton Mifflin.

Clark, G. (2009). The multi-channel cochlear implant: Past, present, and future perspective. *Cochlear Implants International, 10*(S1), 2–13.

Cohen, S., Labadie, R., Dietrich, M., & Haynes, D. (2004). Quality of life in hearing-impaired adults: The role of cochlear implants and hearing aids. *Otolaryngology—Head and Neck Surgery, 131*(4), 413–422.

Djourno, A., & Eyries, C. (1957). Auditory prosthesis by means of a distant electrical stimulation of the sensory nerve with the use of an indwelt coiling. *La Presse Medicale, 65*(part 2), 1417.

Eapen, R. J., & Buchman, C. A. (2009). Bilateral cochlear implantation: Current concepts. *Current Opinion in Otolaryngology & Head and Neck Surgery, 17*(5), 351–355.

Food and Drug Administration. (2009). What is a cochlear implant? Available online: www.fda.gov/MedicalDevices/ProductsandMedicalProcedures/ImplantsandProsthetics/Cochlear Implants/ucm062823.htm. Accessed July 24, 2009.

Geers, A. E. (2004). The ears of the deaf unstopped: Changes associated with cochlear implantation. *Seminars in Hearing, 25*(3), 257–268.

Geers, A. E., Moog, J. S., Biedenstein, J., Brenner, C., & Hayes, H. (2009). Spoken language scores of children using cochlear implants compared to hearing age-mates at school entry. *Journal of Deaf Studies and Deaf Education, 14*(3), 371–385.

Gifford, R. H., Dorman, M. F., Spahr, A. J., Bacon, S. P., Skarzynski, H., & Lorens, A. (2008). Hearing preservation surgery: Psychophysical estimates of cochlear damage in recipients of a short electrode array. *Journal of the Acoustical Society of America, 124*(4), 2164–2173.

Hammes, D. M., Novak, M. A., Rotz, L. A., Willis, M., Edmondson, D. M. & Thomas, J. F. (2002). Early identification and cochlear implantation: Critical factors for spoken language development. *Annals of Otology, Rhinology, and Laryngology Supplement, 189*, 74–78.

Harrington, T. (2009). *FAQ: Audism.* Gallaudet University. Available online: http://library.gallaudet.edu/Library/Deaf_Research_Help/Frequently_Asked_Questions_(FAQs)/Cultural_Social_Medical/Audism.html. Accessed July 17, 2009.

Hedley-Williams, A. J., Sladen, D. P., & Tharpe, A. M. (2003). Programming, care, and troubleshooting of cochlear implants in children. *Topics in Language Disorders, 23*(1), 46–56.

Hirsh, I. J. (1966). The ears of the deaf unstopped. *Volta Review, 68*, 623–633.

House, W. F. (1974). Goals of the cochlear implant. *The Laryngoscope, 84*(6), 1883–1887.

House W. F., & Urban, J. (1973). Long term results of electrode implantation and electronic stimulation of the cochlea in man. *The Annuals of Otology, Rhinology, and Laryngology, 82*(5), 504–517.

James, A. I., & Papsin, B. C. (2004). Cochlear implant surgery at 12 months of age or younger. *Laryngoscope, 114*, 2191–2195.

Klop, W. M., Briaire, J. J., Stiggelbout, A. M., & Frijns, J. H. (2009). Cochlear implant outcomes and quality of life in adults with prelingual deafness. *The Laryngoscope, 117*(11), 1982–1987.

Krueger, B., Joseph, G., & Rost, U. (2008). Performance groups in adult cochlear implant users: Speech perception results from 1984 until today. *Otology and Neurotology, 29*(4), 509–512.

Lane, H. (1992). *The mask of benevolence: Disabling the Deaf community.* New York: Knopf.

Litovsky, R. Y., Johnstone, P. M., & Godar, S. P. (2006). Benefits of bilateral cochlear implants and/or hearing aids in children. *International Journal of Audiology, 45* (Suppl 1), S78–S91.

Loizou, P. C. (1998). Mimicking the human ear. *IEEE Signal Processing Magazine, 15*(5), 101–130.

Loizou, P., Dorman, M., & Tu, Z. (1999). On the number of channels needed to understand speech. *Journal of Acoustical Society of America, 106*(4), 2097–2103.

Luntz, M., Shpak, T., & Weiss, H. (2005). Binaural-bimodal hearing: Concomitant use of unilateral cochlear implant and contralateral hearing aid. *Acta Oto-Laryngologia, 125*(6), 863–869.

Maini, S., Cohen, M. A., Hollow, R., & Briggs, R. (2009). Update on long-term results with auditory brainstem implants in NF2 patients. *Cochlear Implants International, 10*(S1), 33–37.

Matthies, C., Thomas, S., Moshre, M., Lesinski-Schiedat, A., Frohnem, C., Battmer, R.D., Lenarz, T., & Samii, M. (2000). Auditory brainstem implants: Current neurosurgical experiences and perspective. *The Journal of Laryngology & Otology, 114*(Suppl 27), 32–36.

National Association of the Deaf. (2009). Available online: www.nad.org. Accessed July 28, 2009.

National Association of the Deaf. (2000). NAD Position Statement on Cochlear Implants. Available online: www.nad.org/issues/technology/assistive-listening/cochlear-implants. Accessed July 28, 2009.

National Institutes of Deafness and Communication Disorders. (2007). Cochlear implants. Available online: www.nidcd.nih.gov/health/hearing/coch.asp. Accessed July 28, 2009.

Nevins, M., & Chute, P. (1996). *Children with cochlear implants in educational settings.* San Diego, CA: Singular.

Niparko, J. K., & Wilson, B. S. (2000). History of cochlear implants. In J. K. Niparko, K. I. Kirk, N. K. Mellon, A. M. Robbins, D. L. Tucci, & B. S. Wilson (Eds.), *Cochlear implants: Principles and practices* (pp. 103–108). Philadelphia, PA: Lippincott Williams & Wilkins.

Palmer, C. S., Niparko, J. K., Wyatt, J. R., Rothman, M., & de Lissovoy, G. (1999). A prospective study of the cost-utility of the multichannel cochlear implant. *Archives of Otolaryngology Head Neck Surgery, 125*(11), 1221–1228.

Paul, P. (2009). *Language and deafness* (4th ed.). Sudbury, MA: Jones & Bartlett.

Public Broadcasting System. (2006). *Cochlear implants: The debate.* Available online: www.pbs.org/wnet/soundandfury/cochlear/debate10.html. Accessed July 28, 2009.

Pfingst, B. E. (2008). Frontiers of auditory prosthesis research: Implications for clinical practice. *Hearing Research, 242*(1–2), 1–2.

Raine, C. H., Summerfield, Q., Strachan, D. R., Martin, J. M., & Totten, C. (2008). The cost and analysis of nonuse of cochlear implants. *Otology & Neurotology, 29*(2), 221–224.

Snik, A. F., Mylanus, E. A., Proops, D. W., Wolfaardt, J. F., Dent, M., Hodgetts, W. E., Somers, T., Niparko, J. K., Wazen, J. J., Sterkers, O., Cremers, C. W., & Tjellstrom, A. (2004). Consensus statements on the BAHA system: Where do we stand at present? *Annals of Otology, Rhinology, & Laryngology, 114*(12, Suppl 195), 1–12.

Trehub, S. E., Vongpaisal, T., & Nakata, T. (2009). Music in the lives of deaf children with cochlear implants. *Annals of the New York Academy of Science, 1169,* 518–533.

Tye-Murray, N. (2009). *Foundations of aural rehabilitation: Children, adults, and their family members.* Clifton Park, NY: Delmar.

The University of Texas at Dallas News Center. (2009). Engineer working to improve cochlear implants research project targets difficulties users face in noisy environments. Available online: www.utdallas.edu/news/2009/08/13-003.php. Accessed August 14, 2009.

Van de Heyning P., Vermeire, K., Diebl, M., Nopp, P., Anderson I., & De Ridder, D. (2008). Incapacitating unilateral tinnitus in single-sided deafness treated by cochlear implantation. *Annuals of Otology, Rhinology, & Laryngology, 117*(9), 645–652.

Wilson, B. S. (2004). Engineering design of cochlear implants. In F. G. Zeng, A. N. Popper, & R. R. Fay (Eds.), *Cochlear implants: Auditory prostheses and electric hearing* (pp. 14–52). New York: Springer.

Wilson, B. S., & Dorman, M. F. (2008). Cochlear implants: Current designs and future possibilities. *Journal of Rehabilitation Research & Development, 45*(5), 695–730.

Yuen, H.W, Bodmer, D., Smilsky, K., Nedzelski, J.M., & Chen, J.M. (2009). Management of single-sided deafness with the bone-anchored hearing aid. *Otolaryngology—Head and Neck Surgery, 141*(2), 16–23.

Zeng, F (2004). Trends in cochlear implants. *Trends in Amplification, 8*(1), 1–34.

Zeng, F. (2009). The best of 2008: Cochlear implants. *The Hearing Review, 62*(6), 26–28.

Further Readings

Blume, S. (2010). *The artificial ear: Cochlear implants and the culture of deafness.* Piscataway, NJ: Rutgers University Press.

Chute, P., & Nevins, M. E. (2006). *School professionals working with children with cochlear implants.* San Diego, CA: Plural Publishing.

Eisenberg, L. S. (2009). *Clinical management of children with cochlear implants.* San Diego, CA: Plural Publishing.

Loy, B., & Roland, P. (2009). *Cochlear implants: What parents should know.* San Diego, CA: Plural Publishing.

Weber, D. T. (2004). *I danced: A cochlear implant odyssey.* Edina, MN: Beaver's Pond Press.

HEARING, SPEECH, AND LANGUAGE DEVELOPMENT

Everyone born with the normal capacity to learn acquires the ability to listen and speak long before the ability to read and write. Moreover, when the English alphabet was first devised, its letters were based on a consideration of the nature of the sounds in Old English. The origins of the written language lie in the spoken language, not the other way round. It is therefore one of life's ironies that traditionally in present-day education we do not learn about spoken language until well after we have learned the basic properties of the written language. As a result, it is inevitable that we think of speech using the frame of reference which belongs to writing. We even use some of the same terms, and it can come as something of a shock to realize that these terms do not always have the same meaning.

—Crystal (1995, p. 236)

*Despite the rise of email and text messaging, speech remains the main means of human communication. Through speech we can express our thoughts and feelings in a remarkably detailed and subtle way. We can allow other people an almost immediate appreciation of what is going on in our heads. The arrival of speech had a drastic effect on our development as a species, and in many ways made possible the cultures and civilizations that exist in the world today. For humans, therefore, speech is the most important acoustic signal, and the **perception** of speech the most important function of the auditory system.*

—Plack (2005, p. 215)

Key Concepts

After completing this chapter, you should have a basic understanding of:

- The nature and stages of language development
- The nature of the speech process
- Research on speech development and deafness
- Amplification and assistive technology

As indicated by the opening passages, speech remains the most basic and prevalent form of communication for most humans, despite the proliferation of technological devices. In fact, as noted by Pinker (1994) and others (e.g., Chomsky, 2006; Crystal, 1995, 2006), spoken language is the real engine of verbal communication. Reading and written language are built upon or, to put it bluntly, parasitic upon the spoken-language capacities of individuals. As we shall highlight in the next chapter (Chapter 7), strong development in the spoken-language form—via phonology, morphology, syntax, semantics, and pragmatics—influences the acquisition of literacy skills, such as reading and writing in English. We also mention in that chapter that phonology provides access to the development of a spoken language, which we shall expound in this chapter because of its relation to the development of speech.

In human evolution, speech emerged as the most basic and efficient form of communication, probably as a result of the evolution of the physiological properties of the central nervous system (e.g., Boothroyd, 1986; Ling, 1976, 1989, 2001, 2002). Earlier forms of communication may have been nonverbal, involving the use of the hands and body movements. However, it was evidently more efficient to free up the hands for manual activities and to communicate via voice (e.g., Crystal, 1995, 2006; Just & Carpenter, 1987).

How we perceive sounds and what it means to perceive sounds are fascinating phenomena. The peripheral auditory system does its part in breaking down sounds into components and transmitting the various components to the auditory cortex (e.g., Plack, 2005). However, we do not perceive the individual components, nor do we perceive phonemes (discussed later), although we can learn to identify (e.g., blend or segment) them (which seems to be critical for reading, as discussed in Chapter 7). The act of perception of sounds is actually an interpretation process, which involves—at the very least—cognitive and, in some cases, cognitive and social factors (e.g., Ling, 2001, 2002; Plack, 2005).

We bet that you have a zillion questions about this business of speech, hearing, and language. Let us see if we can guess a few of them that we hope to answer in this chapter. For example:

- Is speech the same as language?
- Is language the same as communication?
- What are the nature and stages of language development? What role does phonology play?

■ What is the nature of the speech process?

■ With respect to research, what can we say about the speech development of d/Deaf and hard of hearing students? Does signing interfere with speech development (a controversial issue!)?

■ Has technology—notably amplification and assistive devices—impacted the development of speech in d/Deaf and hard of hearing students?

Obviously, this list of questions is not exhaustive. Nevertheless, we feel the need to immediately address the first one about the relation between speech and language, because it is often misunderstood. In fact, Ling (2001; see also 2002) argues that "Speech skills are strongly associated with superior educational achievements" (p. 147). In our view, this *association* really depends on the development of language.

By now, you should be able to predict the answer to our question: is speech the same as language? And, we shall praise you if you say "no." In essence, speech is not language, but rather a representation of the sounds of language in an arbitrary order (i.e., sequence of sounds to produce words in the language). *Speech* is defined as the verbal means of communicating, which includes articulation (e.g., how speech sounds are made), voice (e.g., using the vocal folds and breathing to support speech production), and fluency (e.g., the rhythm of speech) (American Speech-Language-Hearing Association, 2009). What is produced via the mouth or via the hands (as in signing) is simply a manifestation of what occurs in the brain, particularly the left hemisphere—the seat of the language module (e.g., Crystal, 2006; Fodor, 1983).

Analyses of spoken-language productions via speech, for example, may provide a glimpse or an estimate of the language competency of individuals. But this estimate is not perfect, and it might not even be accurate (e.g., Chomsky, 2006). Chomsky (2006) has argued strongly that linguists and others need to focus on language competency (via introspections, grammaticality judgments, etc., of individuals) rather than language productions to develop a good, working theory of language acquisition (see also the discussion in Paul, 2009). Language productions or utterances are subjected to confounding factors, such as memory issues, affective factors, articulation errors (e.g., the speech representation of language is unintelligible to the listener), fluency of the message, and so on.

We hope that we have convinced you that speech is not language. But then, what is language? What does it mean to say that someone has a level of competency or proficiency in the use of a language? Admittedly, the answers to these questions depend on how language is defined theoretically, how it is examined or studied, and how it is measured—for starters. We will take the easy way out—well, nothing is easy.

In any case, our goal in the next section is to provide a synthesis of the nature and development of language, especially with respect to the language components that we mentioned previously (e.g., phonology, morphology, etc.). To be succinct, *language* can be defined simply (which may be an oxymoron, as we have stated here, because little related to language is simple) as a socially shared rule system that governs a number of areas, including word meaning, how to create new words, how to combine words, and what combinations of words work best in specific situations (American Speech-Language-Hearing Association, 2009).

The Nature and Stages of Language Development

The best way to begin a discussion of language development is to quickly state that there is no best way to begin this discussion. For example, this discussion would vary among the professionals who are describing language; that is, descriptions would vary according to individuals in fields such as linguistics, anthropology, speech and hearing science, psychology, and deaf education (see Paul, 2009). Some individuals would ascribe to a behavior-environmental description, some to a cognitive description, and some to a social description, as well as combinations of these three broad domains. Pick up any book on language acquisition and you will be bombarded with numerous models and theories (e.g., Pence & Justice, 2008).

So, where to begin? We shall adopt an approach that focuses on the development of the language components from birth to maturity—well, at least to age 3 with some general statements on what occurs afterwards. In essence, our plan is this: we describe each component of language (with examples), and then we chart the development of all components (briefly!) in typical individuals.

PHONOLOGY

Succinctly stated, *phonology* is concerned with the rules that govern the production, structure, sequence, and distribution of articulatory elements, either sounds, as in speech, or hand movements, as in signing, of a language (e.g., Crystal, 1995, 2006; Owens, 2004; Pence & Justice, 2008). You will read periodically in this text that *phonology represents the building blocks of a language*. Essentially, this means that to learn or acquire a language, one must access its phonology. We shall be concerned with the phonology of English. Just so you are not confused: *phonology* addresses the rules of sounds or hand movements in a language whereas *phonetics* refers to the science of sounds as produced by speech mechanisms. The nature of speech mechanisms is discussed later.

Let us go to work. In discussing phonology, we shall distinguish two groups of elements: segmentals and suprasegmentals. In English, segmentals entail phonemes, which are abstract entities and are the smallest units that can signal differences in meaning. In short, phonemes can be operationalized as consonants and vowels and as families of distinctive, similar sounds (e.g., consider the /b/ sound in *base*, *superb*, and *disturbance*—i.e., allophones of the phoneme). Suprasegmentals entail prosodic elements such as intonation, rhythms, and pauses. Both segmentals and suprasegmentals are critical for the development of speech and for the development of phonology (Crystal, 1995, 2006; Ling, 1976, 1989, 2001, 2002).

English has about 45 phonemes, give or take one or two, due to dialectical variations. A selected list of phonemes and examples in words are provided in **Table 6-1**.

Humans can produce a wide range of sounds via the manipulations of the articulators (e.g., throat, tongue, teeth, lips) of speech. Only a small range of these sounds are meaningful, and this is arbitrarily defined or confined by the language of the culture in which

Table 6-1	*List of Selected Consonant and Vowel Phonemes of English*	
	Consonants	**Vowels**
	/b/ as in <u>b</u>ase	/a/ as in m<u>a</u>ss
	/d/ as in <u>d</u>og	/e/ as in m<u>a</u>te
	/dz/ as in <u>j</u>et	/i/ as in b<u>ea</u>m
	/f/ as in <u>f</u>og	/I/ as in h<u>i</u>p
	/g/ as in <u>g</u>irl	/u/ as in m<u>oo</u>t
	/h/ as in <u>h</u>appy	/U/ as in b<u>oo</u>t
	/k/ as in <u>c</u>at	/o/ as in b<u>oar</u>d
	/l/ as in <u>l</u>ate	
	/m/ as in <u>m</u>ine	
	/n/ as in <u>n</u>ight	
	/p/ as in <u>p</u>age	
	/r/ as in ba<u>r</u>	
	/s/ as in <u>s</u>et	
	/t/ as in <u>t</u>imid	
	/v/ as in <u>v</u>an	
	/w/ as in <u>w</u>in	
	/wh/ as in <u>wh</u>en	
	/z/ as in <u>z</u>ip	

one resides. So, the specific sounds associated with one language, and thus having meaning, may be meaningless to the ears of a person who knows a different language in which these sounds do not carry meaning (consider Swahili and English). Dialectical variations within a language may cause confusion to some listeners, but they can be understood, sometimes with practice.

Before leaving phonology, we need to make one more point. A working knowledge of phonology, including the suprasegmental aspects such as intonation, stress, and rhythm, also provides the foundation for the development of reading (see Chapter 7), especially given the importance of phonemic awareness (e.g., National Reading Panel, 2000). At best, the National Reading Panel avers that to become good readers children need to be able to blend and segment phonemes, especially in the beginning reading process. Of course, as discussed later in Chapter 7, there is more to reading than phonology, but phonology facilitates the learning of the alphabetic system—the relations between sounds and letters. Does one have to hear in order to learn phonology? This issue is explored briefly in Chapter 7 and again in Chapter 8.

MORPHOLOGY

In the section on phonology, we mentioned phonemes. In this section on morphology, we shall discuss morphemes. *Morphemes* can be described as the smallest segment of speech (or articulatory element) that possesses meaning (Goodluck, 1991; Matthews, 1991). For example, consider the words *girls* and *walked*. The word *girls* contains two morphemes: /girl/ and /s/. It also contains four phonemes associated with the four sounds in the word. The word *walked* contains two morphemes—/walk/ and /ed/—and five phonemes (We shall let you figure that out! The *ed* has one sound, a *t*, and there is a phonological rule for that!).

Morphology is concerned with the structure of words, and it is typically influenced by both phonology and syntax (word order—discussed later). You can see that the phonemes are *combined* to produce morphemes. Again, this combination is governed by rules.

Morphology is important, but it not analogous to phonology, as a building block, for learning a language such as English—as least not for learning the spoken form of the language. We are sure that you will find other scholars who disagree with us. Perhaps, the best evidence for our assertion is the disappointing findings associated with the research on the various English sign systems, none of which has resulted in the adequate development of English for many or even most d/Deaf or hard of hearing students (e.g., Paul, 2009; Trezek, Wang, & Paul, 2010). These sign systems are based predominantly on English morphology. Phonology is not represented but is purported to be acquired through the use of speechreading by students via the simultaneous production of signs and speech by teachers or parents (see Chapter 8).

The influences of syntax on morphology can be seen in English, especially via the use of sentences such as the following (Crystal, 1997, 2006):

1. The boxer *win/won* the fight last week. [Past tense, *won*, is dictated by the phrase *last week*.]

2. The tall boxer *win/wins* the round! [The singular form of *win* is dictated by the noun phrase *The tall boxer* or *boxer*].

In these examples, the influence of syntax (e.g., the surrounding words) refers to items such as tense (past) and number (singular).

The last major issue that we shall discuss about morphology is the use of terms such as *free morpheme* and *bound morpheme*. A *free morpheme* represents the minimum notion of a word and can stand by itself. For example, words that cannot be divided further into other morphemes include *piano*, *tree*, *pen*, and *wow*. This is considered the base form of the word, often called a *root* or *stem* (e.g., see also Crystal, 1995, 1997, 2006).

Bound morphemes are morphemes that cannot occur alone and need to be combined with at least one other morpheme (free or bound) to form a word. We like to think of bound morphemes as affixes such as prefixes (e.g., *ir-*, *re-*, *dis-*) and suffixes (e.g., *-ly*, *-ment*, *-ness*). Prefixes represent one robust way in which new words are added to the language (Crystal, 1995).

However, suffixes are important and quite interesting as well. Suffixes can be categorized into two types: derivational and grammatical (or inflectional). Derivational suffixes (e.g., *-able*) change the meaning of the base form or word as in *movable* from *move*. Another function of suffixes is to indicate the use (grammatical) of a word in a sentence as in plurality (e.g., *pianos*) or past tense (*rated*). These examples are inflectional suffixes or, simply, inflections. It should come as no surprise that derivational suffixes are more difficult than inflectional suffixes. Examples of derivational and inflectional morphemes are provided in **Table 6-2**.

Table 6-2

Examples of Derivational and Inflectional Morphemes

Derivational Morphemes

- Derivational morphology deals with the construction of new words, typically via additions of specific morphemes (e.g., *re-*, *-ment*, *-ness*, and *-less*). Examples include: *rewrite, reice, replace, merriment, judgment, loveliness*, and *clueless.*

- Derivational morphemes may change the meaning of a word, as in *clear* and *unclear*, or indicate the part of speech (form class) of a word, for example, noun suffixes such as *-ance* in *tolerance* and *-dom* in *freedom*. It should be clear that these are examples of different words, each with its own grammatical properties or aspects. Other examples include: *unknown, undo, persistence, maintenance*, and *serfdom.*

Inflectional Morphemes

- Inflectional morphology is the study of word variations, or inflections, such as plurality (girl, girls) and tense (walk—present; walked—past). Thus, inflections refer to changes in the root or base word (i.e., the uninflected, citation form) to express syntactic functions and relationships. These changes do not affect the meaning of the root or base word. Other examples include: *boys, oxen, rated, studied, walking, running*, and *lovely.*

Finally, we like to mention that morphology in conjunction with phonology assists with the acquisition of conventional spellings of words and, possibly, to the understanding of orthography (i.e., in this case, the arrangement of letters in words). Obviously, these language components appear to work in tandem—so to speak. We already mentioned briefly the contributions of syntax to the development or understanding of morphology. Let us explore syntax further in the next section.

SYNTAX

For some linguists, syntax is the most basic component of a language such that (1) it is essential for comprehension and (2) it reflects the structure of the mind (e.g., Chomsky, 2006; Lund, 2003). We shall focus on the former and leave it up to you to explore further the implications of the latter, which entails, among other issues, the concept of innate structures (e.g., Carruthers, Laurence, & Stich, 2005, 2006). Indeed, for a number of linguists and scholars, syntax seems to reflect the essence of a mind having learned language.

Let us return to the first issue: Is syntax essential for comprehension? To examine this, we need a working definition of syntax. *Syntax* is concerned with rules that govern the order or arrangement of words (e.g., Crystal, 1995, 2006). The order or arrangement of words reveals a set of meaningful relationships within and between sentences, focusing on sentence organization and relationships between words.

There is little doubt that order is important. Suppose we have the following list of words: *The, the, girl, pit bull, mauled, was, by.* We can create two different sentences with different meanings:

1. The girl was mauled by the pit bull.

2. The pit bull was mauled by the girl.

Both sentences are syntactically correct, albeit perhaps only the first is plausible.

An infinite number of examples can be offered to demonstrate the centrality or, at the least, the importance of syntax. Consider the following:

1. That John was happy was not obvious to Mary.

2. Walking is good exercise, but I prefer to ride a bike.

3. The boy who kissed the girl ran away.

The limits seem to be our imagination. In fact, this is a major premise; that is, the rules of syntax are finite, but these rules can engender an infinite number of sentences, many of which we have never heard or read before (e.g., Chomsky, 2006; Crystal, 1997, 2006; Lund, 2003). We wager that you have never heard or read any of the following sentences, albeit you may be somewhat familiar with the concepts or ideas.

1. The Reconstruction of the South, which was fraught with corruptions, might have prolonged the acrimonious tensions and attitudes that still exist today between proponents with a Northern or North-mentality and those with a Southern or South-mentality.

2. Faith has several faces, which—at a superficial level—correspond with the definitions in any dictionary, but apparently, do not reflect the deeper meanings of this concept, including the conflation and influence of other terms such as *desire, hope*, or a *fierce, blind loyalty*.

3. *This world is all that there is* is one of the most ridiculous metaphysical statements that has ever been put down in writing to corrupt a generation of future philosophers.

We are quite confident that you can create a few sentences of your own!

Another concept that we want to highlight is the two broad levels of syntactical complexity (obviously, this is a simple rendition because syntax is enormously complex). The two levels are linear and hierarchical structures (e.g., Crystal, 1997; Paul, 2009). Linear structures can be interpreted by the use of a subject–verb–object (SVO) strategy. Consider the following examples:

1. The boy kissed the girl.

2. I want my pipe.

3. My mother loves me.

Hierarchical structures contain embedded elements, which render them difficult and impossible to be interpreted by the use of the SVO strategy. Consider the following examples:

1. The boy who kissed the girl ran away. [Poor readers or listeners assume that the girl ran away.]

2. The light on top of the blue police car turned to the right. [Poor readers or listeners assume that the blue police car turned to the right.]

Hierarchical structures not only require an understanding of syntax (and other elements), but also the ability to hold in memory information from the beginning of the sentence to the end. This might be a rather odd notion to mention here. Nevertheless, it will become clearer in Chapter 7, which posits that the use of a phonological code in working memory facilitates the understanding of sentences, especially hierarchical sentences. And, of course, our ongoing thesis is that phonology is critical for both spoken and written language development. The development of phonology, along with other language components, is facilitated by audition—even though audition may not be mandatory or necessary.

We agree that ample evidence shows that syntax is critical for the comprehension of sentences. Examples of different types of syntactic structures are provided in **Table 6-3**.

Nevertheless, there is a nagging thought running around in our minds (of course, we will NOT discuss the challenges of figurative language!). Let us put this thought in action by asking you to reflect on the following sentence:

The Reconstruction of the South, while not well accepted, had some positive benefits to individuals, who were slaves prior to the Civil War.

Table 6-3

Examples of Syntactic Structures

Structure	Example(s)
Negation	John will *not* go to the store.
	I'm *not* hungry.
Conjunction	John *and* Mary are happy.
	He went to the movies *and* she went to the opera.
Question formation	
Wh- questions	*What* is your name?
	Where do you live?
Yes/No questions	Do you want a cup of coffee?
	Are you mad?
Tag questions	You like me, don't you? (negative tag)
	You are not eating that cookie, are you? (positive tag)
Reflexivization	Katherine did this *herself.*
Passivitization	The ball *was hit* by the girl.
Relativization	The boy *who kissed the girl* ran away.
	The cat *whom the dog* bit yelped.
Disjunction and alternation	The woman wants *either* coffee *or* tea.
	I like coffee, *but* it does not like me.

In general, to understand the complexity of this sentence, one needs more than just knowledge of the syntactic structures of the sentence. Granted, it is important to understand the concept of history, the culture, and other social views of this particular period in time. In addition, it seems to be critical to understand the meanings of the words in the sentence in conjunction with other linguistic and cultural knowledge. We will not delve deeper into the issue of interpretation, including whether one agrees or disagrees with the statement. Our focus here is to delve a little bit into the meanings in the sentence itself; that is, on semantics, another important language component.

SEMANTICS

For some scholars, semantics is the most basic component of a language; that is, semantics is the core and everything else revolves around it (e.g., see discussions in Crystal, 1995, 1997; Paul, 2009). *Semantics* is the study of meaning *in* language (Lyons, 1995; Pence & Justice, 2008). Exchanges between individuals cannot be separated from a context in which there is meaning or understanding of the message that needs to be meaningful.

The concept of meaning is not only difficult to define, it is also difficult to measure. Nevertheless, there is no question that meaning is critical in order to understand language acquisition; whether it is *the* critical notion is debatable. In fact, it might very well be that there cannot be meaning separate from syntax (e.g., Carruthers et al., 2005, 2006; Lund, 2003).

In any case, the notion of meaning in language has several levels: word (or word parts), phrase, sentence, and beyond the sentence (i.e., passages or stories) (e.g., Crystal, 1995, 1997; Pence & Justice, 2008). We maintain that comprehension, whether of speech, print, or other media, is essentially the construction of meaning, or even the construction of reality. One of the most interesting and critical areas within semantics is how children acquire word meanings; that is, the development of their lexicons. Another area of intense interest is how words and other information are organized, stored, and retrieved (e.g., Hiebert & Kamil, 2005; Pence & Justice, 2008; Stahl & Nagy, 2006).

The importance of semantics in the field of reading can be seen with the widespread classroom use of semantic elaboration techniques such as word maps, semantic maps, semantic feature analysis, word webs, and semantic webs (see examples in Heimlich & Pittelman, 1986; Pearson & Johnson, 1978). These devices and others may also be useful in understanding concepts such as synonyms (word with similar meanings—*big, large*), antonyms (words with opposite meanings—*heavy, light*), and analogies (e.g., relationships between words and phrases; *Light is to sun as* _____ *is to lamp*).

One of the most interesting aspects of semantics, with enormous impact for both language and literacy development, is *polysemy*, or words with multiple meanings. For example, consider the various meanings of the word *bank*:

- A place to save or store items (money, food, sperm)
- Land beside a body of water (riverbank, canal or stream bank, etc.)
- To count on (You can bank on that.)

Multimeaning words are part of the overall framework of vocabulary knowledge. Namely, it is critical to possess both breadth (range; large number of words) and depth (multi-meanings, nuances, etc.) of knowledge. Vocabulary knowledge not only contributes positively to reading comprehension but also affects phonological and morphological development as well (e.g., Nagy, 2005; Stahl & Nagy, 2006). In essence, good language users as well as good readers need to be aware of more than just the semantic features of words in order to develop rapid, automatic, word identification skills or to use their mental lexicon as a major source of comprehension in language use.

In short, there is no doubt that semantics is important for both language and literacy development. Semantics is also a major aspect in many theories of cognitive development. There is considerable overlap between cognitive and semantic developments in the scholarly literature on the early language acquisition of children (e.g., see Pence & Justice, 2008). A few scholars even argue that semantics overlaps with the component of pragmatics, which is the last language component to be discussed, in the next section.

Pragmatics

Pragmatics involves the use of language within a social communicative or interactional situation or context (e.g., see Crystal, 1997; Owens, 1996, 2004). We mentioned the notion of overlap between pragmatics and semantics in the previous section. Specifically, both pragmatics and semantics are concerned with the intentions of the language user and the background knowledge about the worlds of both speakers and listeners during social intercourses (e.g., Crystal, 1997; Owens, 1996, 2004).

Unlike the other components discussed thus far, such as phonology, morphology, syntax, and semantics, pragmatics is not a part of language structure. Many children produce pragmatics errors, such as not understanding turn taking, not waiting to speak, having poor conversation openers, or not respecting the topic of conversation (actually, a few of our university students produce these errors as well!). However, these pragmatics errors do not affect the rules of or use of the other language components. Nevertheless, a number of scholars have argued that language develops as a consequent of social and communicative interactions; that is, via the use of the pragmatics domain (e.g., see Owens, 2004; Pence & Justice, 2008).

Children learn to adapt to a listener's knowledge and perspectives by *asking for clarification* or *requesting information* (e.g., Ninio & Snow, 1996; Owens, 2004). Other behaviors that have been delineated in children are as follows: *requesting, labeling, repeating, negating,* and so on (e.g., Owens, 2004; Pence & Justice, 2008; Thompson, Biro, Vethivelu, Pious, & Hatfield, 1987).

Descriptions of some of these behaviors are as follows (Thompson et al., 1987):

> Requesting: Solicitation of a service from a listener.
>
> Repeating: Repetition of part or all of previous adult utterance. Child does not wait for a response.
>
> Negating: Denial, resistance to, or rejection by child of adult statement, request, or question. (pp. 11, 13)

In sum, pragmatics is a serious component that needs to be developed, especially in children with language and reading disabilities. The manner in which pragmatics is connected to the other components of language is the focus of ongoing investigations. It is not uncommon to find that many language intervention programs are heavily focused or influenced by the domain of pragmatics (e.g., Owens, 2004).

Brief Description of Language Development

Now that we have described the major components of language, we can relate a few words about their development; that is, we can chart the development of language, which is truly remarkable when you consider what children learn by the end of their third year (Crystal, 2006; O'Grady, 2005; Pence & Justice, 2008). We provide major highlights with respect to two broad periods of development: prelinguistic and linguistic. Admittedly, this is only a brief rendition; we strongly advise you to read additional sources (e.g., Crystal, 2006; O'Grady, 2005).

PRELINGUISTIC DEVELOPMENT

The development of language begins in a hurry—so to speak (or sign!). During the first few months of life, infants can discriminate between speech sounds, recognizing their mothers' voices immediately, responding differently to their voices than to the voices of other speakers (Crystal, 1997, 2006; Gerken, Jusczyk, & Mandel, 1994; O'Grady, 2005). During this period, infants also become sensitive to the suprasegmental aspects of speech—intonations, pauses, and rhythms—and then to the segmental aspects—vowels and consonants. The rise–fall contour of infant vocalization portends the later development of sentence types such as statements, questions, and explanations.

With respect to production, infants begin to use their voices to control others and to get them to do things (Crystal, 1997, 2006; Gerken et al., 1994; O'Grady, 2005). This can be seen in the variations of cries and sounds, which may correspond to hunger, sleepiness, crankiness, and boredom. In short, infants are learning about the power of language for communication purposes. During this first year, the infant develops the precursors for all language components and proceeds into the one-word stage. The production of the first words marks the beginning of the linguistic period (Crystal, 1997, 2006; O'Grady, 2005; Pence & Justice, 2008).

LINGUISTIC DEVELOPMENT

When the first words are spoken, the nature of these words varies based on the individual, as well as the culture. Nevertheless, the common element seems to be this: the first words typically refer to objects and events that are present in the infant's environment (Crystal, 1997, 2006; Gerken et al., 1994; O'Grady, 2005).

Understanding the child's words during this stage can be challenging and sometimes frustrating for both the child and significant others. The initial words often can only be understood within the contexts in which they are uttered. *Milk* can have several interpretations, ranging from *I want milk* to *The milk is on the floor*, and so on.

Once a number of single words are mastered, children begin combining words to express their ideas. When children begin producing utterances by combining two or more words, this is the beginning of the syntactic development and the start of a rapid growth in language development (Crystal, 1997, 2006; Gerken et al., 1994; O'Grady, 2005). A large amount of individual variation continues with regard to language development, especially with the development of vocabulary knowledge (semantics), and this lasts into the early school years.

In sum, most of the phonologic rules are acquired by 6 to 8 years of age (Crystal, 1997, 2006; Gerken et al., 1994; O'Grady, 2005; Pence & Justice, 2008). By the time they start school, children can engage in lessons involving phonemic awareness and phonics (learning the relations between sounds and letters). Most children internalize much of the grammar of the language by the age of 4 or 5 years, and master nearly all of the grammar by age 9 or 10 (Crystal, 1997, 2006; Gerken et al., 1994; O'Grady, 2005; Pence & Justice, 2008).

The Nature of the Speech Process

Now that you have obtained basic information about the components and the development of language, you are ready to delve into the nature of the speech process. Keep in mind that speech is a manifestation of language; it is not the same as language. To understand the speech process, we need to describe the production of speech sounds via the speech mechanism.

Several authors have different models for describing the mechanisms and production of speech (e.g., Ling, 1976, 2001, 2002; Plack, 2005; Shames & Anderson, 2002). One way to view speech communication is to think of it as a series of stages. Speakers need to construct their ideas and thoughts and code these items in an arbitrarily defined conventional symbol system; that is, language via words and sentences. On the flip side, speakers use their speech/language areas of the brain to perceive and interpret an incoming message or speech input.

To produce speech, the efforts of three broad areas—the respiratory system, the laryngeal system, and the articulatory system—must be coordinated (e.g., Ling, 1976, 1989, 2001, 2002; Plack, 2005; Shames & Anderson, 2002). The respiratory system entails structures such as the lungs, trachea, and bronchial tubes. The laryngeal system involves the larynx, including the vocal folds and the glottis. Finally, the articulatory system involves the following cavities: pharyngeal (throat area), oral (mouth area), and nasal (nose area). These cavities are critical for resonance; that is, the quality associated with voiced sounds (discussed later).

Of course, we need our tongue and lips to assist in this speech process. From another standpoint, the mechanisms that we use for breathing and eating are also used for speaking. It is still a good idea not to speak with your mouth full of food.

In the production of speech, air flows from the respiratory system through the cavities and the articulators. This flow of air is obstructed or constricted along the way through the laryngeal and articulatory systems depending on the sound that we intend to produce (e.g., Ling, 1976, 1989, 2001, 2002; Plack, 2005; Shames & Anderson, 2002).

Before the sound leaves the lips, it is modified or enhanced by the resonant qualities of oral and nasal cavities in the pharyngeal system. For example, the velum can be raised, resulting in the use of the oral cavity alone. This accounts for most of the speech sounds. The velum can be lowered, resulting in a blocked oral cavity, and this leads to nasal sounds such as /m/ and /n/.

In the following sections, we shall focus on the major categories of sources of sound: voicing, frication, and stop-plosion (e.g., Boothroyd, 1986; Shames & Anderson, 2002; Zemlin, 1968).

VOICING

In our view, the most important source of speech sounds is the notion of *voicing*. Voicing occurs in the larynx, particularly via the vibrations or actions of the vocal folds or chords (i.e., two muscular flaps) (e.g., Ling, 1976, 1989, 2001, 2002; Plack, 2005; Shames & Anderson, 2002). The space between the vocal folds is called the glottis.

Here's how this works. As the vocal folds are pulled together, the glottis closes, and this action obstructs the flow of air from the respiratory system. Pressure then builds under the glottis. This pressure forces the glottis to open and the vocal folds to pull apart. Immediately, a pulse of air escapes into the vocal tract. The vibrations of the vocal folds are caused by the simultaneous actions of the air pulses and the opening and closing of the glottis. These vibrations produce *voiced sounds*. As noted by Boothroyd (1986, p. 18): "The air is thus released in brief, repetitive bursts, generating a complex tone, called voicing." You can try this easily: make a *t* sound (unvoiced) and then make the *d* sound (voiced). The major difference between these two sounds is the act of voicing.

We discussed pitch in Chapter 2. Here we can relate that the frequency of the vibration of the vocal folds is called the *fundamental frequency* of voicing, and this frequency is perceived as pitch. Now we can state that the differences that we hear in frequencies across the speech of adults such as men and women and that of children are due to the differences in size and weight of the vocal folds (e.g., Ling, 1976, 1989, 2001, 2002; Plack, 2005; Shames & Anderson, 2002). In general, men's voices are lower on the frequency range than those of women's and, of course, women's are lower than those of children.

Have you wondered why boys' voices change when they reach puberty? We shall let you investigate this question and share your findings with your instructor and classmates. In any case, the variations of frequency during the production of speech are perceived as the intonation (suprasegmental) of speech.

FRICATION

When a random turbulence of air is forced through a narrow opening, we have the phenomenon known as *frication*. This constriction of airflow can occur anywhere along the vocal tract and can be caused by any of the speech mechanisms (e.g., Ling, 1976, 1989, 2001, 2002; Plack, 2005; Shames & Anderson, 2002). The location of a particular narrow opening is labeled the *place of articulation*. There are several places of articulation, including the lips (bilabial), the area between lower lip and upper teeth (labiodental), and the area between the partially closed vocal folds (glottal). Examples of sounds at these areas are illustrated later.

If there is only a random turbulence with no voiced sound (e.g., /f/ and /s/), then these sounds are labeled *voiceless sounds*. Turbulence accompanied by voice (e.g., /v/ and /z/) are labeled *voiced sounds* (e.g., Ling, 1976, 1989, 2001, 2002; Plack, 2005; Shames & Anderson, 2002).

STOP-PLOSION

When the airflow is stopped completely and then released quickly (from the buildup of air pressure), the sound source is labeled *stop-plosion* (e.g., Ling, 1976, 2001; Plack, 2005; Shames & Anderson, 2002). It is possible to completely and briefly obstruct airflow at several locations along the vocal tract (e.g., lips, tongue, vocal folds). Examples of stop-plosives are presented later in the section on classification. Note that these sounds cannot be produced in isolation. Invariably, one also makes a vowel sound when producing this type of sound.

The Speech Sounds

Earlier in this chapter, we discussed the English phonemes, the 45 or so phonemes that refer to the consonants and vowels, or segmentals. In this section, we shall classify the phonemes according to the mechanism of speech production. Consonants are typically classified with respect to the position of articulation, whereas vowels are categorized with respect to tongue positions.

CONSONANTS

The constriction and obstruction of airflow along the vocal tract is primarily responsible for the production of consonants (e.g., Ling, 1976, 1989, 2001, 2002; Plack, 2005; Shames & Anderson, 2002). Several features of articulation differentiate the consonants: place, manner, position, and the absence or presence of voicing (i.e., in general, consonants involve no voice, except for *glides*, discussed later). With respect to the manner of articulation, the following labels are used: *stop-plosive, affricate, fricative, nasal,* and *vowel-like consonants (glides)*. The classification of consonants is provided in **Table 6-4**.

As mentioned previously, in the production of stop-plosive consonants, the articulators stop the air flow and air pressure builds up behind the occlusion (e.g., Ling, 1976, 1989, 2001, 2002; Plack, 2005; Shames & Anderson, 2002). Then, the articulators release the airflow, producing a stop or plosive, as in /p/ or /b/. English has six stop-plosive consonants. Half of these are accompanied by voice; half are not. The stop-plosives are shown in Table 6-4.

English has only two affricates, one voiced and one voiceless (e.g., Ling, 1976, 1989, 2001, 2002; Plack, 2005; Shames & Anderson, 2002). These sounds are similar to stop-plosives except that the air pulses are sustained for a slightly longer period of time. The

Table 6-4

Classification of Consonants

Position	Manner of Articulation					
	Stop	Affricate	Fricative	Nasal	Lateral	Semivowel
Bilabial	*p* in *pat* *b* in *bat*		*wh* in *when*	*m* in *me*		*w* in *wine*
Labiodental			*f* in *fat* *v* in *vine*			
Interdental			*th* in *thin* *th* in *that*			
Apicoalveolar	*t* in *time* *d* in *dog*	*ch* in *choppy* *j* in *jack*	*s* in *site* *z* in *zorro*	*n* in *nice*	*l* in *late*	*r* in *war*
Frontopalatal			*sh* in *shop* *z* in *azure*			*y* in *yo*
Dorsovelar	*k* in *kitchen* *g* in *go*			*ng* in *song*		
Glottal			*h* in *hot*			

Sources: Data based on Creaghead & Newman (1985) and Shelton & Wood (1978).

voiced affricate is the only sound that uses all three types of sound sources, mentioned previously. Affricates are also shown in Table 6-4.

For the production of fricatives, airflow is forced through a narrow opening, resulting in a turbulent stream of noise. English has six voiceless and four voiced fricatives (e.g., Ling, 1976, 1989, 2001, 2002; Plack, 2005; Shames & Anderson, 2002). Resonance is provided by the oral cavity only (see Table 6-4 for examples).

We have already mentioned the nasal sounds (e.g., /m/, /n/, and /ng/). For these sounds, the velum is lowered and the vibrated air flows via the nose only. The nasal cavity is the sole resonator for the three nasal sounds of English (see Table 6-4). Obviously, the only sound source for nasals is voicing.

Finally, we come to the group of vowel-like consonants (e.g., Ling, 1976, 1989, 2001, 2002; Plack, 2005; Shames & Anderson, 2002). These consonants are similar to vowels from one standpoint. The types of vowel-like consonants include a lateral glide and semi-vowel glides. Classifying these consonants is the source of considerable disagreement; however, there seems to be a consensus that there are only four common vowel-like consonants in English (see Table 6-4).

VOWELS

It should be clear by now that vowels involve voicing, the sound source (e.g., Ling, 1976, 1989, 2001, 2002; Plack, 2005; Shames & Anderson, 2002). The oral cavity serves as the sole resonator. In general, the vowels are differentiated predominantly by the placement of the tongue in the mouth. The lips and pharyngeal cavity also play critical roles in the production of vowels. **Table 6-5** illustrates the vowels with respect to tongue placement.

Table 6-5

Classification of Vowels with Respect to Tongue Placement

	Tongue Positions		
	Front	**Center**	**Back**
High	eat it		mood cook
Mid	rate ever	herd cut butter about	coat caw
Low	at mass		rot father

Sources: Data based on Creaghead & Newman (1985) and Shelton & Wood (1978).

Inspection of Table 6-5 reveals that vowels can be classified as *front*, *center*, and *back* in conjunction with *high*, *middle*, or *low*. Other possible combinations are *midfront*, *low front*, *high back*, *midback*, *low back*, and *midcentral*. The vowels depicted in Table 6-5 represent "ideal positions, reflecting isolated sound production, and these ideal positions are rarely reached during running speech" (Shelton & Wood, 1978, p. 68; see also Ling, 1976, 1989, 2001, 2002; Shames & Anderson, 2002). Nevertheless, the classification of vowels is critical for the teaching of vowel production to d/Deaf and hard of hearing children and adolescents.

Vowels can also be classified according to the qualities of *tenseness* and *laxness* (e.g., Ling, 1976, 1989, 2001, 2002; Shames & Anderson, 2002). Tense vowels demand more muscular tension and tongue adjustments than do lax vowels. They are also longer in duration than their lax counterparts. With respect to duration, it is permissible to consider tense vowels as long vowels, as in the words, *rate* and *wine*, whereas lax vowels exemplify short vowels, as in the words, *rat* and *win*.

The last category of vowels to be discussed here is also the most challenging for d/Deaf and hard of hearing students and even for other students with language disabilities or differences: diphthongs (e.g., Ling, 1976, 1989, 2001, 2002; Shames & Anderson, 2002). Diphthongs are often called "double vowels" (Boothroyd, 1986, p. 41). In producing diphthongs, the vocal tract and tongue positions undergo changes, exhibiting more than one dimension or position. For example, the tongue may begin in a position to produce a low or midlong vowel, but end up producing a high short one, exemplifying the two sounds of the diphthong. The vocal tract configuration and the tongue position work together to modify the resonance and quality of the vowel. As noted by Creaghead and Newman (1985): "Two resonances may occur, one blending into another, creating a diphthong" (p. 18). In English, a few common diphthongs are /oy/ as in *boy*, /aU/ as in *now*, and /oU/ as in *flow*.

Connected Speech Production

In our discussion of consonants and vowels in this chapter, we have presented information pertaining to the production of these phonemes in isolation. This is the ideal situation, which—as we mentioned—is necessary for the instruction of the production of vowels. Nevertheless, to completely understand the production of sounds, it is important to discuss the conditions of connected speech production, or what is often called *running speech* (e.g., Ling, 1976, 1989, 2001, 2002; Shames & Anderson, 2002). In our view, the important conditions of running speech are the concepts of intonation, rhythm, and coarticulation. The first two concepts refer to the prosodic system or suprasegmentals (e.g., Ling, 1976, 1989, 2001, 2002; Shames & Anderson, 2002).

Intonation refers to the rise and fall of pitch (perception of frequency) during the production of speech (e.g., Ling, 1976, 1989, 2001, 2002; Plack, 2005; Shames & Anderson, 2002). As such, we can state that intonation represents the various patterns of fundamental frequency produced over a specific period of time during running speech. This speech quality is the result of voiced speech sounds such as vowels and the vowel-like consonants.

Rhythm refers to the timing patterns of speech (e.g., Ling, 1976, 1989, 2001, 2002; Plack, 2005; Shames & Anderson, 2002). That is, it exemplifies the duration of specific sounds, including syllables (e.g., **base**ball, **fi**re). Rhythm is also concerned with the periods of time between stressed sounds and syllables. The duration of the pauses between words also contributes to the rhythm of connected speech.

One of the most important concepts of connected speech is coarticulation. With respect to coarticulation, the production of sounds in a word is influenced by the characteristics of the speech mechanisms needed to produce preceding or following sounds in the word (e.g., Ling, 1976, 1989, 2001, 2002; Shames & Anderson, 2002). Boothroyd (1986) provided an excellent example. In the word *team*, the velum is raised so that the /t/ sound and the /i/ (for *ea*) sound are produced through the oral cavity. In producing the /i/ sound, the velum may be lowered (oral cavity is open) in anticipation of the next sound, /m/, which is nasal. Thus, we coarticulate the two sounds, /i/ and /m/.

Coarticulation may involve the combinations of several sounds, as in the production of diphthongs. Coarticulation is also present with stop-plosives and glides. In one sense, coarticulation presents challenges for teaching the production of words, especially since this is quite different from pronouncing sounds in isolation (e.g., Ling, 1976, 1989, 2001, 2002; Shames & Anderson, 2002).

Research on Speech Development and Deafness

Most students with a hearing loss up to the severe level and a few with a severe-to-profound loss can develop spoken communication via audition with amplification or assistive devices (e.g., Geers, 2006; Ling, 1976, 1989, 2001, 2002; Nicholas & Geers, 2006; Shames & Anderson, 2002; see also the varying perspectives in Spencer & Marschark, 2006). Students in the severe-to-profound range (see Table 1-1 in Chapter 1) may need alternative methods for speech perception and production. These alternative methods may include cued speech/language (Chapter 7), visual phonics (Chapter 7), the use of vision (speechreading; Chapter 8), or touch.

The perception and production of speech do not require the ability to *hear* all speech sounds. Nevertheless, there seems to be a threshold level, or, rather, it seems to be critical to be able to receive (or perceive) a substantial portion of the sounds (e.g., Boothroyd, 1984; Levitt, 1989; Ling, 1976, 1989, 2001, 2002; Shames & Anderson, 2002). The nature of the threshold is still not clear; most likely, it varies from individual to individual.

The speech errors of students who are d/Deaf or hard of hearing are connected to the nature of their impaired perception. In other words, the errors reflect the quality of the speech signal that students receive either through audition or speechreading (Chapter 8), or both. Although several factors can be listed to account for speech errors (e.g., motivation, parental background, social interaction skills, etc.), the predominant factor appears to be degree of hearing impairment.

The greater the hearing loss, generally the less intelligible the speech. Consequently, the greater the hearing loss the more difficult it is for speech to be developed (e.g., Boothroyd, 1984; Levitt, 1989; Ling, 1976, 1989, 2001, 2002; see also the varying perspectives in Spencer & Marschark, 2006). For example, students with a mild hearing loss might have difficulty hearing sibilants such as /f/ and /s/ or stop-plosives such as /p/ without amplification. Those with a severe hearing loss might not perceive voiceless consonants and most of the voiced consonants. These students might also have difficulty with a few vowels. Individuals with a profound hearing loss might perceive only a few low-frequency vowels or nasals, even with the use of amplification systems. These instances are essentially related to the configurations of the students' hearing losses (on the audiogram, as discussed in Chapter 3). In any case, there is little doubt that difficulty with perception contributes immensely to difficulties in production, because these two components are said to be "mirror images."

Wide differences exist among students who are d/Deaf or hard of hearing with respect to the perception and production of speech (e.g., Boothroyd, 1984; Levitt, 1989; Ling, 1976, 1989, 2001, 2002). This issue contributes to the frustration of parents and educators. It is possible to describe the general speech errors, particularly patterns within the segmental (consonants and vowels) and suprasegmental (intonation, rhythm, pauses, etc.) categories.

Quite some time ago, Levitt (1989) cautioned us about the exceptions. His comments are still relevant today (see review in Spencer & Marschark, 2006; see also Boothroyd, 1984; Ling, 1976, 1989, 2001, 2002):

> Exceptions occur at either end of the intelligibility scale; that is, children with very good speech intelligibility (close to 100%) make insufficient errors for a pattern to be discernible and children with very poor speech (intelligibility close to zero) often have gross idiosyncratic errors, many of which are not easily defined in conventional phonetic terms. (p. 30)

Recently, it has become clear that some of these types of "exceptions" may be related to disorders of the auditory system that are not reflected by the information on the audiogram. An example of this is in children who have auditory neuropathy, a hearing disorder characterized by abnormal auditory brainstem results in the presence of cochlear functioning. In general, these children have speech intelligibility that is much poorer than would be predicted by their audiogram (Madden, Rutter, Hilbert, Greinwald, & Choo, 2002).

In the following sections, we discuss speech errors with respect to segmental and suprasegmental categories. Note that these are general patterns or guidelines, not fixed entities. We think that these patterns are robust enough so that instructors can develop adequate speech instructional programs (e.g., Boothroyd, 1984; Levitt, 1989; Ling, 1976, 1989, 2001, 2002).

SUPRASEGMENTAL ERRORS

The importance of the suprasegmental aspects of speech is often forgotten or underestimated. In fact, as mentioned previously, suprasegmental aspects contribute to the development of phonology, which is related to the acquisition of beginning reading skills via phonemic awareness and phonics (e.g., see discussions in Paul, 2009; Trezek et al., 2010; see also Chapter 7). Errors of students who are d/Deaf or hard of hearing have been documented in areas such as respiration, rate, rhythm, stress, pattern, and duration (Erber, 1982; Levitt, 1989; Ling, 1976, 1989, 2001, 2002).

Typically, students with severe-to-profound hearing loss exhibit an excessive prolongation of vowels and other continuant sounds. In addition, they might struggle with the use of inappropriate (prolongation and improperly inserted) pauses in connected speech. Students might also have difficulty with the production of syllables due to their inappropriate utterance rates and their difficulty in producing stressed versus unstressed syllables. Students might also group the syllables improperly.

Other glaring suprasegmental problems include those that affect the pitch and quality of voice (e.g., Boothroyd, 1984; Levitt, 1989; Ling, 1976, 1989, 2001, 2002). It is not unusual to encounter issues of breathiness—either too much or too little—nasality (mostly too little), and inappropriate variations and pauses in pitch. These problems have led educators to label the voice quality of many students with severe-to-profound hearing loss as *breathy* or *tense*. One hypothesis is that the students are struggling with the position and use of the vocal folds during the production of speech. Obviously, without an adequate articulatory–auditory feedback loop, it is difficult for these students to maintain control of their speech mechanisms.

It is easy to see that the problems just described can and do affect the ability of listeners to understand the speech of children who are d/Deaf or hard of hearing. Intonation becomes an issue due to the excessive prolongation of speech sounds and the improper control of voice pitch (e.g., Boothroyd, 1984; Levitt, 1989; Ling, 1976, 1989, 2001, 2002). Other errors result from inadequate breath control and inadequate use of the speech mechanisms. Students seem to have difficulty coordinating their speech articulators and their breathing system.

Ling (1976, 1989, 2001, 2002) has argued vehemently that students need to be taught how to use their speech mechanisms and to coordinate them with the breathing system. However, despite Ling's dictum, these problems seem to persist even after long periods of instruction. In fact, a case can be made that the more successful students might be those who are able to take advantage of their residual hearing through the use of amplification devices such as hearing aids and cochlear implants (e.g., Christiansen & Leigh, 2002; Geers, 2006; Nicholas & Geers, 2006). We shall have more to say about the use of residual hearing with respect to technology and amplification later.

SEGMENTAL ERRORS

It is possible to delineate patterns of segmental errors for students with severe-to-profound hearing loss. For example, the vowel productions of many of these students exhibit insufficient intensity and are often accompanied by excessive aspiration and nasality (e.g., Boothroyd, 1984; Levitt, 1989; Ling, 1976, 1989, 2001, 2002). The common vowel errors that have been categorized entail substitutions, diphthongization, and nasalization. Students might substitute lax vowels for tense vowels (e.g., /I/ or /i/ as in h*i*t and h*ea*t) or even tense vowels for lax vowels. Substitutions of central vowels have been documented (e.g., b*e*t to b*u*t). Students have enormous difficulty producing diphthongs.

Given what we know about vowels, it is permissible to argue that students' difficulty with vowels is related to the difficulty of placing, positioning, or moving their tongues appropriately (e.g., Boothroyd, 1984; Levitt, 1989; Ling, 1976, 1989, 2001, 2002). Interestingly, there seems to be a restricted range of tongue movement that influences the quality and intelligibility of adjacent (to vowels) consonants. If there are vowel errors, they are most likely going to be consonant errors. Thus, educators and therapists need to recognize that adequate vowel production is almost essential for the improvement of the intelligibility of the speech of students with severe-to-profound hearing loss (e.g., Boothroyd, 1984; Levitt, 1989; Ling, 1976, 1989, 2001, 2002).

The most common consonant errors are omissions (e.g., Boothroyd, 1984; Levitt, 1989; Ling, 1976, 2001). Students are likely to omit consonants that are produced near the center or back of the mouth (e.g., /t/, /l/, /k/, /g/) rather than those near the front of the mouth (e.g., /p/, /b/, /f/, /v/, /m/), which can be speechread (see Chapter 8). In addition, consonants that occur in the middle or final position of a word are more likely to be omitted than are those that occur in the beginning positions of words.

Other types of omission errors include verb endings (e.g., -*s*, -*ing*) and unstressed syllables. In fact, it is possible to argue that omissions may include a large number of inflectional and derivational affixes (see previous discussion in the section on morphology). It can also be argued that a number of these errors are due to an inadequate development of language in general (e.g., see discussion in Paul, 2009). However, it is also possible that several or many of these errors are due to perceptual deficiencies. Essentially, the reason for errors involving unstressed affixes and prepositions is because, historically, these sounds are simply difficult to see (speechread) or hear, as noted by Stelmachowicz (2005).

Another pattern of errors that has been documented is substitution (e.g., Boothroyd, 1984; Levitt, 1989; Ling, 1976, 1989, 2001, 2002). It is hard to believe, but students will substitute consonants for vowels and vice versa. In general, the substitutions entail the same place of articulation. For example, students may experience difficulty differentiating voice (/b/) from voiceless (/p/) consonants produced at the same articulatory location. Errors also occur in the manner of production involving high-frequency consonants (e.g., /s/), blends (e.g., /bl/), and clusters (e.g., /str/).

Because students have poor velar (soft palate) control, they tend to produce nasal errors; that is, they often have difficulty differentiating the nasals (/m/, /n/, /ng/) from their voiced counterparts or stops (/b/, /d/, /g/) involving the same place of articulation. Students have problems producing intelligible consonant clusters that involve the use of nasals (e.g., /nd/, /mp/).

There are more patterns of errors. For example, and not surprisingly, students struggle with fricatives and affricates. They will substitute stop consonants for fricatives, especially at the same place of articulation. This becomes a recurring pattern for almost all groups of sounds. Substitutions are often made with sounds that occur at the same place of articulation or that involve the same manner of articulation (e.g., Boothroyd, 1984; Levitt, 1989; Ling, 1976, 1989, 2001, 2002). Note that fricatives are substituted for stops less frequently and that affricates are rarely substituted for other consonants. Affricates, however, are typically substituted for other affricates. In general, similar to suprasegmental errors, the segmental errors are also due to poor control of the speech mechanisms and problems with rhythm or timing.

Levitt (1989) has postulated that lack of effort may be the most common source of error. Obviously, if students perceive that they have enormous difficulty being understood, they might resort to lackadaisical endeavors or just give up. Motivation becomes a major issue in addressing the speech errors of students with severe-to-profound hearing loss. Although this is beyond the scope of this chapter, motivation is certainly impacted by the notion of success. However, informing the students that they are successful (falsely) or overpraising their efforts may also be counterproductive. It is also important for professionals to remain professionals—namely, to keep facial expressions to a minimum when students have produced sounds erroneously. The first author has had firsthand experiences of such behaviors.

The last issue—and a controversial one—is the relationship between signing and the development of speech. The first author has argued previously (Paul & Quigley, 1990) that it is not clear whether the use of a signed system or a sign language has any direct causative effects, either negative or positive, on the development of spoken English. More recently, ample documentation has shown that signed communication is not detrimental to the development of speech skills (e.g., Marschark, 2007; Moores, 2001).

In our view, the issue becomes one of motivation and effort. If students substitute signs for speech or do not make the effort to improve their speech due to the ease of signing, then we are bound to see adverse effects. Nevertheless, these are speculations, because there is no strong empirical evidence for our assertions.

Amplification and Assistive Technology

With respect to the use of residual hearing, we can assert that there has been tremendous progress, considering the explosion of new amplification technologies, as discussed in Chapters 4 and 5. This explosion has positively impacted our current understanding of the development of both segmentals and suprasegmentals in children who are d/Deaf or hard of hearing.

The newer technology options have provided better access to auditory information and have contributed to success in both speech perception and production. In the past, the hearing aid, for example, could not provide much amplification in the higher frequencies. Thus, many of the consonant sounds were difficult to perceive and produce since perception shapes the ability to produce the sounds. Current hearing aid technology has the ability to transpose frequencies so that some of the higher-frequency consonant sounds are audible to the individual with the hearing loss.

This is critical, because even something as simple as being able to detect and perceive the /s/ sound has potentially huge benefits in speech production and perception. Stelmachowicz, Pittman, Hoover, Lewis, and Moeller (2004) pointed out that it is important to recall that the /s/ sound, as one of the most commonly occurring phonemes in the English language, provides information about many linguistic cues, including plurality of nouns, possession, past versus present tense, possessive pronouns, and contractions. It is easy to see how this issue of not perceiving a particular speech sound impacts the acquisition of language concepts. However, this situation is related both to the degree of hearing loss and the bandwidth of the hearing aid response. This means that the frequency response of the earlier hearing aids was limited, which affected the perception of /s/, particularly for women's and children's voices.

Stelmachowicz (2005) suggested also that cochlear implants have impacted the perception of high-frequency sounds, because, theoretically, they have no bandwidth restrictions. Stelmachowicz supported this assertion with the statistic that children with cochlear implants have a 15 to 18% higher production accuracy of /s/ and /z/ sounds when compared with hearing aid users.

Given this information, we should inquire about the success of "oral" programs in developing speech and language skills in children who are d/Deaf or hard of hearing. In addition, we should delve further into the benefits of cochlear implants on these areas, which were mentioned in Chapter 5. In the ensuing sections, we present brief salient highlights of these lines of research. Readers are referred to other sources for more in-depth information (e.g., Marschark, 2007; Moores, 2001; Paul, 2009; Spencer & Marschark, 2006).

RESEARCH ON ORALISM

Historically, it has been difficult to offer general findings or recommendations for effective oral methods in the development of speech and language skills for children who are d/Deaf or hard of hearing. This is also the case for assessing the effectiveness of specific approaches to remedying speech problems once patterns of errors have been discovered (e.g., see discussions in Beattie, 2006; Paul, 2009). Many programs have been recommended in the past with general descriptions of their methods. However, little evidence supported the overall effectiveness of the programs.

A number of sources have provided suggestions for the teaching of speech and language, both with and without amplification (e.g., Erber, 1982; Ling, 1976, 2001, 2002). This does not mean that these sources are without merit; however, there is a clear need for more systematic, scientific research, particularly for parents or professionals who are looking for a "cookbook" of how to develop hearing and speech skills. In recent years, programs (such as the Central Institute for the Deaf) have attempted to incorporate more systematic research to evaluate their methods for developing speech perception and production in children with hearing loss.

COCHLEAR IMPLANTS

In Chapters 4 and 5, we provided basic information and discussed some of the research results associated with the use of hearing aids and cochlear implants. It has become clear that assistive devices are instrumental, almost mandatory, in developing speech, hearing, and language skills in children who are d/Deaf or hard of hearing (e.g., Geers, 2006; Nicholas & Geers, 2006). In this section, we offer a few additional highlights on the merits of cochlear implants because there seems to be an increase in research in this area.

The benefits of cochlear implants have been documented in several publications (e.g., Christiansen & Leigh, 2002; Geers & Moog, 1994; Nevins & Chute, 1996; see also the varying perspectives in Spencer & Marschark, 2006, and Chapter 5 of this text). Researchers have attempted several types of comparisons. For example, children with cochlear implants have been compared to children with typical hearing, to children with hearing aids, and to children with no amplification devices. The specific variables explored were speech production, speech perception, English language and literacy skills involving vocabulary knowledge, working memory (see Chapter 7), suprasegmentals (the discussion in this chapter), and comprehension (e.g., Burkholder & Pisoni, 2006; Fagan, Pisoni, Horn, & Dillon, 2007; Geers, 2006; James, Rajput, Brinton, & Goswami, 2008; Marschark, Rhoten, & Fabich, 2007; Most & Peled, 2007; Vermeulen, van Bon, Schreuder, Knoors, & Snik, 2007).

Interesting and significant findings have been reported, especially with the development of the multichannel cochlear implantations (see Chapter 5; see also Miyamoto, Svirsky, & Robbins, 1997; Tye-Murray, Spencer, & Woodworth, 1995; Tyler, Fryauf-Bertschy, Gantz, Kelsay, & Woodworth, 1997). These positive findings do not mean that the cochlear implant is an all-encompassing factor; however, the implant does seem to assist with the development of speech, language, and literacy. Nevertheless, it should be clear that there is much more to consider in the development of language and literacy than just the ability to hear the speech signal. The benefits are not due *solely* to the use of cochlear implants, or any other assistive device for that matter.

Despite the positive trends documented in the various research studies, the findings need to be interpreted with some caution. The main reason for this assertion is that there seems to be variability of results across children due to lack of control (or no data available) on several important factors such as age at onset of the hearing impairment, etiology of the hearing impairment, age at implementation of the implant, the quality of the management program, mode of communication of the children, consistency in the use of the device, and even attitudes of the users or parents. This calls for the establishment of more rigorous scientific investigations so that we can obtain a clearer picture of the benefits of cochlear implantations with respect to the development of speech, language, and literacy.

Finally, even with an improvement in research, it should be highlighted that it is extremely difficult to impact the oral language development of d/Deaf children with implants. More often than not, the performance of these children is not always commensurate to that of their peers with typical hearing. In our view, the future is still looking bright for the continued development of and benefits associated with assistive devices, especially cochlear implants. Nevertheless, it is still necessary to combine the use of the assistive device with effective speech, language, and literacy methods (e.g., see discussion in Paul, 2009).

Summary of Major Points

Our goal in this chapter was to discuss the interrelations among hearing, speech, and language development. In addition, we provided some basic information on language and language development, the speech mechanisms, and research on the speech development and patterns of children who are d/Deaf or hard of hearing. We hope that we were able to answer or partially answer most of your questions that you created at the beginning of the chapter. If not, we encourage you to read some of the references cited and/or to dialogue with your instructor and classmates.

The overall intent of this chapter was to provide a brief introduction to the *Key Concepts*, as follows:

■ The nature and stages of language development

■ The nature of the speech process

■ Research on speech development and deafness

■ Amplification and assistive technology

With respect to the nature and stages of language development, we remarked that

■ Descriptions of language development vary according to individuals in fields such as linguistics, anthropology, speech and hearing science, psychology, and deaf education.

■ Some individuals ascribe to a behavior-environmental description, some to a cognitive description, and some to a social description, as well as combinations of these three broad domains.

■ Phonology is concerned with the rules that govern the production, structure, sequence, and distribution of articulatory elements, either sounds, as in speech, or hand movements as in signing, of a language.

■ Phonology represents the building blocks of a language.

■ Morphology is concerned with the structure of words, and it is typically influenced by both phonology and syntax.

■ Morphemes can be described as the smallest segment of speech (or articulatory element) that possesses meaning.

■ Morphology in conjunction with phonology assists with the acquisition of conventional spellings of words and, possibly, to the understanding of orthography.

■ For some linguists, syntax is the most basic component of a language such that (1) it is essential for comprehension and (2) it reflects the structure of the mind.

■ Syntax is concerned with rules that govern the order or arrangement of words.

- The two levels of syntax discussed are linear and hierarchical structures.

- Semantics is the study of meaning *in* language.

- The concept of meaning is not only difficult to define, but it is also difficult to measure.

- Pragmatics involves the use of language within a social communicative or interactional situation or context.

- The two major stages of language development are prelinguistic and linguistic.

- During the first year, the infant develops the precursors for all language components and proceeds into the one-word stage. The production of the first words marks the beginning of the linguistic period.

- Most children internalize much of the grammar of the language by the age of 4 or 5 years and master nearly all of the grammar by age 9 or 10.

With respect to the nature of the speech process, it was stated that

- To produce speech, we have the efforts of—in one model—three broad areas—the respiratory system, the laryngeal system, and the articulatory system.

- The respiratory system entails structures such as lungs, trachea, and the bronchial tubes. The laryngeal system involves the larynx—including the vocal folds and the glottis. Finally, the articulatory system involves all the cavities—pharyngeal (throat area), oral (mouth area), and nasal (nose area).

- In the production of speech, air flows from the respiratory system through the cavities and the articulators. This flow of air is actually obstructed or constricted along the way through the laryngeal and articulatory systems, depending on the *sound* that we intend to produce.

- Before the sound leaves the lips, it is modified or enhanced by the resonant qualities of oral and nasal cavities in the pharyngeal system.

- The major categories of sources of sound are voicing, frication, and stop-plosion.

- Voicing occurs in the larynx, particularly via the vibrations or actions of the vocal folds or chords (i.e., two muscular flaps).

- When a random turbulence of air is forced through a narrow opening, we have the phenomenon known as frication. This constriction of airflow can occur anywhere along the vocal tract and can be caused by any of the speech mechanisms.

- When the airflow is stopped completely and then released quickly (from the build-up of air pressure), this sound source is labeled stop-plosion.

- The constriction and obstruction of airflow along the vocal tract is mainly responsible for the production of consonants.

- Several features of articulation differentiate the consonants: place, manner, position, and the absence or presence of voicing.

- In general, the differentiation of the vowels is determined predominantly by the placement of the tongue in the mouth. The lips and pharyngeal cavity also play critical roles in the production of vowels.

- Vowels can also be classified according to the qualities of tenseness and laxness.

- To completely understand the production of sounds, it is important to discuss the conditions of connected speech production, or what is often called *running speech*.

- The important conditions of running speech are the concepts of intonation, rhythm, and coarticulation.

Research on speech development and deafness reveals that

- Most students with hearing impairment up to the severe level and some with severe-to-profound impairment can develop spoken communication via audition with amplification or assistive devices.

- Students in the severe-to-profound range often need alternative methods for speech perception and production. These alternative methods may include cued speech/language, visual phonics, or the use of vision (speechreading), and touch.

- The perception and production of speech do not require the ability to hear all speech sounds. Nevertheless, there seems to be a threshold level, or rather, it seems to be critical to be able to receive (or perceive) a substantial portion of the sounds.

- It appears that the speech errors of students who are d/Deaf or hard of hearing are connected to the nature of their impaired perception. In other words, the errors reflect the quality of the speech signal that students receive either through audition or speechreading, or both.

- Although several factors can be listed to account for speech errors (e.g., motivation, parental background, social interaction skills, etc.), the predominant factor appears to be the degree of hearing impairment.

- There are wide individual differences among students who are d/Deaf or hard of hearing with respect to the perception and production of speech. Nevertheless, it is possible to describe the general speech errors, particularly patterns within the segmental (consonants and vowels) and suprasegmental (intonation, rhythm, pauses, etc.) categories.

- Errors of students who are d/Deaf or hard of hearing have been documented in areas such as respiration, rate, rhythm, stress, pattern, and duration; that is, suprasegmental errors.

- It is possible to delineate patterns of segmental errors for students with severe-to-profound hearing impairment. For example, the vowel productions of many of these students exhibit insufficient intensity and are often accompanied by excessive aspiration and nasality.

- The common vowel errors that have been categorized entail substitutions, diphthongization, and nasalization.

- Ample documentation demonstrates that signed communication is not detrimental to the development of speech skills.

In considering amplification and assistive technology, we remarked that

- It has been difficult to offer general findings or recommendations for effective oral methods in the development of speech and language skills for children who are d/Deaf or hard of hearing. This is also the case for assessing the effectiveness of specific approaches to remedying speech problems once patterns of errors have been discovered.

- Issues have arisen with the descriptions of programs and the design of rigorous scientific research experiments.

- It has become clear that assistive devices are instrumental, almost mandatory, in developing speech, hearing, and language skills in children who are d/Deaf or hard of hearing.

- The benefits of cochlear implants have been well documented. The specific variables that have been explored include speech production, speech perception, English language and literacy skills involving vocabulary knowledge, working memory, suprasegmentals, and comprehension.

- Interesting and significant findings have been reported, especially with the development of the multichannel cochlear implantation, along with bimodal amplification and bilateral cochlear implantation. Positive findings do not mean that the cochlear implant is an all-encompassing factor; however, the implant does seem to assist with the development of speech, language, and literacy.

- Rigorous scientific investigations must be conducted so that we can obtain a clearer picture of the benefits of cochlear implantations.

- It is still necessary to combine the use of the assistive device with effective speech, language, and literacy methods.

By now, it is hoped that you can see the interrelations among speech, hearing, and language, especially for a phonemic-based language such as English. The journey continues in the next chapter as we discuss these interrelations with English literacy; that is, the development of reading and writing skills. We suspect that there will not be many surprises for you, concerning the relations between knowledge of the language of English and the ability to read and write in English. However, the acquisition of English literacy skills is an extremely complex phenomenon. In fact, we are betting that there will be a few surprises in store for you.

Chapter Questions

Note: Some answers to the questions can be found in the chapter; however, others have a variety of possible responses based on students' backgrounds and experiences.

1. This chapter briefly examined the five major components of a language. List and describe each component. Do the authors feel that one component is most important? Why or why not?

2. Provide a brief description of each of the following terms:

   a. Inflectional morphology

   b. Derivational morphology

   c. Phonemes

   d. Morphemes

3. List the prosodic features associated with the phonological system of a spoken language. Why are these features important?

4. This chapter examined two major types of syntactic relations: linear and hierarchical. Describe each category and provide two examples of each.

5. Discuss a few of the major developmental milestones for both the prelinguistic and linguistic periods of language development.

6. In this chapter, it was argued repeatedly that phonology is the building block of any language. What does this mean? Does it have implications for the development of a language, or even of literacy (reading and writing)?

7. What are the three major systems involved in the production of sounds? What provides the resonance for sounds?

8. List and briefly describe the three categories of sound source that are responsible for producing consonants and vowels.

9. Provide one example (using a word) for the following categories of consonants and vowels. The first example has been done for you.

   Consonant: stop-plosive: /b/ as in *baseball*.

   a. Nasal

   b. Affricate

   c. Fricative

   Vowel: high front: /i/ as in *meat*

   a. Low front

   b. High back

   c. Midfront

10. Describe briefly the following concepts of connected speech:

    a. Intonation

    b. Coarticulation

11. Describe a few (at least three) segmental and suprasegmental patterns of error of d/Deaf or hard of hearing children. Do we have sufficient research to recommend effective approaches for teaching speech? Why or why not?

12. How would you describe the current status of the research on cochlear implantation?

13. If you had an opportunity to converse with the authors, what burning questions would you ask them? Share and discuss these questions with your instructor and classmates.

Challenge Questions

Note: Complete answers are not in the text. Additional research/reading is required. In some cases, reading further or elsewhere in the text might provide some information to guide a response to a particular question.

1. In this chapter, it was argued that speech is not equal to language. What does this mean? What do you think is the relationship of speech to language? Is speech necessary for the development of language? Why or why not? Is this question the same as asking what the relationship of signs is to a sign language?

2. Now, what are your views on cochlear implants? Can you support your views with theoretical and/or research data? Is there a positive linear relationship between cochlear implants and achievement? Why or why not? Does this mean that cochlear implants are an all-encompassing factor? Why or why not? [Yes, we have asked this question previously!]

3. Do you think that advances in technology such as digital hearing aids or cochlear implants will eradicate the Deaf culture? Why or why not? Should this even be a consideration? What are the implications? [We promise not to ask this question again either! Now that you have read this far, your views might have evolved.]

Suggested Activities

1. Interview teachers and clinicians in your area. Ask these professionals to comment on the following questions:

    ■ Is speech or sign equal to language? Why or why not?

    ■ Did you take courses on language and language development as part of your educational preparation? Were these courses helpful to you in your career? Why or why not?

- Can you describe the speech errors of d/Deaf or hard of hearing children and adolescents? Do you work to improve the speech of these individuals? If yes, what do you do? If no, why not?

Share your findings with your instructor and the rest of your classmates.

2. Select a partner (or two!) from your class. With your partner, select a language component—phonology, morphology, syntax, semantics, or pragmatics—and conduct a review of the literature on this component. Discuss the research history and background and provide several examples of the component. Discuss the relation of the component to the development of speech and language. Discuss the developmental milestones with respect to children up to the age of 10. Share your findings on all above activities with your instructor and the rest of your classmates.

3. Select a classmate (or two) and perform the following tasks:

- Identify the phonemes in the following words: *cat, computer, football, hotdog, jam, iron,* and *December.*

- Identify the morphemes (bound or free) in the following words: *girls, remarkable, debrief, understand, walking, argument,* and *reconstruction.*

- Provide three examples (i.e., in sentences) each for the following syntactic structures: *determiners, wh- questions, passive voice (verbs),* and *relative clauses.*

Share your findings with your instructor and the rest of your classmates.

References

American Speech-Language-Hearing Association. (2009). What is language? What is speech? Available online: www.asha.org/public/speech/development/language_speech.htm. Accessed August 28, 2009.

Beattie, R. (2006). The oral methods and spoken language acquisition. In P. Spencer & M. Marschark (Eds.), *Advances in the spoken language development of deaf and hard of hearing children* (pp. 103–135). New York: Oxford University Press.

Boothroyd, A. (1984). Auditory perception of speech contrasts by subjects with sensorineural hearing loss. *Journal of Speech and Hearing Research, 27,* 134–144.

Boothroyd, A. (1986). *Speech acoustics and perception.* Austin, TX: Pro-Ed.

Burkholder, R., & Pisoni, D. (2006). Working memory capacity, verbal rehearsal speed, and scanning in deaf children with cochlear implants. In P. Spencer & M. Marschark (Eds.), *Advances in the spoken language development of deaf and hard of hearing children* (pp. 328–357). New York: Oxford University Press.

Carruthers, P., Laurence, S., & Stich, S. (Eds.). (2005). *The innate mind: Structure and contents.* New York: Oxford University Press.

Carruthers, P., Laurence, S., & Stich, S. (Eds.). (2006). *The innate mind: Volume 2: Culture and cognition.* New York: Oxford University Press.

Chomsky, N. (2006). *Language and mind* (3rd ed.). New York: Cambridge University Press.

Christiansen, J., & Leigh, I. (2002). *Cochlear implants in children: Ethics and choices.* Washington, DC: Gallaudet University Press.

Creaghead, N., & Newman, P. (1985). Articulatory phonetics and phonology. In P. Newman, N. Creaghead, & W. Secord (Eds.), *Assessment and remediation of articulatory and phonological disorders* (pp. 13–39). Columbus, OH: Merrill.

Crystal, D. (1995). *The Cambridge encyclopedia of the English language.* New York: Cambridge University Press.

Crystal, D. (1997). *The Cambridge encyclopedia of language* (2nd ed.). New York: Cambridge University Press.

Crystal, D. (2006). *How language works.* London, England: Penguin Books.

Erber, N. (1982). *Auditory training.* Washington, DC: Alexander Graham Bell Association for the Deaf.

Fagan, M., Pisoni, D., Horn, D., & Dillon, C. (2007). Neuropsychological correlates of vocabulary, reading, and working memory in deaf children with cochlear implants. *Journal of Deaf Studies and Deaf Education, 12*(4), 461–471.

Fodor, J. (1983). *The modularity of mind: An essay on faculty psychology.* Boston: MIT Press.

Geers, A. (2006). Spoken language in children with cochlear implants. In P. Spencer & M. Marschark (Eds.), *Advances in the spoken language development of deaf and hard of hearing children* (pp. 244–270). New York: Oxford University Press.

Geers, A., & Moog, J. (1994). Effectiveness of cochlear implants and tactile aids for deaf children: The sensory aids study at Central Institute for the Deaf. *Volta Review, 96*(5).

Gerken, L., Jusczyk, P., & Mandel, D. (1994). When prosody fails to cue syntactic structure: 9-months-olds' sensitivity to phonological versus syntactic phrases. *Cognition, 51*(3), 237–265.

Goodluck, H. (1991). *Language acquisition: A linguistic introduction.* Cambridge, MA: Blackwell.

Heimlich, J., & Pittelman, S. (1986). *Semantic mapping: Classroom applications.* Newark, DE: International Reading Association.

Hiebert, E., & Kamil, M. (2005). *Teaching and learning vocabulary: Bringing research to practice.* Mahwah, NJ: Erlbaum.

James, D., Rajput, K., Brinton, J., & Goswami, U. (2008). Phonological awareness, vocabulary, and word reading in children who use cochlear implants: Does age of implantation explain individual variability in performance outcomes and growth? *Journal of Deaf Studies and Deaf Education, 13*(1), 117–137.

Just, M. A., & Carpenter, P. A. (1987). *The psychology of reading and language comprehension.* Boston: Allyn & Bacon.

Levitt, H. (1989). Speech and hearing in communication. In M. Wang, H. Reynolds, and H. Walberg (Eds.), *The handbook of special education: Research and practice* (Vol. 3) (23–45). Oxford, England: Pergamon.

Ling, D. (1976). *Speech and the hearing-impaired child: Theory and practice.* Washington, DC: Alexander Graham Bell Association for the Deaf.

Ling, D. (1989). *Aural habilitation: The foundation of verbal learning in hearing-impaired children* (2nd ed.). Washington, DC: Alexander Graham Bell Association for the Deaf.

Ling, D. (2001). Speech development for children who are hearing impaired. In R. Hull (Ed.), *Aural rehabilitation: Serving children and adults* (4th ed., pp. 145–165). San Diego: Singular/Thomson Learning.

Ling, D. (2002). *Speech and the hearing-impaired child: Theory and practice* (2nd ed.). Washington, DC: Alexander Graham Bell Association for the Deaf.

Lund, N. (2003). *Language and thought.* New York: Routledge.

Lyons, J. (1995). *Linguistic semantics: An introduction.* New York: Cambridge University Press.

Madden, C., Rutter, M., Hilbert, L., Greinwald, J. H., & Choo, D. I. (2002). Clinical and audiologic features in auditory neuropathy. *Archives of Otolaryngology—Head & Neck Surgery, 128*(9), 1026–1030.

Marschark, M. (2007). *Raising and educating a deaf child: A comprehensive guide to the choices, controversies, and decisions faced by parents and educators* (2nd ed.). New York: Oxford University Press.

Marschark, M., Rhoten, C., & Fabich, M. (2007). Effects of cochlear implants on children's reading and academic achievement. *Journal of Deaf Studies and Deaf Education, 12*(3), 269–282.

Matthews, P. (1991). *Morphology* (2nd ed.). Boston, MA: Cambridge University Press.

Miyamoto, R., Svirsky, M., & Robbins, A. (1997). Enhancement of expressive language in prelingually deaf children with cochlear implants. *Acta Oto-Laryngologica, 117*(2), 154–157.

Moores, D. (2001). *Educating the deaf: Psychology, principles, and practices* (5th ed.). Boston: Houghton-Mifflin.

Most, T., & Peled, M. (2007). Perception of suprasegmental features of speech by children with cochlear implants and children with hearing aids. *Journal of Deaf Studies and Deaf Education, 12*(3), 350–361.

Nagy, W. (2005). Why vocabulary instruction needs to be long-term and comprehensive. In E. Hiebert & M. Kamil (Eds.), *Teaching and learning vocabulary: Bringing research to practice* (pp. 27–44). Mahwah, NJ: Erlbaum.

National Reading Panel. (2000). *Report of the National Reading Panel: Teaching children to read—An evidence-based assessment of the scientific research literature on reading and its implications for reading instruction.* Jessup, MD: National Institute for Literacy at EDPubs.

Nevins, M., & Chute, P. (1996). *Children with cochlear implants in educational settings.* San Diego: Singular.

Nicholas, J., & Geers, A. (2006). The process and early outcomes of cochlear implantation of three years of age. In P. Spencer & M. Marschark (Eds.), *Advances in the spoken language development of deaf and hard of hearing children* (pp. 271–297). New York: Oxford University Press.

Ninio, A., & Snow, C. (1996). *Pragmatic development.* Boulder, CO: Westview.

O'Grady, W. (2005). *How children learn language.* New York: Cambridge University Press.

Owens, R. (1996). *Language development: An introduction* (4th ed.). Boston: Allyn & Bacon.

Owens, R. (2004). *Language disorders: A functional approach to assessment and intervention* (4th ed.). Boston: Pearson Education.

Paul, P. (2009). *Language and deafness* (4th ed.). Sudbury, MA: Jones & Bartlett.

Paul, P., & Quigley, S. (1990). *Education and deafness.* White Plains, NY: Longman.

Pearson, P. D., & Johnson, D. (1978). *Teaching reading comprehension.* New York: Holt, Rinehart, & Winston.

Pence, K., & Justice, L. (2008). *Language development from theory to practice.* Upper Saddle River, NJ: Pearson/Merrill Prentice Hall.

Pinker, S. (1994). *The language instinct: How the mind creates language.* New York: William Morrow & Company.

Plack, C. (2005). *The sense of hearing.* Mahwah, NJ: Erlbaum.

Shames, G., & Anderson, N. (2002). *Human communication disorders: An introduction* (6th ed.). Boston: Allyn & Bacon.

Shelton, R., & Wood, C. (1978). Speech mechanisms and production. In P. Skinner and R. Shelton (Eds.), *Speech, language, and hearing: Normal processes and disorders* (pp. 54–77). Reading, MA: Addison-Wesley.

Spencer, P., & Marschark, M. (Eds.). (2006). *Advances in the spoken language development of deaf and hard of hearing children*. New York: Oxford University Press.

Stahl, S., & Nagy, W. (2006). *Teaching word meanings*. Mahwah, NJ: Erlbaum.

Stelmachowicz, P. G. (2005). Optimizing amplification for infants and young children. *Proceedings of the 2nd European Pediatric Conference: Sounds for a new generation*. Amsterdam, The Netherlands, October 24–25.

Stelmachowicz, P. G., Pittman, A. L., Hoover, B. M., Lewis, D. E., & Moeller, M. P. (2004). The importance of high-frequency audibility in the speech and language development of children with hearing loss. *Archives of Otolaryngology Head and Neck Surgery, 130*(5), 556–562.

Thompson, M., Biro, P., Vethivelu, S., Pious, C., & Hatfield, N. (1987). *Language assessment of hearing-impaired school age children*. Seattle, WA: University of Washington Press.

Trezek, B. J., Wang, Y., & Paul, P. (2010). *Reading and deafness: Theory, research, and practice*. Clifton Park, NY: Delmar/Cengage Learning.

Tye-Murray, N., Spencer, L., & Woodworth, G. (1995). Acquisition of speech by children who have prolonged cochlear implant experience. *Journal of Speech and Hearing Research, 38*, 327–337.

Tyler, R., Fryauf-Bertschy, H., Gantz, B., Kelsay, D., & Woodworth, G. (1997). Speech perception in prelingually implanted children after four years. *Advances in Oto-Rhino-Laryngology, 52*, 187–192.

Vermeulen, A., van Bon, W., Schreuder, R., Knoors, H., & Snik, A. (2007). Reading comprehension of deaf children with cochlear implants. *Journal of Deaf Studies and Deaf Education, 12*(3), 283–302.

Zemlin, W. (1968). *Speech and hearing science: Anatomy and physiology*. Englewood Cliffs, NJ: Prentice-Hall.

Further Readings

Boothroyd, A. (1976). *The role of hearing in education of the deaf*. Northampton, MA: Clarke School for the Deaf.

Chomsky, N. (1975). *Reflections on language*. New York: Pantheon Books.

Cole, E. B., & Flexer, C. A. (2006). *Children with hearing loss: Developing listening and talking—birth to six*. San Diego: Plural.

Dodd, B., & Campbell, R. (Eds.). (1987). *Hearing by eye*. London, England: Erlbaum.

Flexer, C. (1999). *Facilitating hearing and listening in young children* (2nd ed.). San Diego: Plural.

Nittrouer, S. (2009). *Early development of children with hearing loss*. San Diego: Plural.

HEARING, LANGUAGE, AND LITERACY

Spoken language may be described from several viewpoints in terms of receptive and expressive components; sensory, cognitive, and motor components; or phonology, morphology, syntax, semantics, and pragmatics. It is obvious that hearing has a direct influence on the receptive and sensory components of spoken language processing and on the learning of the phonology (the sounds) of the language. . . . Hearing may have less influence on spoken language learning after the child has begun to read and write.

—Blamey (2003, p. 233)

. . . serious delays in core language functions like expressive vocabulary, syntax, and semantics put a child at high risk for difficulties with more advanced reading skills, like reading comprehension. This is due to a complex interaction of factors that, so far, have not been teased apart. Core language functions are a product of heredity, "shared environment," and "unshared environment," such as a school system. There is certainly compelling evidence implicating educational practice in this equation.

—McGuinness (2005, p. 12)

Key Concepts

After completing this chapter, readers should have a basic understanding of:

- The development of English literacy
- The reciprocal relations within and between language and literacy
- The interrelations among phonology, working memory, and reading

- The concept and implications of cued speech/language
- The concept and implications of visual phonics (see-the-sound)

Taken together, the two opening passages make a strong case for the interrelations among hearing, language, and literacy—especially with respect to the development of English. We are certain that this is not a "eureka" revelation for you or for professionals in our field. In fact, it might be deemed as axiomatic that this is the case.

One danger, of course, is overstating the position. We are not saying that one must *hear* in order to learn a spoken language; that is, to perceive the message or to speak the language. Other interesting avenues may be considered, for example, the effects of the English sign systems (not discussed here, but see Paul, 2009) and the effects of speechreading and auditory training/learning (discussed in Chapter 8 and mentioned in Blamey, 2003, as well). Nevertheless, the hearing process does contribute to the development of spoken English (e.g., Blamey, 2003; Northern & Downs, 2002; Plack, 2005).

We even agree somewhat with the statement by Blamey (2003) in the opening passage that hearing may play a lesser role in this development after a child learns to read and write. However, there is more to this complicated position. For starters, it depends on what is meant by *reading* and *writing*. To provide a preview of what is to come in this chapter, consider this: we doubt seriously that an individual will learn more about the English language if his or her reading or writing is narrow or limited and if he or she does not increase his or her understanding of major concepts associated with the majority culture of society (e.g., see Hirsch, 1987; Hirsch, Kett, & Trefil, 2002; Paul, 2009; Trezek, Wang, & Paul, 2010). And, we bet that there is an argument brewing about this controversial statement. We are also certain that there is enormous dissension regarding what Hirsch (e.g., 1987; Hirsch et al., 2002) has termed *cultural literacy*.

Another point that we are also *not* saying is this: one must hear in order to learn to read and write English. However, again, hearing does contribute or can contribute to the development of English literacy. As discussed later, it is not merely the act of hearing that is critical. In fact, it is the development of the articulatory (speaking)–auditory (hearing) loop that contributes immensely to this process, starting with the development of the spoken component of English, particularly the domain of phonology.

The real danger is *understating* the importance of knowing the language of English for the purposes of reading and writing English. We are not referring to the elements of speech; that is, articulation of speech sounds, voice, or fluency, as discussed in Chapter 6. In fact, intelligible speech is not really critical, albeit it does help (e.g., Adams, 1990; Paul, 2009; Snow, Burns, & Griffin, 1998).

To understand our points, you need to reread the passage by McGuinness (2005) and to think again about the concept of cultural literacy (e.g., Hirsch, 1987; Hirsch et al., 2002). To put it briefly, for now, much of the English literacy problems of d/Deaf or hard of hearing students can be attributed to their poor development of the language of English. This means the inadequate development of the components of English, such as morphology, syntax, semantics, pragmatics, and, especially, phonology.

The difficulties become compounded if students have inadequate prior or background knowledge about the topics of print or even about the culture of mainstream society (i.e., cultural literacy), which are often a part of the school content areas. We agree with McGuinness (2005) that the precise reasons for this phenomenon are not clear, but there seems to be little doubt that the overall assertions are accurate (e.g., see research reviews in Paul, 2009; Trezek et al., 2010). Finally, we should not forget the problem of general language and cognitive comprehension issues, which impede the development of metacognitive, inferencing, and even literate thought skills necessary for advanced reading and reflection (e.g., see McGuinness, 2005; Paul, 2009; Trezek et al., 2010).

This brings us back to the concept of hearing and the interrelations among hearing, language, and literacy. Now is the time for you to think of possible questions for which you want answers after completing this chapter. A sample might be the following:

- What is reading/writing? How does an individual develop these skills?

- Are there reciprocal relations within and between language and literacy?

- Why is phonology considered to be important for the development of English language and literacy skills? Is it possible to bypass the phonological component [Note: In fact, this is what many American Sign Language-English bilingual–bicultural programs attempt to do]?

- What is working memory? How is this related to phonology and reading?

- Are there alternatives to the development of English language and literacy if one cannot employ the function of hearing adequately? Specifically, what is cued speech/language? What is visual phonics? What is the research effectiveness of cued speech/language and visual phonics?

You might have other questions as you read along; however, we doubt that we will be able to answer all of your questions. We are certain, however, that you will think differently about the interrelations among hearing, language, and literacy after reading this chapter. In fact, we wonder, even if one can read or write well, whether audition or hearing might represent the most productive or feasible avenue for which a chunk of information, including clarifications of information, can be obtained. We are not denigrating the use of the English sign systems or even American Sign Language. In any case, much of the available information in our American society is in spoken or written English rendered via face-to-face or in print. In essence, we think that it is critical to *know* English as a first or second language. We shall begin with the development of English literacy skills.

English Literacy

In Chapter 6, we discussed, briefly, the development of a spoken language such as English from birth to maturity. The goal was to provide some background for understanding the speech development issues of d/Deaf or hard of hearing children. It is certainly possible (albeit a real challenge) to develop English via the use of a sign system or cued speech/language (e.g., see Paul, 2009; Trezek et al., 2010). However, one of the major difficulties is for children to develop a deep, intuitive understanding of phonology as part of their overall competence in English.

To state it again, phonology is the building blocks for accessing and developing other components of a phonemic language such as English. In addition, phonology is also a critical aspect of the beginning process of literacy and for the subsequent development of higher-level reading skills, including conventional spelling skills. Whether it is possible to develop phonology without *hearing* is debatable. The importance of phonology for literacy can be gleaned explicitly and implicitly from the subsequent paragraphs.

NATURE OF READING

Providing a definition or description of *reading* that would be widely accepted is an impossible—well, formidable—task. In fact, debates on this endeavor have been occurring for over 150 years (Bartine, 1989, 1992). At best, we can state that reading is a complex entity that involves language, cognitive, and affective factors. More interesting, if someone is said to be a good reader, we should ask: A good reader of what? Newspapers? Textbooks? Poetry? Novels? Is there such as thing as a good reader in general, or must this concept be restricted to a specific genre? These are not easy questions to answer.

One may be adept at reading fiction or other narrative materials, but not skilled in reading expository materials such as textbooks. In fact, during the pinnacle of the whole language movement many teachers seemed to have avoided using expository materials relevant to content areas or disciplines; that is, reading across the content areas. This may have contributed to weaknesses and problems for a generation of students (e.g., see discussions in Paul, 2008; Pearson, 2004).

Although no widely accepted theoretical model can account for the reading acquisition process, several models do exist (e.g., Adams, 1990; Carlisle & Rice, 2002; McGuinness, 2004; Snow et al., 1998). A simple rendition of some current models and descriptions is provided in **Table 7-1**.

Despite our best efforts—and some scholars just will not give up this pursuit—we have not discovered a single factor (i.e., a "magic bullet") that can account for the range of difficulties that impede the development of skilled readers. Nevertheless, scholars and researchers have expended an enormous amount of attention and energy on the area of phonological processing/awareness. This area can best be described as the ability to understand the sound structure of words (i.e., phonemes) and the relationships between the sounds (phonemes; consonants and vowels) and letters (graphemes).

In an opaque language such as English, a specific letter or letters may have several sounds (consider the letter *a* in words such as *rat, rate*) or a particular sound or sounds may be represented by several different letters (consider /c/, as in cake and cease). Now it is time for us to ask a few provoking questions: Is hearing—that is, the ability to hear—critical for awareness of these distinctions? How about the differences between the pronunciations of *resume* (to go again or a vita), *contract* (an agreement or to obtain something), and *the* (definite or indefinite)? What about the different pronunciations of the past tense of *d*, as in *rated* (sounds like a *d*), and *walked* (sounds like a *t*)? Does hearing contribute to a better understanding of the phonology of English? Does hearing contribute to the reading

Table 7-1	*Selected Points of Three Major Literacy Frameworks and Models Within the Cognitive Framework*

Cognitive Information-Processing Framework

- Reading and writing consist of similar underlying processes, including a number of subprocesses.

- Lower-level processes should become automatic and fluent so that readers/writers can concentrate on higher-level processes associated with the construction of meaning.

Naturalism Framework

- A heavy focus is placed on the individual; for example, it is the individual who must interpret the world and construct his or her own personal meaning via reading and writing activities.

- Strong emphasis is placed on child-centered or child-directed literacy activities. Formal or teacher-controlled instruction, especially of specific skills, is deemphasized or discouraged.

Social Constructivism Framework

- The promotion of the view that all knowledge, particularly human knowledge, is socially constructed.

- It is argued that language, cognition, and literacy are not entities unto themselves; rather, they are manifestations of social and cultural processes.

Broad Models Within the Cognitive Framework

Bottom-Up or Text-Based Models
- There is a great deal of emphasis on the recognition (identification) of letters and words.

- The process begins with the perception of letters and words on the page, proceeds through the analyses at several successive levels involving larger units such as phrases and sentences, and culminates with the construction of meaning at the top; that is, in the readers' minds.

- The models have demonstrated the importance of knowledge of the alphabetic system.

- The use of context clues in a deliberate manner actually plays a minor role in lexical access in highly literate readers.

(continues)

Table 7-1	*Selected Points of Three Major Literacy Frameworks and Models Within the Cognitive Framework (continued)*

Top-Down or Reader-Based Models

- The only purpose of reading is comprehension, and this should be emphasized from the beginning.

- Reading is said to begin with information that is in the readers' heads, not with what is on the printed page.

- In one top-down model, reading acquisition is similar to language acquisition.

- Models have shown that reading is a predictive process and that an adequate knowledge of the culture and, specifically, the language in which one is trying to read, are important.

Interactive Models

- These models emphasize the reader as an active information processor whose goal is to construct a model of what the text means.

- Comprehension is driven by preexisting concepts in the readers' heads as well as by the information from the text.

- The construction of meaning requires the development and coordination of both bottom-up and top-down skills and occurs at many different levels of analysis, such as lexical, syntactic, schematic, planning, and interpretative.

Source: Adapted from Bernhardt (1991) and Samuels & Kamil (1984). This table, with a few adaptations, is taken from Paul (2009, pp. 271–272).

process? Can you simply *memorize* all of these distinctions without hearing them? This is more complicated than what we have presented here. A sample of the complexity of the opaqueness of English is illustrated in **Table 7-2**.

Returning to the concept of phonology, it is clear that slow, inconsistent development in this area results in an incomplete, inaccurate understanding of the alphabetic system (sounds and their relations to letters). We do not mean to imply that phonological and phonemic awareness alone are sufficient for improving the plight of many struggling readers. In fact, it is possible to overstate the importance of phonology, especially if we proceed

Table
7-2

Examples of the Opaqueness of English

Sounds Operationalized as Different Letters

/i/ as in meet, meat, me, Fritos

/s/ as in see, cease, mess

/oo/ as in blue, blew, food

Letters Operationalized as Different Sounds

/r/ as in sir, farther, more

/c/ as in kite, cease

/y/ as in rye, toy, yo-yo

beyond the primary years of developing reading skills (e.g., Nation, 2005; Scarborough, 2005; Snowling, 2005).

As has been argued, to develop mature or proficient reading skills, teachers and clinicians need to devote attention to other language-based areas, such as fluency (reading quickly and accurately), vocabulary (meanings of words), and text comprehension (constructing meaning; making inferences, etc.) (e.g., Carlisle & Rice, 2002; McGuinness, 2004, 2005; National Reading Panel, 2000). In discussing the reading process, the focus should be balanced; that is, teachers and clinicians should emphasize the underpinnings and skills associated with both form (e.g., access to print skills or decoding) and meaning (e.g., comprehension and metacognitive skills) (e.g., Adams, 1990; Carlisle & Rice, 2002; Paul, 2003, 2009; Pearson, 2004).

In essence, all readers tend to oscillate between form and meaning, and this oscillation depends on readers' skills, experiences, and purposes. To obtain reading fluency—the point at which word identification becomes automatic and almost effortless and the point at which most energy and time can be spent on comprehending and interpreting the message—children need increased experiences with print as well as deeper and more extensive growth in language variables such as vocabulary and syntax. Children also need a broad, extensive familiarity of other variables and topics associated with their majority culture (cultural literacy, again!). This increase in knowledge and experiences supports their ability to identify and understand words and concepts and strengthens the reciprocal relations between word identification and reading comprehension (Adams, 1990; Catts & Kamhi, 2005; Chall, 1996; McGuinness, 2004, 2005; Snow et al., 1998).

EARLY LITERACY DEVELOPMENT

It is important to highlight a few of the points we have presented, and we shall do this in our discussion of the early stages of the development of reading in this section. In the emerging literacy stage, children interact with print and their caretakers (e.g., National Reading Panel, 2000; Snow et al., 1998; Sulzby & Teale, 1987, 2003). Eventually, children understand that print (i.e., orthography) is drastically different from pictures (e.g., Ehri, 1991; Snowling & Hulme, 2005). They figure out that words are composed of letters, which represent sounds. Even the ability to spell (particularly conventional spelling) requires some understanding of these relationships.

One important milestone is the understanding of the concept of a word. During the pre-school years, children begin the use of words in phrases and sentences and as entities whose sounds are arbitrarily related to their meanings (e.g., Adams, 1990, 1994; Crystal, 2006; McGuinness, 2004; Snow et al., 1998). Then, they make distinctions between words and determine their referents. They move on to grasping (intuitively or tacitly) the notions of various grammatical functions and forms, such as nouns, verbs, and adjectives, and function words, such as articles, conjunctions, and prepositions. This *metalinguistic* process continues until children can attend to and analyze the internal phonological structure of spoken words (or their representative equivalents).

As they move through childhood, children understand that certain kinds of intonations (e.g., inflection, stress, prosody) and wording are used with books and other written materials. Children who are read to frequently and enjoy such reading begin to recite selected words, phrases, or longer discourses. One of the most important processes is playing with sounds. Children play with the sounds of words (via repetitions, sound games, etc.), and this deepens their understanding and appreciation of the phonological component of English.

Eventually, children are able to engage in conversations with peers and adults, especially for sharing the contents of literate materials such as books and magazines. It cannot be overstated that these early experiences with sounds via the articulatory–auditory loop provide not only a strong foundation for the development of spoken English, but also a bridge to the development of English literacy skills.

Before leaving this section on reading, we think it is critical to reemphasize that reading involves both decoding (i.e., word identification) and comprehension (e.g., text comprehension, vocabulary, prior knowledge, metacognition). We also want to highlight the interesting close relationship between listening comprehension and text/print comprehension.

We have stressed the importance of phonology for developing decoding or word identification skills and, consequently, the facilitation of comprehension. Although this is the case, we do not want to overstate it. It might be instructive to relate a story about John Milton that has been presented in several scholarly works (e.g., see Nation, 2005). Milton, who became blind, was not able to read and enjoy his favorite classics in Greek and Latin. So he came up with an ingenious idea: he taught his daughters to read Greek and Latin and, subsequently, they read the classics to him. Although the daughters could read (i.e., *decode*) Greek and Latin words, they had no understanding of what they were reading to their father. This should drive home the notion that there is more to comprehension than word identification skills.

The same can be said for the relationship between listening and print comprehension. Ample research shows that children who do poorly on print comprehension also do poorly on listening comprehension; that is, they have poor language comprehension skills (e.g., see review in Nation, 2005). It is tempting to blame the print comprehension difficulties on poor oral language development, which obviously accounts for poor listening comprehension skills. Essentially, these children seem to have poor phonological skills, which is reasonable; however, they also have problems in other language areas. In fact, the difficulties in the broader language areas contribute to both listening and print comprehension problems. This does not mean that hearing and phonology are not important; it simply means that there are other language issues to consider.

NATURE OF WRITING

Now that you have a basic understanding of reading, we can proceed to the notion of writing. Of course, defining or describing *writing* is just as difficult as doing the same for reading. Writing, similar to reading, is not a unitary skill; that is, there is no single all-encompassing factor or variable that can account for or explain all of written language development. It has also been argued that reading and writing share underlying processes (Adams, 1990; Snow et al., 1998; Tierney & Pearson, 1983). In other words, reading facilitates the development of writing, and writing facilitates the development of reading. The specific facilitative aspects of both reading and writing are still being debated and investigated.

What exactly does it mean to state that someone is a good writer? This is the same issue that we had previously with our discussion of reading. If someone is said to be a good writer, we should ask: A good writer of what? Newspaper or magazine articles? Textbooks? Poetry? Novels? Letters? Is there such as thing as a good writer in general, or must this concept be restricted to a specific genre? Again, similar to reading, one might be adept at writing in an expository manner (scholarly articles, books, etc.), but not in a narrative manner (e.g., fiction pieces, poetry, etc.). Examples of expository and narrative passages are presented in **Table 7-3**.

Let us return to the reciprocal relations between reading and writing. In our view, good readers have the potential to become good writers. This means that good writers (of a particular genre) are already good readers (of the same genre). Let us take this one step further. If one does not read well, it is not likely that one can write well. If one does not write well, one may or may not be a good reader. Obviously, this is a complex relationship (e.g., Adams, 1990; Snow et al., 1998; see also the review in Paul, 2009).

In essence, the foundations for being a good reader must be fairly, but not completely, established before one can become a good writer. We do not deny that reading and writing can develop simultaneously—especially during the emergent literacy years. However, it seems that a specific level of proficiency in writing cannot be higher than the corresponding level of proficiency in reading.

Table 7-3

Example of Expository and Narrative Passages

Expository Passage

The comparative analysis of writing systems sheds considerable light on what the human mind can or cannot remember, and how human memory and language determine the way writing systems are designed. This knowledge helps us understand how a particular writing system can and cannot be taught.

Comparative analysis came of age when there was a sufficient body of evidence to provide a complete succession of forms protowriting to full-blown writing systems. (McGuinness, 2004, p. 11)

Narrative Passage

"A wicked birth … monstrous … evil … "

The elderly man had come out of the shadows so suddenly that Dr. Frederick Treves had not been aware of him until he heard the shaking voice. He turned abruptly, trying to see the man by the poor light of the smoking oil lamps. He could just make out a ravaged face, the lips trembling, the eyes glazed with horror.

"I beg your pardon?" said Treves politely. "Did you speak to me?" (Sparks, 1980, p. 1)

Thus, there is more to writing than just the ability to read, just as there is more to reading than just knowing a language in the conversational or oral form. And, finally, there is more to language than just proficiency or competency in the phonological component of that language. Nevertheless, you should be able to see the interrelations among hearing (and speaking), language, and literacy development. Before leaving the notion of writing, we think it is instructive for our readers to be aware of certain developmental milestones, especially with respect to the chronological age levels of children and adolescents. In the next section, we discuss, briefly, the developmental stages of writing.

DEVELOPMENT OF WRITING

It is not difficult to find data that support the emergent literacy concept; that is, that the early acquisition of reading and writing occurs in tandem with the emerging language development of children. One can see the steady, incremental increases in quantity and quality during this period (e.g., Klein, 1985; Routman, 2005; Ruddell & Haggard, 1985; Snow et al., 1998; Williams, 2004). In fact, the early writings of children seem to resemble the level of their corresponding spoken language.

The scribblings of children reflect these early attempts to write (e.g., Avery, 2002; Harste, Burke, & Woodward, 1982; Sulzby & Teale, 1987, 2003; Williams, 2004). Via marks on the page, children explore the functions and purposes of print. It is interesting to listen to children's interpretations of their marks, which are often difficult to decipher. These written expressions (i.e., marks and scribbles) are similar to the playing-with-sound stage in children's development of phonology (i.e., phonological awareness activities, such as saying *rat-tat-tat* and other rhyming ditties) that was mentioned previously (Bear, Invernizzi, Templeton, & Johnston, 2007; Snow et al., 1998). In other words, children are exploring the notion of putting something (their ideas, etc.) down on paper (or on the computer screen!). Only later do these marks or scribbles become words, phrases, or sentences, namely, the progression into a more mature writing stage. **Table 7-4** provides a few brief descriptions of the development of writing from preschool to about the second grade.

Beginning about age 9, we see what can be called a small explosion in the written language development, especially in the use of certain language variables and more complex and longer language constructions. Interestingly, this development seems to occur in tandem

Table 7-4

The Development of Writing

Grade Level	Description of Writing
Preschool	Scribbles with and without drawings; produces letter-like forms; produces random letter strings; writing is different from drawing
Late preschool to mid-kindergarten	Produces writing that is somewhat readable; produces conventional letters; engages in syllabic writing
Mid-kindergarten to mid-first grade	Produces texts that are relatively simple and can be read—partially—by others; experiences difficulty in writing (both lower- and upper-level issues); has the concept of a sentence
Late first to second grade	Writing improves; uses phrases; produces extended and coherent text

Source: Based on information in Bear, Invernizzi, Templeton, & Johnston (2007); Snow et al. (1998). Taken with slight adaptations from Paul (2009, p. 332).

with the increase of language and cognitive demands of reading materials; that is, at about the third- or fourth-grade level. Children gain control over the use and understanding of embedded sentences involving, for example, relative clauses: *The boy who kissed the girl ran away. The lion whom the mouse scared roared loudly.*

Although this growth in clauses mirrors its increasing use in the spoken language of children, the written domains of children are still more complex and intricate than their spoken domains. In other words, children's use of more complex syntactic structures occurs more often or is more prevalent in their writings than in their spoken language utterances. This is not difficult to understand. More mature writing or written language utterances do not simply reflect more mature spoken language utterance. We do not merely write the way we speak. We can, of course, do this, but more likely we produce more complex and intricate written language structures than we typically use in our face-to-face dialogues or conversations. Spoken language development assists with the development of written language; nevertheless, written language takes on a life of its own.

Relations Between Spoken and Written Language

Now that you have a basic understanding of reading and writing, we should reiterate and expand on a major concept, *reciprocity*, which has also been espoused by the National Reading Panel (2000) and by other sources (e.g., see discussion in Paul, 2008, 2009). It is possible to observe similarities and differences between the contents of spoken (i.e., oral) and written language productions. More interesting, however, we can argue that there is a strong relationship between these two entities; although, as we mentioned previously, the exact nature of the connection is still not complete or clear.

Remarkably, some scholars have highlighted the written language productions of d/Deaf or hard of hearing children—children with severe-to-profound hearing loss—to illustrate the intricate, complex, reciprocal link. The following passage by Danielewicz (cited in Ruddell & Haggard, 1985) is still relevant today (e.g., see discussions in McGuinness, 2004, 2005; Snow et al., 1998; Treiman, 2006):

> Danielewicz's extensive review...suggests that children progress through stages of writing development in which they (1) *unify* spoken and written language, making few distinctions between the two; (2) *distinguish* between spoken and written language by reducing coordinating conjunctions; (3) *strip* features of spoken language from written productions; and (4) *add* features typically associated with written language. (Ruddell & Haggard, 1985, p. 68)

In essence, we feel that a deeper understanding of the written language development of children requires a deeper understanding of the intricate and complex relations between oral (i.e., spoken) and written components of the *same* language. There is little doubt in our minds that children need to achieve proficiency in the primary (i.e., oral or conversational) form of the language of print via the internalization of phonology, morphology, syntax, and semantics (e.g., see also McGuinness, 2004, 2005). This internalization, fueled by hearing (and speech), contributes to the development of both reading and writing skills.

To reiterate, a few important early childhood skills include an understanding of letter names and shapes, phonemic awareness, and interest in literacy (e.g., Ehri, 2006; Nicholson & Ng, 2006). Children do need to develop comprehension and metacognitive skills, and this process can begin during the preschool years (e.g., National Reading Panel, 2000; McGuinness, 2004, 2005). But, this all begins with a development of phonology and other general language skills, which sets in motion the reciprocity between language and literacy. The reciprocity also extends to reading and writing. As aptly stated by Wang, Lee, and Paul (2010):

> Reading and writing (i.e., decoding and encoding) are essentially a mirror image of one another (McGuinness, 2004, 2005). The reading difficulties of many students who are deaf or hard of hearing in the United States also lead to their low writing skills. There is a reciprocal relationship between lower level (e.g., grammar, spelling punctuation, etc.) and higher level (e.g., purpose, audience, etc.) skills in writing. Access to the lower level skills requires, at the least, an understanding of phonology (and morphology) of the spoken language (or language of print). We can emphatically state that good readers have the potential to become good writers. Good writers are almost always good readers. In this sense, there is also reciprocity between reading and writing.

Interrelations Among Phonology, Working Memory, and Reading

Reciprocity impacts nearly all of reading and writing development. One of the most interesting lines of reciprocity research is one that demonstrates the interrelations among phonology, working memory, and reading. This complex interrelationship—albeit controversial—can be found in the literature on d/Deaf children (e.g., Paul, 2009; Trezek et al., 2010), children in other special education programs, and children with language and reading disabilities (e.g., Catts & Kamhi, 2005; McGuinness, 2004, 2005; Snowling & Hulme, 2005; Stanovich, 1991, 1992). We shall present only basic information here.

One impetus for examining this interrelation is the question posed by McGuinness (2004): How do children decode words in print? It is assumed, of course, that when children look at the letters and words that they need to engage in a decoding process. The assumption is that readers—all readers—need to convert the letters on the page into phonological abstract equivalents as the beginning stage of the comprehension process. Furthermore, it is assumed that this conversion process has two aspects: a visual process (i.e., fixating on letters) and a phonological translation/decoding (e.g., Adams, 1990; Snow et al., 1998; Snowling & Hulme, 2005).

As stated by Adams (1990), visual processing initiates the spark of identification and other associated processes, which include phonological, orthographic, syntactic, and semantic (meaning) information. As is discussed later, this conversion process is extremely controversial with respect to children who are d/Deaf or hard of hearing. Nevertheless, we surmise that you will be in for a surprise when you become familiar with the gist of the research findings (e.g., Paul, 2003, 2009; Trezek et al., 2010; Wang, Trezek, Luckner, & Paul, 2008).

This conversion process is said to occur in short-term (working) memory if one ascribes to a stage-of-processing view of reading, which involves sensory register, working memory, and long-term memory (e.g., see the discussions in Paul, 2009; Paul & Jackson, 1993; Trezek et al., 2010). The conversion involves the use of what is termed a *phonological code*; that is, converting letters to their phonological equivalents (actually, phonemic equivalents). The use of a phonological code is deemed to be most efficient for facilitating the reading process, mainly because it fits or matches the structure of the language of print, English in this case, which is a phoneme-based language.

In short, readers understand that words can be segmented into phonemes (i.e., vowels and consonants). This segmentation process assists with word identification and, subsequently, comprehension. The real issue is the cognitive representation of phonological and other information, not the peripheral hearing of such information. This is critical to keep in mind as we discuss the merits of alternative systems such as cued speech/language and visual phonics. In essence, success in reading or the development of mature reading skills is driven, in part, by phonological knowledge (e.g., Perfetti & Sandak, 2000; see also Mayer, 2007; Paul, 2003).

Arguments for the use of a phonological code in reading, especially beginning reading, are so controversial, and perhaps distasteful, that a number of researchers and scholars in deafness have attempted to dismiss this assertion or argue for alternative means other than phonology (e.g., Israelite, Ewoldt, & Hoffmeister, 1992; Yurkowski & Ewoldt, 1986; see reviews in Allen et al., 2009; Paul, 2003; Paul, Wang, Trezek, Luckner, 2009; Wang et al., 2008). A few scholars have argued that it does not play a predominant or efficient role at the word level (e.g., Miller, 2006). The real efficiency of the use of a phonological code can be seen in research documenting comprehension beyond the word level, as discussed in the ensuing section.

Internal Coding Strategies and Deafness

In the research on d/Deaf or hard of hearing individuals, at least five major types of internal coding strategies in working memory have been proffered: sign (e.g., Bellugi, Klima, & Siple, 1974/1975), dactylic (e.g., Locke & Locke, 1971), phonological-based (e.g., reviews in Conrad, 1979; Hanson, 1989), visual (e.g., Blanton, Nunnally, & Odom, 1967), and multiple (e.g., Lichtenstein, 1983, 1984, 1985, 1998; MacSweeney, Campbell, & Donlan, 1996). **Table 7-5** provides a brief description of each type of internal coding strategy.

To describe the strategies that d/Deaf individuals are using, researchers have had to develop ingenious techniques that consider the features of the tasks and the errors or responses produced by the participants, who are attempting to remember selected pieces of information. For example, the use of a sign code can be inferred if individuals produce

	Table 7-5

Description of Internal Coding Strategies

Type of Code	Description
Visual (graphemic, print)	Based on configuration of print words
	Sample confusion error: *tip* for *tap*
Sign	American Sign Language or English signs
	Sample confusion error: *train* for *short*
Dactylic	Fingerspelling
	Sample confusion error: *n* for *m*
Phonological	Articulatory movements (e.g., lips); representation of auditory impressions
	Sample confusion error: *blue* for *dew*
Multiple	Various combinations of the coding strategies.

Source: Taken with slight adaptations from Paul (2009, p. 310).

confusion errors based on the similarities between two similar signs, such as the sign for *short* and the sign for *train*.

Admittedly, open issues exist regarding the use of a phonological code in d/Deaf or hard of hearing students. For example, a number of studies have not examined this entity in word identification or in actual reading tasks and thus are not *direct* investigations of the use of this code (Stanovich, 1991). Even if researchers show that this code is used during reading, it is not always clear whether readers possess phonological awareness prior to the reading task or have acquired such awareness after the reading task (e.g., before or after word identification; e.g., Leybaert & Alegria, 1993; Pearson, 2004). Most of these studies have been conducted on older readers, such as high-school or college-age d/Deaf adolescents, some of whom have already become good readers. There is a need to examine the coding strategies of beginning, younger readers.

In spite of the caveats, the bulk of the findings indicate that individuals who are d/Deaf or hard of hearing and who use predominantly a phonological-based code in working memory tend to be better readers than other students who use predominantly a nonphonological-based code (e.g., Hanson, 1989; LaSasso & Metzger, 1998; Leybaert, 1993, 2005; Mayer, 2007; Paul, 2003; 2009; Paul et al., 2009; Trezek et al., 2010; Wang et al., 2008). In addition, the merits of phonological coding are not only evident at the word level (i.e., lexical retrieval), but also for connected structures, as in complex English syntax (e.g., Kelly, 1996; Lichtenstein, 1998). Deaf adolescent readers who use a phonological code seem to have less difficulty making simultaneous use of syntactic and semantic information at the sentence level and beyond; that is, the use of the code in working memory assists the readers in holding critical pieces of information in working memory so that they can work on the comprehension of the sentence.

It is clear that many d/Deaf students do not use phonological coding as efficiently as good readers who are hearing (e.g., Miller, 2006). This does not mean that this type of coding is irrelevant (Paul et al., 2009; Wang et al., 2008). In addition, as discussed in the ensuing sections, this might mean that alternative means to enhance the use of this code are important. In any case, the role of phonology with respect to decoding is considered to be an important factor in the use of information in working memory, especially for beginning reading development (e.g., Dyer, MacSweeney, Szczerbinski, Green, & Campbell, 2003; Nielsen & Luetke-Stahlman, 2002; Mayer, 2007; Paul et al., 2009; Wang et al., 2010).

Alternative Approaches for Representing Phonology

You have survived our summary of the research on working memory. Thus far, we have discussed the relationship between oral language and written language and have shown that phonology plays a major role in both the development of a spoken language and its written counterpart. Although phonology is not all that is needed, we think that if the graphophonemic components of reading are not addressed, then this will impact word identification (i.e., access to form) and contribute to the difficulty of developing comprehension skills.

Now let us assume that the new amplification systems (Chapters 4 and 5) are not sufficient by themselves—at least, at this point in time. What else can be done? Wang et al. (2008; see also Paul et al., 2009) have conducted a review of the literature and have averred that only two approaches have been relatively successful in developing phonological skills or awareness in d/Deaf or hard of hearing children: cued speech/language and visual phonics. We examine both notions in the ensuing paragraphs.

You should keep in mind that developing phonological skills is not the same as developing competence in phonology, one of the major components of a language (e.g., see Paul, 2009). Proficiency in phonology entails a number of skills, such as an understanding of both segmental (consonants and vowels) and suprasegmental (intonation, rhythm, prosody) aspects (see discussions of these areas in Chapter 6). To presume that the use of cued speech/language or even visual phonics is sufficient for the development of phonology, especially in children who are struggling with English, is an overgeneralization. Clearly, cued speech/language and visual phonics can help, and it might be that visual phonics holds the most promise (e.g., Morrison, Trezek, & Paul, 2008; Trezek & Malmgren, 2005; Trezek & Wang, 2006; Trezek, Wang, Woods, Gampp, & Paul, 2007; Wang et al., 2008).

DESCRIPTION OF CUED SPEECH/LANGUAGE

Cornett (1967, 1984), the creator of cued speech (now referred to as *cued speech/language*), considered the daunting task of assisting children who are d/Deaf to develop a spoken language via the use of a visual mechanism. Cornett recognized that a number of d/Deaf children were not succeeding through the traditional oral method, which tended to focus on the development of speech and speechreading skills (e.g., see discussion in Paul, 2009). More interesting, this scholar understood the challenges of learning to speechread— namely, the fact that several sounds, or groups of letters, look alike on the lips. For example, the letters *m*, *p*, and *b*, as in *mane*, *pane*, and *bane*, respectively, are difficult to disambiguate either in isolation or even in the context of running speech.

Cornett devised an interesting system of hand signs/symbols to address these ambiguities (see also Hage & Leybaert, 2006). His goal was to develop an approach that permits a rapid, automatic, natural development and use of the spoken language in most home environments. Cornett knew that in order to learn a spoken language d/Deaf children needed to access the phonology of that language.

In essence, Cornett's system entails the use of eight handshapes, with each handshape representing a cluster of letters to supplement the information on the lips. The eight handshapes are used in four positions either on or near the face, and there are also vowel positions that are near the face. It should be emphasized that Cornett only focused on the segmentals (consonants and vowels) of the phonological system. The cued speech/language symbols are shown in **Figure 7-1**.

Each handshape represents a group of consonants, and each group consists of consonantal letters that can be disambiguated by speechreading. For example, as can be seen in Figure 7-1, one handshape refers to /m/, /f/, and /t/, which are distinguishable visually. In fact, Cornett separated /m/, /p/, and /b/ and other similar clusters into different handshapes based on the ability to differentiate these letters visually; that is, /m/ is associated with one handshape, /p/ with another, and /b/ with a third. To discern a consonant among the three in a group, the viewer needs to observe the lips of the speaker in conjunction with the consonant hand cues.

To represent vowels, Cornett created symbols for hand positions, which are placed near or on the face. The movements of the handshapes and the use of vowel positions produce words, which result from the pairings of consonants and vowels. Thus, it is possible to represent all the sounds of a specific language, including pronunciations associated with dialects. Vowel diphthongs (e.g., *oi* as in *boy*) are executed by a sequence of two different vowel locations.

There is more to phonology than just consonants and vowels. What seemed to be missing from Cornett's system or, rather, assumed to be received via speechreading, was the suprasegmentals. Suprasegmentals represent phonological items such as intonation, rhythm,

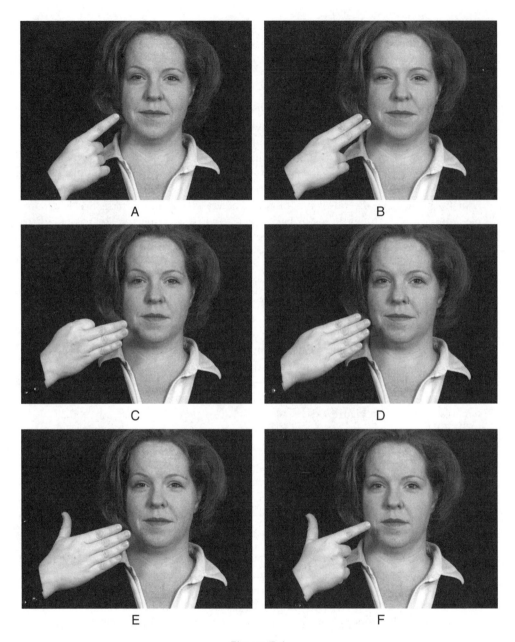

Figure 7-1

Handshapes and Positions of Cued Speech/Language

*Handshape and consonants: **A:** /d/, /p/, /zh/. **B:** /k/, /v/, /tH/, /z/. **C:** /h/, /s/, /r/. **D:** /b/, /n/, /wh/. **E:** /m/, /f/, /t/. **F:** /l/, /sh/, /w/. **G:** /g/, /j/, /th/. **H:** /ng/, /y/, /ch/.*

*Location for vowels. **1:** Corner of mouth. **2:** Tip of chin. **3:** Center of neck. **4:** Noncontact (about four inches to side of chin).*

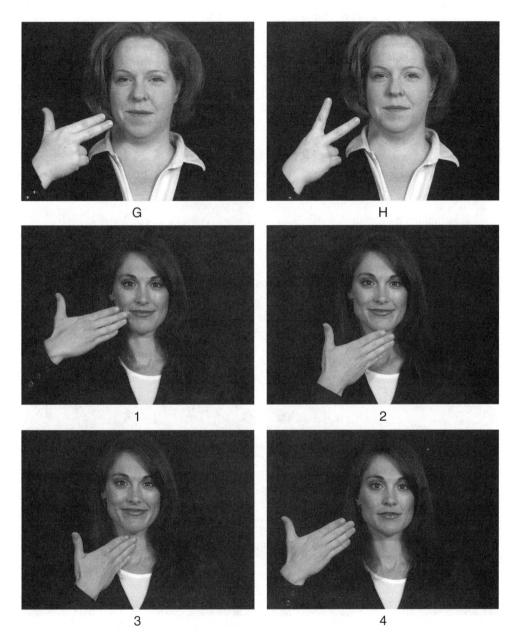

G   H

1   2

3   4

Figure 7-1
Continued

and other prosodic features. Children need to access, at the least, both the segmentals and suprasegmentals.

This situation was clarified by the work of Fleetwood and Metzger (1998), who coined the term *cuem*, which is roughly analogous to, but not the same as, a speech sound. These scholars argued that the cuems consisted of both segmentals and suprasegmentals, the latter of which were symbolized by what they called nonmanual signals, or NMS. The NMS is executed by mouth movements used to produce consonants and vowels.

In American English, Fleetwood and Metzger identified seven NMS for the consonants and three NMS for the vowels. In **Figure 7-2**, two NMS are illustrated. NMS A involves bilabial compression associated with the consonant phonemes /p/, /b/, and /m/ and refers to the mouth movements that accompany the production of these sounds. NMS B involves the upper teeth and lower lip for the consonant phonemes /v/ and /f/.

The combination of the handshape and NMS assists the viewer in distinguishing among the group of phonemes associated with the same handshape. For example, let us again consider the handshape for /m/, /f/, and /t/. A distinct NMS is associated with each of these three phonemes, and the particular NMS assists the viewer with the disambiguation process. In a similar manner, a specific handshape or hand placement may assist viewers in distinguishing phonemes (e.g., /m/, /p/, /b/) that share the same NMS.

One of the most interesting points made by Fleetwood and Metzger (1998) is that this representation of segmentals and suprasegmentals is sufficient enough such that there is

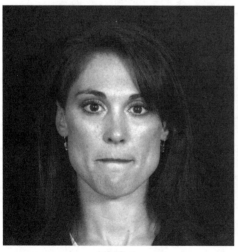
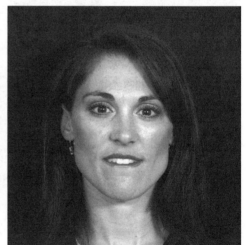

NMS A   NMS B

Figure 7-2

Examples of Nonmanual Signals of Cued Speech/Language

Nonmanual signal (NMS) A involves bilabial compression associated with the consonant phonemes /p/, /b/, and /m/. NMS B involves upper teeth and lower lip for the consonant phonemenes /v/ and /f/.

no need for sound or an acoustic signal to accompany the combined movements. In fact, these scholars asserted that the cued articulators can represent the same range of abstract phonemic values as do the speech articulators, including the suprasegmental aspects such as intonation, stress, and rhythm. If this representation is indeed adequate, then recipients should be able to develop both phonological and phonemic awareness.

As is discussed in the ensuing section, there seems to be some success in the development of literacy for some children exposed to cued speech/language, especially with respect to the more recent studies. Nevertheless, some scholars do not think that cued speech/language can be as efficient as visual phonics (e.g., see discussions in Trezek et al., 2010; Wang et al., 2008). The reason is this: cued speech/language does not represent the *individual* phonemes as does visual phonics (discussed later). Rather, cued speech/language represents a cluster of phonemes that need to be disambiguated by NMS or by speechreading skills. Despite this criticism, cued speech/language has engendered some fascinating results. It should also be remarked that cued speech/language has been adapted or adjusted such that it is being used in more than 56 languages (Cornett & Daisey, 1992).

RESEARCH ON CUED SPEECH/LANGUAGE

Early studies were conducted prior to the formulation and clarification of NMS and before the revelation of connecting this symbol system to the development of reading and writing skills. Because of the influence of traditional oral approaches and their emphasis on speech and speechreading, these early research efforts focused on improvement of speech reception and speech intelligibility.

In two early investigations (Clarke & Ling, 1976; Ling & Clarke, 1975), researchers examined students' speech receptive abilities. As expected, students performed significantly better on cued stimuli than on noncued stimuli. Cued words were easier to understand than the longer stimuli—cued phrases and cued sentences. Cued phrases were easier than cued sentences. Even more interesting, the students' speech errors in this study exhibited certain patterns, which made it possible to develop a remedial program to address the errors.

These early results on speech reception have been reiterated in later investigations (e.g., see Nicholls & Ling, 1982). In fact, there has been much success for some children and adults in improving their visual speech reception and speechreading skills. There has also been success associated with the use of cued speech for some children with cochlear implants (e.g., for a good review on phonology and cued speech/language, see LaSasso & Metzger, 1998; Leybaert, 2005).

Most of the recent publications and research on cued speech/language have centered on the development of specific English reading skills. Cornett (1991) has argued that cued speech/language can play a major role in the development of phonological awareness and, subsequently, reading achievement. Evidence suggests that cued speech/language is sufficient for some d/Deaf individuals to develop the use of a phonological code in short-term memory and representations of phonological information cognitively (see Leybaert, 2005; Leybaert & Charlier, 1996). And, the evidence seems to suggest that cued speech/language is effective for facilitating the development of reading (see reviews and discussions in Hage

& Leybaert, 2006; LaSasso & Crain, 2003; LaSasso & Metzger, 1998; Leybaert, 2005; Torres, Moreno-Torres, & Santana, 2006).

Cued speech/language has also been used with students with symptoms of autism, Down syndrome, deaf-blindness, cerebral palsy, and auditory processing deficits. It has even been used by general education teachers for phonics instruction and by speech therapists for articulation therapy (National Cued Speech Association, 2007). Despite these successes, cued speech/language is still not widely used with children who are d/Deaf or hard of hearing, especially in the United States.

Whether cued speech/language is an efficient method for representing the phonological and phonemic aspects of a language is still open to debate and research. It must be determined whether cued speech/language is consistently sufficient for developing phonological and phonemic awareness in beginning reading stages and for developing these areas adequately enough to facilitate the more advanced acquisition of reading in English. In our view, similar to any other approach or method, we do not feel that cued speech/language is a panacea, especially for all or most d/Deaf or hard of hearing children and adolescents.

DESCRIPTION OF VISUAL PHONICS

Another approach to developing phonology or, rather, the sounds of a language as well as the possible relations between letters and sounds, is *visual phonics*, also known as *see-the-sound* (Morrison et al., 2008). Visual phonics can be described as a multisensory approach involving visual, motor, and kinesthetic capabilities. This system can be used to help children with articulation as well as with phonological and phonemic development.

See-the-sound/visual phonics (STS/VP) has two types of representations: hand signs and line drawings (e.g., Morrison et al., 2008). The hand signs correspond to the sounds (i.e., phonemes) of a language. English has anywhere from 43 to 45 hand signals, reflecting the number of phonemes (consonants and vowels) in American English (see Chapter 6). The hand signs are easy for most children to learn, although adults find them challenging. The hand signs are purported to reflect the movements of the articulators in producing the sound. Clearly, this is a debatable issue; however, some research indicates that the hand signs are most likely performed in a reinforcing manner (Morrison et al., 2008; Paul, 2009). A few of the hand signs for visual phonics are depicted in **Figure 7-3**.

To produce a word such as *cat*, one would need the hand signs for three phonemes: /k/, /a/, and /t/. It should be emphasized that the hand signs corresponds to individual sounds, not a cluster of letters, as in cued speech/language (see Figure 7-1). In addition, this approach enables children to *see* (no pun intended!) that certain sounds are similar in certain words. Later, children learn that certain sounds are represented by more than one letter, as is the case for an opaque language such as English (e.g., consider *cake, cease*). Children also learn that certain letters can have more than one sound (e.g., consider the *a* in *rat, rate,* and *father*).

The second type of representation entails the use of line drawings that correspond with the phonemes represented by the hand signs. Thus, in English, 43 to 45 different symbols look or resemble schematically each corresponding hand sign. The line drawings provide

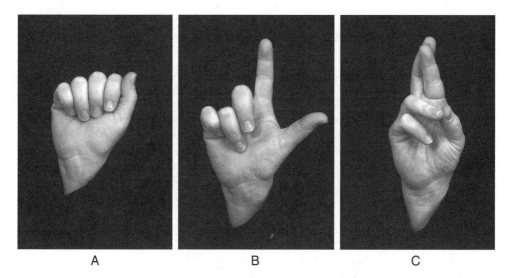

Figure 7-3
Three Examples of Handshapes for Visual Phonics

(A) This is the handshape for the long a sound.
(B) This is the handshape for the l sound.
(C) This is the handshape for the r sound.
For more details, see Waddy-Smith & Wilson (2003)

visual support for making the phoneme–grapheme links and are placed under letters in print that correspond to each phoneme. Children learn to connect the line drawings to the previously learned hand cues for the phonemes and, essentially, to associate the phonemes with the letters. The line drawings are particularly facilitative for complex vowels, silent letters, and digraphs that frequently confuse struggling readers.

Taken together, the hand signs and the line drawings show the relationships between the sounds of the languages and their corresponding letters; that is, the alphabetic system upon which the English language is based. STP/VP can be used as part of a phonics lesson, especially for children who need a multisensory approach to assist them in remembering the phoneme–grapheme relationships.

STS/VP was used initially with children and adolescents who are deaf (i.e., profound hearing impairment; see Chapter 1). This approach seems to address the issue of teaching sounds (and letters) to individuals who do not have the ability to hear sounds accurately or completely. Although much of the research has been done on children who are d/Deaf or hard of hearing (the work of Trezek, discussed in the following section), recent research has documented the effectiveness of STP/VP with children who are hearing and are struggling readers experiencing difficulty with phonological and phonemic-awareness tasks (e.g., Cihon, Gardner, Morrison, & Paul, 2008).

For a more detailed description of visual phonics, including research results, you are referred to the work of Waddy-Smith and Wilson (2003).

RESEARCH ON VISUAL PHONICS

STS/VP has been in existence for more than 25 years, yet its effectiveness has been documented only recently—specifically in the first decade of 2000 (e.g., see discussion in Morrison et al., 2008). Trezek and her collaborators have conducted a consistent and systematic line of inquiry on visual phonics with children who are d/Deaf or hard of hearing. In essence, Trezek has shown—and research reviews have substantiated the assertion (e.g., Paul, 2009; Trezek et al., 2010; Wang et al., 2008)—that phonology is critical for reading development and that it is possible to improve d/Deaf or hard of hearing children's understanding of letter–sound relationships.

In an initial study, Trezek and Malmgren (2005) used STS/VP with d/Deaf and hard of hearing students at the middle-school level (i.e., sixth through eighth grade). The students performed well with respect to the use of phonological skills after instruction. These benefits existed regardless of the degree of hearing loss; that is, positive effects were found for individuals with all degrees of hearing loss, and there were no significant differences associated with hearing loss. Interestingly, once students learned to associate the STS/VP hand signal with the corresponding sound, the hand signal alone was sufficient for assisting the students in remembering the articulation of the sound.

In a later study, Trezek and Wang (2006) investigated the beginning reading skills of children who were d/Deaf or hard of hearing and who were in kindergarten and first grade. The instructional period was eight months long. Three subtests of the Wechsler Individual Achievement Test-II (WIAT-II)—Word Reading, Pseudoword Decoding, and Reading Comprehension—were administered as part of a pretest/posttest experimental design. Again, positive results were reported; that is, the children demonstrated significant gains on all three measures that were used.

Trezek et al. (2007) also investigated the reading development of d/Deaf and hard of hearing children in kindergarten and first grade. This study occurred over the course of a typical school year. Six subtests of the Dominie Reading and Writing Assessment Portfolio were administered: Sentence Writing Phoneme, Sentence Writing Spelling, Phonemic Awareness Segmentation, Phonemic Awareness Deletion, Phonics Onsets, and Phonics Rimes. As expected, Trezek et al. reported positive significant differences (i.e., gains) for all six measures of reading.

Taken together, the studies by Trezek and her colleagues indicate the possibility and feasibility of developing phonological and phonemic awareness in children who are d/Deaf or hard of hearing, regardless of the level of hearing impairment. It is also remarkable that this line of research has shown that it is possible to use STS/VP as part of phonics instruction, especially during the beginning years of reading instruction. In essence, it appears that the STS/VP system can facilitate the acquisition of phonological and phonemic awareness skills in d/Deaf or hard of hearing students.

With a line of research with typical hearing children in progress (e.g., Cihon et al., 2008), STS/VP may also be a successful tool to develop skills in other struggling readers who have difficulty via traditional instructional approaches. However, keep in mind that despite this success with the development of phonology via STS/VP, struggling readers also need instruction in all other components of language as well as in specific *reading* areas, such as prior knowledge, vocabulary, and metacognition. In short, STS/VP seems to have great potential to serve as an efficient alternative method or mode for developing phonological and phonemic awareness in d/Deaf or hard of hearing children and adolescents.

BRIEF SUMMARY: CUED SPEECH/LANGUAGE AND VISUAL PHONICS

We have expended a considerable amount of space to the descriptions and research on both cued speech/language and visual phonics. We felt that it was necessary to provide adequate details to support the assertions of these two promising interventions for children who are d/Deaf or hard of hearing. In fact, we bet that there will be an increase in research on the effectiveness of visual phonics, and there will be an increase in the debate on this method as well. These debates will revolve around the controversy of phonology—a domain of the English language that simply cannot be avoided in the process of developing both language and literacy skills.

Summary of Major Points

We certainly hope that this chapter was able to provide some background and insights into the interrelations among hearing, language, and literacy. Admittedly, we have only scratched the surface. We also hope that we were able to answer or partially answer many of the questions that you generated at the beginning of the chapter. If not, it would be to your benefit to read some of the references cited and/or to dialogue with your instructor.

The overall intent of this chapter was to provide a brief introduction to *Key Concepts*, as follows:

- The development of English literacy
- The reciprocal relations within and between language and literacy
- The interrelations among phonology, working memory, and reading
- The concept and implications of cued speech/language
- The concept and implications of visual phonics (see-the-sound/visual phonics)

With respect to English literacy, the major points were
- Phonology is a critical aspect of the beginning process of literacy and for the subsequent development of higher-level reading skills, including conventional spelling skills.

- To develop mature or proficient reading skills, teachers and clinicians need to devote attention to other language-based areas, such as fluency (reading quickly and accurately) vocabulary (meanings of words) and text comprehension (constructing meaning).

- In discussing the reading process, the focus should be balanced; that is, teachers and clinicians should emphasize the underpinnings and skills associated with both form (e.g., access to print skills or decoding) and meaning (e.g., comprehension and metacognitive skills).

- Writing, similar to reading, is not a unitary skill; that is, there is no single all-encompassing factor or variable that can account for or explain all of written language development.

- Reading and writing have a reciprocal, facilitative relationship. In other words, reading facilitates the development of writing, and writing facilitates the development of reading. The specific facilitative aspects of both reading and writing are still being debated and investigated.

- There is more to writing than just the ability to read, just as there is more to reading than just knowing a language in the conversation or oral form.

With respect to reciprocal relations for language and literacy, it was highlighted that

- A strong relationship exists between language and literacy, although the exact nature of this connection is not fully or adequately understood.

- Children need to achieve proficiency in the primary (i.e., oral or conversational) form of the language of print via the internalization of phonology, morphology, syntax, and semantics. This internalization, fueled by hearing (and speech), contributes to the development of both reading and writing skills.

With respect to the interrelations among phonology, working memory, and reading, it was remarked that

- The assumption is that readers—all readers—need to convert the letters on the page into phonological abstract equivalents at the beginning stage of the comprehension process.

- As stated by Adams (1990), visual processing initiates the spark of identification and other associated processes, which include phonological, orthographic, syntactic, and semantic (meaning) information.

- This conversion process is said to occur in short-term (working) memory if one ascribes to a stage-of-processing view of reading, which involves sensory register, working memory, and long-term memory.

- The use of a phonological code is deemed to be most efficient for facilitating the reading process, mainly because it fits or matches the structure of the language of print, English in this case, which is a phonemic-based language.

- In the research on d/Deaf or hard of hearing individuals, at least five major types of internal coding in working memory have been proffered: sign, dactylic, phonological-based, visual, and multiple.

- In spite of the caveats, the bulk of the findings indicate that individuals who are d/Deaf or hard of hearing and who use predominantly a phonological-based code in working memory tend to be better readers than students who use predominantly a nonphonological-based code.

With respect to cued speech/language, it was stated that

- Each handshape in cued speech/language represents a group of consonants, and each group consists of consonantal letters that can be disambiguated by speechreading.

- Vowels are represented by hand positions, which are placed near or on the face. Vowel diphthongs (e.g., *oi* as in *boy*) are executed by a sequence of two different vowel locations.

- The movements of the handshapes and the use of vowel positions produce words, which result from the pairings of consonants and vowels. Thus, it is possible to represent all the sounds of a specific language, including pronunciations associated with dialects.

- The nonmanual signals (NMS) are executed by mouth movements used to produce consonants and vowels. The combination of the handshape and NMS assists the viewer in distinguishing among the group of phonemes associated with the same handshape.

- Because of the influence of traditional oral approaches and their emphasis on speech and speechreading, early research efforts focused on improvement of speech reception and speech intelligibility. In fact, much success has been achieved for some children and adults in improving their visual speech reception and speechreading skills. Success has also been found with the use of cued speech/language for some children with cochlear implants.

- Most of the recent publications and research on cued speech/language have centered on the effects of cued speech/language on the development of specific English reading skills. Evidence suggests that cued speech/language is sufficient for some d/Deaf individuals to develop the use of a phonological code in short-term memory and representations of phonological information cognitively.

With respect to visual phonics, it was stated that

■ Visual phonics can be described as a multisensory approach involving visual, motor, and kinesthetic capabilities. This system can be used to help children with articulation as well as with phonological and phonemic development.

■ See-the-sound/visual phonics (STS/VP) has two types of representations: hand signs and line drawings. The hand signs correspond to the sounds (i.e., phonemes) of a language. The hand signs are purported to reflect the movements of the articulators in producing the sound. The line drawings correspond with the phonemes represented by the hand signs. Taken together, the hand signs and the line drawings show the relationships between the sounds of the languages and their corresponding letters; that is, the alphabetic system upon which the English language is based.

■ Although much of the research has been done on children who are d/Deaf or hard of hearing, recent research has documented the effectiveness of STP/VP with children who are hearing and are struggling readers experiencing difficulty with phonological and phonemic awareness tasks.

■ Trezek and her collaborators have conducted a consistent and systematic line of inquiry on visual phonics with children who are d/Deaf or hard of hearing. In essence, Trezek has shown—and research reviews have substantiated the assertion—that phonology is critical for reading development and that it is possible to improve d/Deaf or hard of hearing children's understanding of letter–sound relationships.

Now, you have arrived this far in the book, we certainly hope that you have a good understanding of the essentials of speech, hearing, language, and literacy. You should consider this information in light of what you obtained from the chapters on amplification. You should now be able to appreciate the science and art of speechreading and auditory training/learning, the topics of the next chapter.

 ## *Chapter Questions*

Note: *Some answers to the questions can be found in the chapter; however, others have a variety of possible responses based on the students' backgrounds and experiences.*

1. The authors included two passages at the beginning of the chapter that focus on the interrelations among hearing, language, and literacy. In discussing or interpreting these passages, the authors cautioned that it is possible to overstate the position. What did they mean by this? The authors also mentioned that it is possible to understate the position. What did they mean by this?

2. What is the authors' definition or description of *reading*? Why is it difficult to define or describe reading?

3. Why is phonology considered to be critical for the development of beginning reading skills? Is it possible to overstate the importance of phonology? Why or why not?

4. Describe a few (about three) major highlights of the section "Early Literacy Development."

5. What is the authors' definition or description of *writing*? Why is it difficult to define or describe writing?

6. What does it mean to say that there is a reciprocal relation between reading and writing?

7. Describe a few (about five) major highlights of the section "Development of Writing." Include statements about the relationship between spoken and written language.

8. What is *decoding*?

9. What coding strategies are used by d/Deaf or hard of hearing children and adolescents? Which strategy (or strategies) is considered to be most effective? Why is this the case?

10. Describe cued speech/language. Be sure to discuss both handshapes and NMS.

11. Describe a few (about three) major highlights of the section "Research on Cued Speech/Language."

12. Describe visual phonics.

13. Discuss a few (up to three) major highlights of the section "Research on Visual Phonics."

14. If you had an opportunity to converse with the authors, what burning questions would you ask them? Share and discuss these questions with your instructor and classmates.

Challenge Questions

Note: *Complete answers are not in the text. Additional research/reading is required. In some cases, reading further or elsewhere in the text might provide some information to guide the response to a particular question.*

1. One of the most controversial questions for scholars studying deafness is whether reading is the same for d/Deaf children as it is for hearing children. Do d/Deaf children develop and acquire reading skills in the same manner as do children with typical hearing? Given the way reading was discussed in this chapter, what are your thoughts? Do you think that the answer to this question has implications for the teaching of reading to children and adolescents who are d/Deaf or hard of hearing?

2. Obtain a sample of the written language productions of a few d/Deaf and hard of hearing children and adolescents in your area from the schools. Inspect the writing samples carefully. Are there errors? Can you describe the errors? What do you think you would need to know in order to describe the errors?

3. The chapter discusses reciprocal relationships. Do you think there is a reciprocal relationship between listening comprehension (i.e., listening or watching a story) and reading comprehension (i.e., reading the story yourself)? Why or why not? Do you think that this relationship changes as one grows older? Why or why not?

Suggested Activities

1. Select a partner (or two) from your class and do an in-depth report on cued speech/language or visual phonics. Information and references in the chapter can be used to provide guidance. Summarize the research on your particular area. Discuss its relationship to the development of English language and English literacy. Find out if cued speech/language or visual phonics is used in your area. If so, observe the activities and include this in your report. Share with your instructor and the rest of your class the information and insights gained from this activity.

2. Interview teachers of the d/Deaf or hard of hearing in your area and obtain perspectives on the manner in which they teach reading and writing in their classrooms. How is this instruction different from what occurs in the general education classrooms? How are reading and writing assessed? Share with your instructor and the rest of your class the information and insights gained from this activity.

References

Adams, M. (1990). *Beginning to read: Thinking and learning about print.* Cambridge, MA: MIT Press.

Adams, M. (1994). Phonics and beginning reading instruction. In F. Lehr & J. Osborn (Eds.), *Reading, language, and literacy: Instruction for the twenty-first century* (pp. 3–23). Hillsdale, NJ: Erlbaum.

Allen, T., Clark, M. D., del Giudice, A., Koo, D., Lieberman, A., Mayberry, R., & Miller, P. (2009). Phonology and reading: A response to Wang, Trezek, Luckner, and Paul. *American Annals of the Deaf, 154*(4), 338–345.

Avery, C. (2002). *And with a light touch: Learning about reading, writing and teaching with first graders.* Portsmouth, NH: Heinemann.

Bartine, D. (1989). *Early English reading theory: Origins of current debates.* Columbia, SC: University of South Carolina Press.

Bartine, D. (1992). *Reading, criticism, and culture: Theory and teaching in the United States and England, 1820–1950.* Columbia, SC: University of South Carolina Press.

Bear, D., Invernizzi, M., Templeton, S., & Johnston, F. (2007). *Words their way: Words study for phonics, vocabulary, and spelling instruction* (4th ed.). Upper Saddle River, NJ: Pearson.

Bellugi, U., Klima, E., & Siple, P. (1974/1975). Remembering in signs. *Cognition, 3*(2), 93–125.

Bernhardt, E. (1991). *Reading development in a second language.* Norwood, NJ: Ablex.

Blamey, P. (2003). Development of spoken language by deaf children. In M. Marschark & P. Spencer (Eds.), *Oxford handbook of deaf studies, language, and education* (pp. 232–246). New York: Oxford University Press.

Blanton, R., Nunnally, J., & Odom, P. (1967). Graphemic, phonetic, and associative factors in the verbal behavior of deaf and hearing subjects. *Journal of Speech and Hearing Research, 10*, 225–231.

Carlisle, J., & Rice, M. (2002). *Improving reading comprehension: Research-based principles and practices.* Baltimore, MD: York Press.

Catts, H., & Kamhi, A. (2005). *Language and reading disabilities* (2nd ed.). Boston: Pearson/Allyn & Bacon.

Chall, J. S. (1996). *Stages of reading development* (2nd ed.). New York: McGraw-Hill.

Cihon, T., Gardner, R., Morrison, D., & Paul, P. (2008). Using visual phonics as a strategic intervention to increase literacy behaviors for kindergarten students at-risk for reading failure. *The Journal of Early and Intensive Behavior Intervention, 5*(3), 138–155.

Clarke, B., & Ling, D. (1976). The effects of using cued speech: A follow-up study. *Volta Review, 78*, 23–35.

Conrad, R. (1979). *The deaf school child.* London, England: Harper & Row.

Cornett, R. O. (1967). Cued speech. *American Annals of the Deaf, 112*, 3–13.

Cornett, R. O. (1984). Book review: Language and deafness. *Cued Speech News, 17*(3), 5.

Cornett, R. O. (1991). A model for ASL/English bilingualism. In S. Polowe-Aldersley, P. Schragle, V. Armour, & J. Polowe (Eds.), *Proceedings of the 55th Biennial Meeting of CAID and the 63rd Annual Meeting of CEASD* (pp. 33–39). New Orleans, LA: Convention of American Instructors of the Deaf.

Cornett, R. O., & Daisey, M. (1992). *The Cued Speech resource book for parents of deaf children.* Raleigh, NC: National Cued Speech Corporation.

Crystal, D. (2006). *How language works.* London, England: Penguin Books.

Dyer, A., MacSweeney, M., Szczerbinski, M., Green, L., & Campbell, R. (2003). Predictors of reading delay in deaf adolescents: The relative contributions of rapid automatized naming speed and phonological awareness and decoding. *Journal of Deaf Studies and Deaf Education, 8*(3), 215–229.

Ehri, L. (1991). Development of the ability to read words. In R. Barr, M. Kamil, P. Mosenthal, & P. D. Pearson (Eds.), *Handbook of reading research* (2nd ed., pp. 383–417). White Plains, NY: Longman.

Ehri, L. (2006). Alphabetics instruction helps students learn to read. In R. M. Joshi & P. G. Aaron (Eds.), *Handbook of orthography and literacy* (pp. 649–677). Mahwah, NJ: Erlbaum.

Fleetwood, E., & Metzger, M. (1998). *Cued language structure: An analysis of cued American English based on linguistic principles.* Silver Spring, MD: Calliope Press.

Hage, C., & Leybaert, J. (2006). The effect of cued speech on the development of spoken language. In P. Spencer & M. Marschark (Eds.), *Advances in the spoken language development of deaf and hard of hearing children* (pp. 193–211). New York: Oxford University Press.

Hanson, V. (1989). Phonology and reading: Evidence from profoundly deaf readers. In D. Shankweiler & I. Lieberman (Eds.), *Phonology and reading disability: Solving the reading puzzle* (pp. 69–89). Ann Arbor, MI: University of Michigan Press.

Harste, J., Burke, C., & Woodward, V. (1982). Children's language and world: Initial encounters with print. In J. Langer & M. T. Smith-Burke (Eds.), *Reader meets author/Bridging the gap* (pp. 105–131). Newark, DE: International Reading Association.

Hirsch, E. D. (1987). *Cultural literacy: What every American needs to know.* Boston: Houghton Mifflin.

Hirsch, E. D., Kett, J., & Trefil, J. (Eds.). (2002). *The new dictionary of cultural literacy* (3rd ed.). Boston: Houghton Mifflin.

Israelite, N., Ewoldt, C., & Hoffmeister, R. (1992). *Bilingual–bicultural education for deaf and hard of hearing students.* Toronto, Ontario: MGS Publications Services.

Kelly, L. (1996). The interaction of syntactic competence and vocabulary during reading by deaf students. *Journal of Deaf Studies & Deaf Education, 1*(1), 75–90.

Klein, M. (1985). *The development of writing in children: Pre-K through grade 8.* Englewood Cliffs, NJ: Prentice Hall.

LaSasso, C., & Crain, K. L. (2003). Research and theory support Cued Speech. *Odyssey, 5*(1), 30–35.

LaSasso, C., & Metzger, M. (1998). An alternate route for preparing deaf children for BiBi programs: The home language as L1 and cued speech for conveying traditionally-spoken languages. *Journal of Deaf Studies and Deaf Education, 3*(4), 265–289.

Leybaert, J. (1993). Reading in the deaf: The roles of phonological codes. In M. Marschark & M. D. Clark (Eds.), *Psychological perspectives on deafness* (pp. 269–309). Hillsdale, NJ: Erlbaum.

Leybaert, J. (2005). Learning to read with a hearing impairment. In M. Snowling & C. Hulme (Eds.), *The science of reading: A handbook* (pp. 379–396). Malden, MA: Blackwell.

Leybaert, J., & Alegria, J. (1993). Is word processing involuntary in deaf children? *British Journal of Developmental Psychology, 11,* 1–29.

Leybaert, J., & Charlier, B. (1996). Visual speech in the head: The effect of cued-speech on rhyming, remembering, and spelling. *Journal of Deaf Studies and Deaf Education (JDSDE), 1*(4), 234–248.

Lichtenstein, E. (1983). *The relationships between reading processes and English skills of deaf students.* Unpublished manuscript. Rochester, NY: National Technical Institute for the Deaf.

Lichtenstein, E. (1984). Deaf working memory processes and English language skills. In D. Martin (Ed.), *International symposium on cognition, education, and deafness: Working papers* (Vol. 2, pp. 331–360). Washington, DC: Gallaudet University Press.

Lichtenstein, E. (1985). Deaf working memory processes and English language skills. In D. Martin (Ed.), *Cognition, education, and deafness: Directions for research and instruction* (pp. 111–114). Washington, DC: Gallaudet University Press.

Lichtenstein, E. (1998). The relationships between reading processes and English skills of deaf college students. *Journal of Deaf Studies & Deaf Education, 3*(2), 80–134.

Ling, D., & Clarke, B. (1975). Cued speech: An evaluative study. *American Annals of the Deaf, 120,* 480–488.

Locke, J., & Locke, V. (1971). Deaf children's phonetic, visual, and dactylic coding in a grapheme recall task. *Journal of Experimental Psychology, 89,* 142–146.

MacSweeney, M., Campbell, R., & Donlan, C. (1996). Varieties of short-term memory coding in deaf teenagers. *Journal of Deaf Studies and Deaf Education, 1*(4), 249–262.

Mayer, C. (2007). What really matters in the early literacy development of deaf children. *Journal of Deaf Studies and Deaf Education, 12*(4), 411–431.

McGuinness, D. (2004). *Early reading instruction: What science really tells us about how to teach reading.* Cambridge, MA: MIT Press.

McGuinness, D. (2005). *Language development and learning to read: The scientific study of how language development affects reading skill.* Cambridge, MA: MIT Press.

Miller, P. (2006). What the processing of real words and pseudohomophones can tell us about the development of orthographic knowledge in prelingually deafened individuals. *Journal of Deaf Studies and Deaf Education, 11*(1), 21–38.

Morrison, D., Trezek, B., & Paul, P. (2008). Can you see that sound? A rationale for a multisensory intervention tool for struggling readers. *Balanced Reading Instruction, 15*(1), 11–26.

Nation, K. (2005). Connections between language and reading in children with poor reading comprehension. In H. Catts & A. Kamhi (Eds.), *The connections between language and reading disabilities* (pp. 41–54). Mahwah, NJ: Erlbaum.

National Cued Speech Association. (2007, October 13). *Special Populations*. Retrieved October 13, 2007, from http://www.cuedspeech.org/sub/cued/uses.asp.

National Reading Panel. (2000). *Report of the National Reading Panel: Teaching children to read—An evidence-based assessment of the scientific research literature on reading and its implications for reading instruction*. Jessup, MD: National Institute for Literacy at EDPubs.

Nicholls, G., & Ling, D. (1982). Cued speech and the reception of spoken language. *Journal of Speech and Hearing Research, 25*, 262–269.

Nicholson, T., & Ng, G. L. (2006). The case for teaching phonemic awareness and simple phonics to preschoolers. In R. M. Joshi & P. G. Aaron (Eds.), *Handbook of orthography and literacy* (pp. 637–648). Mahwah, NJ: Erlbaum.

Nielsen, D. C., & Luetke-Stahlman, B. (2002). Phonological awareness: One key to the reading proficiency of deaf children. *American Annals of the Deaf, 147*(3), 11–19.

Northern, J., & Downs, M. (2002). *Hearing in children* (5th ed.). Baltimore, MD: Lippincott Williams & Wilkins.

Paul, P. (1998). *Literacy and deafness: The development of reading, writing, and literate thought*. Needham Heights, MA: Allyn & Bacon.

Paul, P. (2003). Processes and components of reading. In M. Marschark & P. Spencer (Eds.), *Handbook of deaf studies, language, and education* (pp. 97–109). New York: Oxford University Press.

Paul, P. (2008). Introduction: Reading and children with disabilities. Reading and children with disabilities. *Balanced Reading Instruction, 15*(2), 1–12.

Paul, P. (2009). *Language and deafness* (4th ed.). Sudbury, MA: Jones & Bartlett.

Paul, P., & Jackson, D. (1993). *Toward a psychology of deafness: Theoretical and empirical perspectives* (pp. 215–235). Needham Heights, MA: Allyn & Bacon.

Paul, P., Wang, Y., Trezek, B., & Luckner, J. (2009). Phonology is necessary, but not sufficient: A rejoinder. *American Annals of the Deaf, 154*(4), 346–356.

Pearson, P. D. (2004). The reading wars. *Educational Policy, 18*(1), 216–252.

Perfetti, C., & Sandak, R. (2000). Reading optimally builds on spoken language: Implications for deaf readers. *Journal of Deaf Studies and Deaf Education, 5*, 32–50.

Plack, C. (2005). *The sense of hearing*. Mahwah, NJ: Erlbaum.

Routman, R. (2005). *Writing essentials: Raising expectations and results while simplifying teaching*. Portsmouth, NH: Heinemann.

Ruddell, R., & Haggard, M. (1985). Oral and written language acquisition and the reading process. In H. Singer & R. Ruddell (Eds.), *Theoretical models and processes of reading* (3rd ed., pp. 63–80). Newark, DE: International Reading Association.

Samuels, S. J., & Kamil, M. (1984). Models of the reading process. In P. D. Pearson, R. Barr, M. Kamil, & P. Mosenthal (Eds.), *Handbook of reading research* (pp. 185–224). White Plains, NY: Longman.

Scarborough, H. (2005). Developmental relationships between language and reading: Reconciling a beautiful hypothesis with some ugly facts. In H. Catts & A. Kamhi (Eds.), *The connections between language and reading disabilities* (pp. 3–24). Mahwah, NJ: Erlbaum.

Snow, C., Burns, S., & Griffin, P. (Eds.). (1998). *Preventing reading difficulties in young children*. Washington, DC: National Academy Press.

Snowling, M. (2005). Literacy outcomes for children with oral language impairments: Developmental interactions between language skills and learning to read. In H. Catts & A. Kamhi (Eds.), *The connections between language and reading disabilities* (pp. 55–75). Mahwah, NJ: Erlbaum.

Snowling, M., & Hulme, C. (Eds.). (2005). *The science of reading: A handbook*. Malden, MA: Blackwell.

Sparks, C. (1980). *The elephant man*. New York: Ballantine Books.

Stanovich, K. (1991). Word recognition: Changing perspectives. In R. Barr, M. Kamil, P. Mosenthal, & P. D. Pearson (Eds.), *Handbook of reading research* (2nd ed., pp. 418–452). White Plains, NY: Longman.

Stanovich, K. (1992). Speculations on the causes and consequences of individual differences in early reading acquisition. In P. Gough, L. Ehri, & R. Treiman (Eds.), *Reading acquisition* (pp. 307–342). Hillsdale, NJ: Erlbaum.

Sulzby, E., & Teale, W. (1987). *Young children's storybook reading: Longitudinal study of parent-child interaction and children's independent functioning*. Final Report to the Spencer Foundation. University of Michigan, Ann Arbor.

Sulzby, E., & Teale, W. (2003). The development of the young child and the emergence of literacy. In J. Flood, D. Lapp, J. Squire, & J. Jensen (Eds.), *Handbook of research on teaching the English language arts* (2nd ed., pp. 300–313). Mahwah, NJ: Erlbaum.

Tierney, R., & Pearson, P. D. (1983). Toward a composing model of reading. *Language Arts, 60*, 568–580.

Torres, S., Moreno-Torres, I., & Santana, R. (2006). Quantitative and qualitative evaluation of linguistic input support to a prelingually deaf child with cued speech: A case study. *Journal of Deaf Studies and Deaf Education, 11*(4), 438–448.

Treiman, R. (2006). Knowledge about letters as a foundation for reading and spelling. In R. M. Joshi & P. G. Aaron (Eds.), *Handbook of orthography and literacy* (pp. 581–599). Mahwah, NJ: Erlbaum.

Trezek, B., & Malmgren, K. (2005). The efficacy of utilizing a phonics treatment package with middle school deaf and hard-of-hearing students. *Journal of Deaf Studies and Deaf Education, 10*(3), 257–271.

Trezek, B., & Wang, Y. (2006). Implications of utilizing a phonics-based reading curriculum with children who are deaf or hard of hearing. *Journal of Deaf Studies and Deaf Education, 11*(2), 202–213.

Trezek, B. J., Wang, Y., & Paul, P. (2010). *Reading and deafness: Theory, research, and practice*. Clifton Park, NY: Delmar/Cengage Learning.

Trezek, B. J., Wang, Y., Woods, D. G., Gampp, T. L., & Paul, P. (2007). Using visual phonics to supplement beginning reading instruction for students who are deaf/hard of hearing. *Journal of Deaf Studies and Deaf Education, 12*(3), 373–384.

Waddy-Smith, B., & Wilson, V. (2003). *See that sound! Visual phonics helps deaf and hard of hearing students develop reading skills*. Retrieved July 23, 2009, from http://clerccenter2.gallaudet.edu/KidsWorldDeafNet/e-docs/Keys/see.html.

Wang, Y., Lee, C., & Paul, P. V. (2010). An understanding of the literacy levels of students who are deaf/hard-of-hearing in the United States, China, and South Korea. *L1 Educational Studies in Language and Literature, 10*(1), 87–98.

Wang, Y., Trezek, B., Luckner, J., & Paul, P. (2008). The role of phonology and phonological-related skills in reading instruction for students who are deaf or hard of hearing. *American Annals of the Deaf, 153*(4), 396–407.

Williams, C. (2004). Emergent literacy of deaf children. *Journal of Deaf Studies and Deaf Education, 9*(4), 352–365.

Yurkowski, P., & Ewoldt, C. (1986). A case for the semantic processing of the deaf reader. *American Annals of the Deaf, 131*, 243–247.

Further Readings

Bailey, A. (Ed.). (2007). *The language demands of school: Putting academic English to the test.* New Haven, CT: Yale University Press.

Bernstein, D., & Tiegerman-Farber, E. (2004). *Language and communication disorders in children* (5th ed.). Boston: Allyn & Bacon.

Chall, J., Jacobs, V., & Baldwin, L. (1990). *The reading crisis: Why poor children fall behind.* Cambridge, MA: Harvard University Press.

Chomsky, N. (2006). *Language and mind* (3rd ed.). New York: Cambridge University Press.

Pinker, S. (1994). *The language instinct: How the mind creates language.* New York: William Morrow & Company.

SPEECHREADING AND AUDITORY DEVELOPMENT

. . . those who study the book may, by watching others' lips, be able to understand what is said. So the student must not look upon the lessons, explanations, and remarks as things to be memorized, but only as things to make the subject in hand clear and so help the ultimate end. So, too, the systems of symbols used in the book are a means to the ultimate end and not an end in themselves. Therefore I would say to the student, do not let the apparent amount and difficulty of the work (due to present unfamiliarity with it) discourage you or turn you aside from the study. Take only a little at a time, and results are certain. Do not forget, too, that results will not come overnight; there will be no miracle. If you were taking music lessons, you would expect to practice faithfully and with the combined result of time and practice to bring perfection. So must it be with any study, and lipreading is no exception.

—Nitchie (1902/1979, p. 1)

All respondents emphasize the primary importance of using audition to the greatest degree possible; however, there is also acknowledgement of the secondary use of vision (at least as a back-up). Disagreement seems to center around the exact nature of the training procedures, in issues such as when visual cues should be introduced, in exactly what manner, and to what degree they should be allowed in training and natural situations. . . . An auditory approach has benefits and goals that include four areas: maximal use of listening abilities, intelligible spoken language, integration in regular educational settings and mainstream society, and fostering independence.

—Cole & Gregory (1986, pp. 9–10)

Key Concepts

After completing this chapter, you should have a basic understanding of:

- The nature and study of speechreading

- The nature and study of auditory development

- Implications for instruction and further research

We mentioned previously in this book that one of the most challenging goals for educators and clinicians is to assist children and adolescents in accessing and developing the basic foundations of the oral component of English or, in other words, oral language ability and comprehension (e.g., Bader, 2001; Luetke-Stahlman, 1999; see also the discussions in Spencer & Marschark, 2006). On one level, individuals need to be able to access the sounds of English (i.e., phonological development) in order to acquire English. As discussed in Chapters 6 and 7, the use of oral language ability, particularly phonological skills, is instrumental—but not sufficient—for the development of English literacy; that is, reading and writing skills. Access to phonology and other components is also necessary for acquiring the spoken or conversational form of English (e.g., Crystal, 1995, 1997, 2006; Wang, Trezek, Luckner, & Paul, 2008).

This conflation of oral and written language should not be surprising after your reading of the previous two chapters. Even though there are differences between oral and written language, it is best to remember the insights of Sticht and James (1984):

> . . . these **unique** properties of the written language should not lead to approaches to teaching reading, especially early reading, which deny the fundamental **commonalities** among oral and written language that have been achieved through the ages by "one of the greatest and most momentous triumphs of the human mind," the alphabet. (p. 315)

In essence, the differences between oral and written language do not undermine the need to develop oral language skills. Traditionally, the three major components of oral language that have been the focus of development with children who are d/Deaf or hard of hearing are speech, speechreading, and auditory development (also known as auditory training/learning) (e.g., see discussions in Ling, 1989, 2001, 2002; Paul, 2009). In Chapter 7, we indicated that alternative methods might be needed to assist children and adolescents with these oral language components (e.g., cued speech/language and visual phonics). In addition, we remarked that such development can be aided by the use of amplification systems such as digital hearing aids and cochlear implants (e.g., see discussions in Harrison, 2006; Spencer & Marschark, 2006; see also Chapters 4 and 5).

The crux of this matter needs to be highlighted—often repeatedly: even with the use of amplification systems, the oral language correlates—namely, speech, speechreading, and auditory development—still need to be learned or, for the most part, subjected to intensive direct intervention techniques (e.g., Bader, 2001; Harrison, 2006; Luetke-Stahlman, 1999; Paul, 2009). This learning process is often referred to as *aural habilitation*, or the learning of new "aural" (i.e., listening) skills, in children and as *aural rehabilitation*, or "relearning" of listening skills, in adults.

Listening comprehension (or listening skill), to be specific, does not develop simply because one can hear or speak. In addition, listening comprehension (which has been termed *auding* in Sticht & James, 1984) is essential for the development of literacy skills in English (e.g., Cain & Oakhill, 2007; Nation, 2005). As noted in Chapter 5 and as will be stated again in Chapter 10, cochlear implantation—the combination of an appropriately programmed device along with an *intensive* and *systematic* program of aural habilitation and/or rehabilitation—has provided a strong model for success in developing skills for functional listening and learning.

Bader (2001) argues that children who are d/Deaf or hard of hearing need to develop a *listening attitude*, or what we call a *listening consciousness*. In short, children need to learn to be aware of sound stimuli, especially speech stimuli, in their environment. Children need to be tuned in to the possibility of sounds that might be present. This is most important for children who are learning to use hearing aids, cochlear implants, or assistive listening devices.

Flexer (1999) suggests that facilitating listening skills does not begin until the child has been fit with appropriate amplification and has had medical-related issues (e.g., otitis media) diagnosed and managed. In addition, she states that the primary listening environment needs to be addressed (e.g., controlled for noise or the use of assistive technology, such as an FM system, discussed in Chapter 4, has been utilized).

In this chapter, we focus on the development of oral language components via the use of speechreading and auditory development. We should emphasize that such development is an essential part of early intervention, described in detail in the next chapter (Chapter 9). In this chapter, we shall focus on the nature and study of both speechreading and auditory development and offer a few guidelines with respect to instruction and further research.

Prior to proceeding, we encourage you to construct questions that you think should be or can be answered by the information in this chapter. For example, you might inquire:

- What is speechreading? Is this similar to or different from lip reading?

- How has research on speechreading been conducted?

- How can speechreading be developed?

- Are there any consistent instructional guidelines for instruction in speechreading?

- What is auditory development? How can audition be developed?

- Are there any consistent instructional guidelines for instruction in auditory development?

- What are the foci for further research on speechreading and auditory development?

Perhaps you have already formed some conceptions regarding these questions based on the two passages at the beginning of this chapter. Not only are there disagreements on the nature of these notions, but there are also disagreements on the manner in which they should be investigated and developed. We shall push you further with the following, additional questions:

- Are speechreading and auditory development skills dependent on both science (i.e., research) and art (i.e., personal idiosyncrasies)?

- How much can we develop these entities, even with the use of modern amplification systems?

- Is development (and, consequently, the skill, itself) a reflection of perception only, or must it be consider in light of other cognitive skills?

Although we cannot promise to answer all of these questions completely, or even to your satisfaction, we hope that we can provide enough insights to stimulate further reading, discussion, and even research. We strongly encourage you to review or to recall what we have said so far, in previous chapters, about the interrelations among hearing, speech, language, and literacy. Let us continue this discussion with a description of speechreading.

The Nature of Speechreading

It should come as no surprise that there is no consensus on the definition or description of speechreading (e.g., Jeffers & Barley, 1971; O'Neill & Oyer, 1981; Silverman & Kricos, 1990; see also the discussions in Paul, 2009; Trezek, Wang, & Paul, 2010). Simply stated, speechreading refers to the process of understanding a spoken message (Berger, 1972; De Filippo & Sims, 1988; Dodd & Campbell, 1987; Jeffers & Barley, 1971; O'Neill & Oyer, 1981; Silverman & Kricos, 1990). This general description is similar to what has been proffered for reading, namely that reading is understanding the printed message or written language (e.g., see discussions in Israel & Duffy, 2009).

Obviously, this simple description understates the complicated process and development of speechreading. Traditionally, the label *lip reading* has been used to describe this process. However, the comprehension of the spoken message seems to involve more than just reading the lips, albeit the lips do provide a substantial or the overwhelming bulk of the information. Interestingly, the eyes and their surrounding areas are also important or at least complement the message (e.g., see Paul, 1988, 2009).

Historically, several debates have focused on the manner in which speechreading should be developed. Much of the discussion has focused on the role of audition (Berger, 1972; De Filippo & Sims, 1988; Dodd & Campbell, 1987; Jeffers & Barley, 1971; O'Neill & Oyer, 1981; Silverman & Kricos, 1990). It is often argued that there should be a continuing understanding of the process of speechreading with or without the aid of amplification. In light of the proliferation and ubiquity of amplification systems, this seems to be an outdated comparison. Nevertheless, as argued by Paul (2009), research is still necessary in this area so that educators can understand the contribution and role of perception, without audition, to the speechreading process. It is expected that much of the research will emphasize speechreading in conjunction with amplification. There is little doubt that speechreading skill can be enhanced by audition or residual hearing.

Before proceeding, we think it is instructive for you to participate in a speechreading test. Select someone from your class to be the speaker and have that person mouth naturally, with no voice, the following sentences in random order (or create additional sentences).

- The fat man ran fast, and this surprised me.

- What is your name?

- The taxi comes every hour.

- I cannot stand her.

- That John is a maniac was obvious to Marcy.

Now, compare your responses to the actual sentences above. What words did you miss? Why do you think you missed those words? Do you think it would have helped if you knew the topic of the sentence (this works better for a short passage)? How do you think you would have performed if you had to speechread a paragraph? A passage? All day long?

We dare you to watch television with both the sound and the captions inactivated. You either will become extremely frustrated and fatigued or you will appreciate the task of many children who are d/Deaf or hard of hearing (or both and more!). Speechreading is not easy; it can be learned or improved, but it is still a subtle art (Silverman & Kricos, 1990).

Because of the subtlety of speechreading, it has been extremely difficult to conduct research on children and adolescents. In fact, after an intense period of research in the 1960s, 1970s, and 1980s, there have been sporadic investigations (e.g., see review in Paul, 2009). We invite you to think about the possible components involved in speechreading. In fact, in discussing the exploration of speechreading, the paradigm developed by O'Neill and Oyer (1981) has been most productive, as explicated in the following section.

Components of Speechreading

What do you think might be the major components of speechreading? In examining the concept of speechreading, O'Neill and Oyer (1981) proposed four broad areas: speaker-sender, environment, lip reader-receiver, and code-stimulus. For the most part, the speaker-sender variable refers to the factors of the speaker that impact the comprehension of the lip reader-receiver. A few of these conditions are associated with the delivery of the speech signal, such as type and rate of articulation, and speech features, such as coarticulation and nasality. The speaker's style (e.g., prosody) is also important, especially if there is the presence of a specific dialect or use of regional terms.

Another important speaker-sender variable is the characteristics of the speaker's face. For example, effects might be due to conditions such as the size and movement of the lips. Even the use of facial expressions (or lack of expressions) might affect speechreading ability. Another area on which there is little or no research, to the best of our knowledge, is the relationship between the speaker and receiver; that is, personality issues or conflicts. It would seem that whether the receiver is interested in the speaker-sender would also have an effect on the receiver's ability to perceive the message.

Factors associated with the environment include lighting; distractions, visual and auditory; and the distance between the speaker-sender and the speechreader-receiver. The noise level of the room, as discussed in Chapter 2, can be an impediment to the speechreader, who is dependent on amplification or residual hearing. Reducing extraneous noise or reverberation is a critical task.

The viewing angle of the speaker-sender and the speechreader-receiver represents another critical factor. Typically, we can consider the vertical and horizontal dimensions. For example, if the speechreader is seated in a chair and the speaker is standing directly in front of the speechreader, the angle can be described as 35 degrees vertical, 0 degrees horizontal. If both the speechreader and speaker are seated in chairs and facing each other, this can be described as 0 degrees vertical and horizontal. It is sometimes overlooked that the angle of vision is important for classroom situations involving d/Deaf and hard of hearing children.

O'Neill and Oyer (1981) and others (Berger, 1972; De Filippo & Sims, 1988; Dodd & Campbell, 1987; Jeffers & Barley, 1971; Silverman & Kricos, 1990) have remarked that the speechreader-receiver (i.e., in their words, *lip reader-receiver*) is the most complex category to explore. Silverman and Kricos (1990) have implied that it might indeed be this category that contributes most to the difficulty of developing adequate speechreading assessments and tends to give the impression that speechreading is still pretty much of a subtle art. A few speechreader-receiver factors include prior or world knowledge; affective issues, such as motivation or interest; language and cognitive competence; and visual perceptual abilities.

Another complex domain in this category is the interactions among the speechreader-receiver factors. Silverman and Kricos (1990) make this point eloquently:

> Pertinent are orientation to the specific situation in which oral exchange is taking place; concentration which may be vulnerable to fatigue after long periods of looking; alertness to changes in subject of conversation; interest in subject of conversation; background of the speechreader's information, the wider the better; emotional set and sociability that freely encourage association with others and provide opportunity for practice in speechreading, obsessive fear of making mistakes, or conversely, to be undaunted by them; motivation and perseverance; approval or avoidance; and the speechreader's language competency, whether hearing-impaired child or adult. (p. 24)

The content, quantity, and quality of the spoken message reflect another major category, labeled *code-stimulus*. A few factors in this category include the visibility of the speech sounds, rate of speaking, the difficulty level of vocabulary, and length and types of sentences and connected discourse (i.e., across sentences). Similar to the speechreader-receiver domain, these factors have caused difficulty with the development of adequate and complete speechreading assessments. The challenges range from the types and length of words to the use of sentences or short passages.

One of the major sources of difficulties in speechreading development is the visibility of sounds, which is, for the most part, a perceptual issue. For example, many words look similar on the lips, which, we bet, caused problems for you in the speechreading test, previously administered (e.g., see discussions in Berger, 1972; De Filippo & Sims, 1988; Dodd & Campbell, 1987; Jeffers & Barley, 1971; O'Neill & Oyer, 1981; Silverman & Kricos, 1990). For example, consider the articulatory movements associated with the beginning letters of words such as *ball*, *pall*, and *mall*. The /b/, /p/, and /m/ look similar on the lips. Other similar-looking clusters of letters include /f/ and /v/and that of /t/ and /d/. Of course, another challenge is homonyms, particularly homophones such as *mane* and *main*, *pane* and *pain*, *tale* and *tail*, and so on.

It should be clear that speechreading is a complex activity. What seems to puzzle a number of people is that speechreading skill is dependent, in part, on language ability. All things considered, it is not uncommon for a number of individuals who are hearing to actually perform better on a speechreading task than individuals who are d/Deaf or hard of hearing. **Table 8-1** lists the main points relative to the components of speechreading.

Research on Speechreading

Given the purported importance of speechreading, even as an alternative approach, to the development of English, particularly of the phonological component, it is somewhat surprising that there have not been a preponderant number of investigations (see reviews and discussions in Luetke-Stahlman, 1999; Paul, 2009; see also a strong discussion of the limitations of speechreading in Wang et al., 2008). More important, the research on children and adolescents who are d/Deaf or hard of hearing is extremely limited.

Specifically, researchers have not adhered to the suggestion of Moeller (in Luetke-Stahlman, 1999) that there should be formal and informal assessments administered in a variety of settings and that such assessments should provide strengths and areas of improvement similar to criterion-referenced or diagnostic tests (see discussions of diagnostic and related tests in Anastasi & Urbina, 1997; Borg & Gall, 1983). Most speechreading tests are designed for the observer to render general qualitative remarks about the speechreader-receiver (e.g., good, average, fair, poor), rather than to prescribe or diagnose specific instructional lessons. In essence, Moeller is arguing for a link between assessment and speechreading instruction. This principle has been argued vehemently elsewhere for all children, including those who are d/Deaf or hard of hearing (e.g., see Pearson & Stallman, 1994; Trezek et al., 2010).

With respect to the framework of O'Neill and Oyer (1981), discussed previously, researchers have examined the relationships between training techniques and the improvement of speechreading skills (e.g., Black, O'Reilly, & Peck, 1963; Crawford, Dancer, Pittenger, 1986; Squires & Dancer, 1986). Specifically, few studies have examined the effects of speechreading and vibrotactile aid training (i.e., the use of devices worn by a person with a hearing loss that represent sound energy in vibrations). Effects from other aids and approaches, such as cochlear implants and cued speech/language, have also been documented (see also the review in Paul, 2009; Wang et al., 2008).

Other researchers have attempted to delineate the relationships of factors such as age, gender, and education and speechreading ability (e.g., Dancer, Krain, Thompson, Davis, & Glenn, 1994). Finally, a number of investigations have attempted to describe the relations between (and among) speechreading and other pertinent educational variables such as academic achievement, age at onset of hearing impairment, degree of hearing impairment,

Table 8-1	

The Nature and Components of Speechreading

Nature of Speechreading

- There is no consensus on the definition or description of speechreading.

- Speechreading refers to the process of understanding a spoken message.

- Traditionally, the label *lip reading* has been used to describe this process. However, the comprehension of the spoken message seems to involve more than just reading the lips.

- It is often argued that there should be a continuing understanding of the process of speechreading with or without the aid of amplification.

- Speechreading is not easy; it can be learned or improved, but it is still a subtle art.

Components of Speechreading

- O'Neill and Oyer (1981) proposed four broad areas: speaker-sender, environment, lip reader-receiver, and code-stimulus.

- The speaker-sender variable refers to the factors of the speaker that impact the comprehension of the lip reader-receiver. A few of these conditions are associated with the delivery of the speech signal, such as type and rate of articulation, and speech features, such as coarticulation and nasality.

- Factors associated with the environment include lighting; distractions, visual and auditory; and distance between the speaker-sender and the speechreader-receiver.

- A few speechreader-receiver factors include prior or world knowledge; affective issues, such as motivation or interest; language and cognitive competence; and visual perceptual abilities. The speechreader-receiver area is the most difficult to investigate.

- The content, quantity, and quality of the spoken message reflect another major category, labeled *code-stimulus*. A few factors in this category include the visibility of the speech sounds, rate of speaking, the difficulty level of vocabulary, and length and types of sentences and connected discourse (i.e., across sentences).

intelligence, linguistic skills, perceptual skills, and personality traits (e.g., see De Filippo & Sims, 1988; Farwell, 1976; Paul, 1988, 2009).

Unfortunately, these paradigms have not changed much, even in light of the research on other domains, such as language and literacy development (e.g., see Luetke-Stahlman, 1999; Marschark, Lang, & Alberini, 2002; Moores, 2001; Paul, 2009; Trezek et al., 2010). More complex, comprehensive paradigms are needed, but such research is hampered by the availability of good speechreading tests, as discussed later. There is also a need to investigate speechreading in conjunction with domains such as auditory development and speech (e.g., see Luetke-Stahlman, 1999; see also the discussions in Ling, 1989, 2002; Stoker & Ling, 1992).

Nevertheless, it is possible to proffer some general—albeit cautious—findings. However, as noted by Paul (2009), it is not feasible to provide clear, unambiguous guidelines for the development of speechreading skills, even in classroom situations. This does not mean that there are no implications for the types of instructional strategies that might have a positive effect on speech production and perception in children, especially in conjunction with sensory aids such as cochlear implants and digital hearing aids.

To provide an example of what we mean by general findings, we quote the summary passage by the research of Dancer and colleagues (1994) on adults, which seems to be relevant and representative of such research:

1. There were not statistically-significant effects of education on the speechreading scores of this sample of 50 persons, which consisted of higher than average socioeconomic individuals ranging in age from 20–69 and having no hearing or vision complaints.

2. There was a statistically-significant effect of gender on speechreading scores: females scored higher than males.

3. There was a statistically-significant interaction between gender and practice on speechreading performance: females increased their performance from a first to a second trial; males did not.

4. There was a statistically-significant effect of age group on speechreading scores in females: 30- and 40-year old females scored higher than the other age groups. (p. 35)

What is the future for explorations in speechreading? First of all, we know that the findings on adults cannot be generalized indiscriminately to younger populations such as children and adolescents (e.g., Dancer et al., 1994; Samar & Sims, 1983; Shepherd, 1982; Spradlin, Dancer, & Monfils, 1989). It has been documented that children can speechread short, syntactically simple sentences more easily than the long complex sentences, especially those that involve embedded elements such as relative clauses (e.g., *The boy who kissed the girl ran away*). In fact, children seem to have fewer difficulties with subject-verb-object (S-V-O) constructions (e.g., *The girl is happy*). Ironically, this situation seems to mirror d/Deaf and hard of hearing children's understanding of syntax in English as well (e.g., see discussion of the research of Quigley and collaborators in Paul, 2001, 2009); that is, children and adolescents understand sentences of the S-V-O constructions better than those that do not follow this order (e.g., *The boy who kissed the girl ran away. The dog was bit by the cat.*).

Just as there is a critical period for the development of auditory skills, current research has suggested that there may be an early optimal stage for the development of visual perceptual skills that contributes to improved speechreading skills. Infants demonstrate a strong ability to make visual discriminations. Weikum and her colleagues (2007) found that 4- to 6-month-old infants can visually discriminate one language from another; however, by age 8 months, this ability is diminished. It was suggested that the infants' sensitivity to visual language discrimination decreases at this age, unless the child is learning more than one language at that time. These findings suggest that sensitivity to speechreading skills may occur earlier than previously determined and may involve different mechanisms for children than for adults.

Because there seems to be a wide gap between knowledge of speechreading and how this translates into practice, there has been a call for more sophisticated research designs. Multidisciplinary and multifaceted approaches are needed that take into account the interactive effects of numerous variables, especially those delineated within the O'Neill and Oyer framework, that have been studied in previous speechreading studies.

Future research in speechreading is likely to involve the use of the computer and other technology. For example, some of the more recently developed analytic approaches to speechreading have utilized computer-based applications such as Computer-Aided Speechreading Training (CAST) (Pichora-Fuller & Benguerel, 1991) and Computerized Laser Videodisc Programs for Training Speechreading and Assertive Communication Behaviors (Tye-Murray, Tyler, Bong, & Nares, 1988). As noted by Gagne and Jennings (2000), although the computerized programs that focus on speechreading have not been the panacea that was expected with regard to improving speech-perception competencies for individuals with hearing loss, they certainly provide additional training for those motivated to improve these skills.

We also need new directions or foci in explorations in speechreading. For example, it is often forgotten that the perception of suprasegmental or prosodic aspects (i.e., pitch, loudness, rate, and stress) contribute to the understanding or perception of syllables (or combination of segmental aspects) (e.g., see Ling, 1976; 2002; Sanders, 1982). During development, infants become aware of the rhythm and prosodic aspects of speech prior to the segmental aspects. Does this awareness, or its subsequent development, contribute to speechreading ability?

For analogical purposes, consider the differences in fingerspelling patterns between children who know American Sign Language (ASL) and those with a range of knowledge of English, including English phonology and morphology. The rate and rhythm of the fingerspelling of children who know English reflect the phonological and morphological properties of English. This is not necessarily the case for the fingerspelling of children for whom ASL is the first or only language. Does this type of fingerspelling pattern contribute to speechreading ability? What are the effects of working with children who know ASL as a first language on the development of speechreading skills?

Another interesting area for future investigations is to focus on pragmatics and examine, for instance, communicative interaction breakdowns. Consider the occurrences of errors between the speaker-sender and the listener-receiver. In essence, both parties might engage in strategies to remedy the situation. Both persons might decide on a plan of action, individually, and/or one that entails a dynamic interplay between them (i.e., dialoguing back and forth for clarification purposes). These techniques seem to reflect what actually occurs during speechreading situations; however, there is difficulty in addressing or examining them. Consider the issue of topic shifts or the difficulty of information—both of which are impacted by variables such as prior knowledge and inferencing (e.g., see discussions in Paul, 1988, 2009).

One of the most challenging domains for future researchers is to decide on the appropriateness and completeness of an adequate speechreading assessment. This challenge seems to be similar to those involved in constructing language or literacy assessments; that is, it is not likely that there will ever be one complete test of speechreading or, at least, a test that can be administered in one sitting or fits all situations involving speechreading. In essence, there seems to be the need for multiple tests.

With respect to assessment, Silverman and Kricos (1990) offered an eloquent summary, which is still relevant:

> Since existing speechreading tests fail to provide completely reliable and valid information, it has been suggested that a battery might consist of a number of tests including a measure of consonant recognition, word discrimination, identification of everyday sentences, and comprehension of connected speech. One notes with irony, however, that this battery approach differs little from Conklin's 1917 proposal for speechreading measurement. (p. 31)

Table 8-2 provides a brief summary of points relative to research on speechreading.

Facilitation of Speechreading Skills

Now that you have a fairly decent understanding of the challenges of speechreading, we shall offer some suggestions for facilitating speechreading development. Ironically, we may not have progressed much further than the potpourri of lessons offered by Nitchie (1902/1979), quoted at the beginning of this chapter. In his little book are 35 lessons, ranging from simple to complex (actually, extremely complex). Many of these activities probably seem ludicrous to the modern mind. For example, Nitchie recommended the following activity:

> Using the mirror, turn the following into English.
> So-na el-ep st-ag ep-mo-tg-rn tg-so ag-lo-it el-tg tf-el ls-ag (p. 125)

And this goes on and on for more than a half page. Apparently, it is the beginning of a passage taken from one of Robert Louis Stevenson's writings (*The Amateur Emigrant*). The disambiguation of this passage, as written, depends on the reader's understanding of lip

<table>

Table
8-2

Research on Speechreading

Research Points and Findings

- Research is necessary on the contribution and role of perception, without audition, to the speechreading process.

- Given the purported importance of speechreading, even as an alternative approach, to the development of English, particularly of the phonological component, it is somewhat surprising that there has not been a preponderant amount of investigations.

- There should be formal and informal assessments administered in a variety of settings and such assessments should provide strengths and areas of improvement similar to criterion-referenced or diagnostic tests.

- Studies have examined the effects of speechreading and vibrotactile aid training. Effects from other aids and approaches, such as cochlear implants and cued speech/language, have also been documented.

- Other researchers have attempted to delineate the relationships of factors such as age, gender, and education and speechreading ability.

- A number of investigations have attempted to describe the relationships between (and among) speechreading and other pertinent educational variables such as academic achievement, age at onset of hearing impairment, degree of hearing impairment, intelligence, linguistic skills, perceptual skills, and personality traits.

- More complex, comprehensive paradigms are needed, but such research is hampered by the availability of good speechreading tests. There is also a need to investigate speechreading in conjunction with other domains, such as auditory development and speech.

- It is not feasible to provide clear, unambiguous guidelines for the development of speechreading skills, even in classroom situations.

- The findings on adults cannot be generalized indiscriminately to younger populations such as adolescents and children.

- Children can speechread short, syntactically simple sentences more easily than long complex sentences, especially those that involve embedded elements such as relative clauses (e.g., *The boy who kissed the girl ran away*). In fact, children seem to have fewer difficulties with subject-verb-object (S-V-O) constructions (e.g., *The girl is happy*).

</table>

movements and the production of sounds (i.e., articulators), presumably while working with a mirror. It takes practice and ingenuity, but we will have to break down and check out Stevenson's book later since this is beyond our ken.

A few practical suggestions (or facilitators) for classroom use of speechreading activities have been offered by Luetke-Stahlman (1999), and these are based on the model of O'Neill and Oyer (1981) discussed throughout this chapter:

1. **English language proficiency**. Short phrases known by the student are easier and should be practiced first. Practice individual words later.

2. **Viewing angle of the speaker**. Speechreading at 0 degrees (in front of the student) is easiest and should be practiced first, then 45 degrees, and then 90 degrees (to the student's side).

3. **Visibility of the speaker**. The more visible the upper torso of the speaker, the easier it is to speechread.

4. **Rate of speech**. A slower-than-average rate of speech has been found to be the easiest to speechread. Practice with normal rates of speech should occur later.

5. **Familiarity and age of the speaker**. Knowing the personality of people (relatives and close friends) makes it easier to understand them. Young children with immature language might be more difficult to speechread than those in at least third grade.

6. **Distance from the speaker**. The closer, the better. Training is most meaningful when it is done at distances most representative of typical daily conversational situations (between 4 and 10 feet).

7. **Lighting on the speaker**. Typical classroom lighting is sufficient for optimum speechreading. Bright light, glare, or an overhead projection light behind a speaker can black out or darken his or her face for the student who is D/HH and can make speechreading difficult.

8. **Visual distractions**. Certain characteristics of people or the apparel that they wear can affect speechreading. Adults working with students who are D/HH should not wear dark glasses; have a beard or mustache; wear long, dangling earrings; have long, flowing hair that covers part of the face; move hands or objects in front of the face; or speak with a pencil or other object in the mouth. (pp. 110–111)

Luetke-Stahlman (1999) and others (e.g., Bader, 2001) have averred that speechreading activities should be integrated with other areas such as speech and auditory development to maximize development. In essence, it is proffered that there are intricate, facilitative interactions among speech, speechreading, and audition—a point also made in this chapter and in earlier chapters. The development of audition is undertaken in the next section.

Auditory Development

It should come as no surprise that the development of audition in children who are d/Deaf or hard of hearing proceeds through stages that are similar to children who have typical hearing (Bader, 2001; Ling, 1989, 2002; for a variety of views, see Spencer & Marschark,

2006). This is similar to the qualitative-similarity hypothesis, which has been applied to the development of language and literacy (e.g., see discussions in Paul, 2008, 2009). Bader (2001) briefly describes this process as follows:

> During the first year of life, infants develop an affective bond with parents, who reinforce the infants' social, motor, and vocal responses to auditory events. As parents attach communicative intent to these responses, an infant begins to associate sounds with their source and meaning. For at least a full year, toddlers then attempt verbal reproductions of the sounds they have heard. Those sounds include their own babble . . . important to integrating the auditory and kinesthetic feedback functions in the brain. The development of that auditory feedback mechanism is the means by which children learn to approximate adult forms of spoken language. Naturally, more speech dimensions are available to children with more hearing and to those children who are appropriately amplified. (p. 118)

The facilitation, assessment, and remediation of audition can be discussed with respect to the chronological age periods of children and adolescents such as birth to 3, 3 to 5, and so on. If access to the auditory signal is limited or distorted, then many children will have difficulty with the development of speech perception and speech discrimination abilities (e.g., Bader, 2001; Ling, 1986, 1989, 2002; Luetke-Stahlman, 1999). Given the fact that speech is a continuous auditory signal, a number of children experience difficulty in recognizing differences (sometimes minimal) in patterns of speech with respect to features such as time (e.g., pauses or gaps), intensity, and pitch. This can result in difficulties in discriminating between sounds, syllables, words, and phrases at various levels. Discrimination difficulties can lead to difficulties with language comprehension (e.g., Bader, 2001; Erber, 1982; Sanders, 1982)

With respect to discrimination, children need to be able to discern a speech signal from background noise, to distinguish between voice and voiceless sounds, and so on. The various types of challenges are related to the degree of hearing impairment, to some extent; however, the correlation is not always clear-cut. In Chapter 6, we described the speech perception and production difficulties of students with hearing losses from mild to profound. These findings have been modified with improvements in technology, such as cochlear implants or hearing aids with frequency transposition. As noted by Flexer (1999), it is critical to remember that "any type and degree of hearing impairment can present a significant barrier to an infant's or child's ability to receive information from the environment" (p. 6).

The development of audition has been labeled *auditory learning* (e.g., see discussion in Cole & Gregory, 1986; Osberger, 1990). Regardless of how it is labeled, and despite the differences of opinions in educators and researchers (see passage at the head of this chapter), auditory training/learning refers to the use of techniques to assist children in their development of audition or to maximize use of residual hearing.

Many of the concepts and ideas for developing audition are based on the work of early pioneers such as Erber (1982), Ling (1976, 2002), and Sanders (1982) (see discussions in Bader, 2001; Luetke-Stahlman, 1999). In fact, the model of Erber (1982) has been used (and elaborated on) to assess and facilitate auditory development. This model focuses on four concepts—detection, discrimination, identification, and comprehension—to be discussed in the ensuing paragraphs. Comprehension is not only the highest skill, but also the desired goal of auditory training/learning activities. The other three levels—detection, discrimination, and identification—are important but are not sufficient for the development of listening comprehension skills.

DETECTION

Detection is the first stage and refers to the awareness or absence of a sound (e.g., Bader, 2001; Erber, 1982; Sanders, 1982). Any test of detection simply requires the child to respond on an awareness level—is there a sound or not? The basic task used in pure tone audiometry is also a detection task, as outlined in Chapter 3. Children with amplification devices (hearing aids, etc.) may need to learn to tune in to the possibility that a sound can be heard or that a sound might be present. In other words, they need to learn to respond to a sound that they have never heard before.

Three common detection assessment tools are the Six Sound Hearing Test (Ling, 1976, 2002), the GASP (Glendonald School for the Deaf Auditory Screening Procedure) Subtest 1 (Erber, 1982), and the MAIS (Meaningful Auditory Integration Scale) (Robbins, Svirsky, Osberger, & Pisoni, 1996). Readers can consult sources for complete descriptions of each assessment.

We shall focus here on the Six Sound Hearing Test as an example because it is widely used due to its simplicity. The Ling 6 Sound Test entails phonemes of low, middle, and high frequencies that replicate the broad speech sound spectrum utilized in conventional audiometry testing, similar to the range in the pure tone audiogram (see Chapter 3). Ling (1976) first introduced this test in 1976, known then as the Ling 5 Sound Test. Since that time, the number of phonemes included in the test has been expanded to 6 ([m], [ah], [oo], [ee], [sh], and [s]).

The Ling Test can be administered several times throughout the day to determine the status of a student's amplification or listening device, the challenges of listening in different acoustic environments, or the ability of the student to hear in a particular seat in the classroom (Ling, 1976, 2002). The listening or amplification device of the student can be manipulated such that the student can detect (not necessarily discriminate or identify) each of these sounds at some distance or situation while the teacher maintains or presents the sounds at a consistent volume level. Thus, the maximum distance from teacher and student can be established. The six sounds are typically presented in a random order. An example of the Ling Test, presenting the sounds up to a distance of 20 feet, is illustrated in **Table 8-3**.

The Six Sound Test can also be used for discrimination and identification purposes, and discrimination is discussed in the next section.

DISCRIMINATION

Discrimination refers to the ability to distinguish between different sounds (Bader, 2001; Ling, 1976, 2002). Children learn to discriminate between suprasegmentals initially, prior

Table
8-3

The Ling 6 Sound Test

THE LING 6 SOUND TEST
Recording Form

CHILD'S NAME: _____

INTERVENTIONIST: _____

DATE: _____

INSTRUCTIONS: *CIRCLE THE SOUNDS DETECTED*

DISTANCE SOUNDS DETECTED

Distance	Sounds
3 inches	/oo/ /ah/ /ee/ /s/ /sh/ /m/
6 inches	/oo/ /ah/ /ee/ /s/ /sh/ /m/
1 foot	/oo/ /ah/ /ee/ /s/ /sh/ /m/
2 feet	/oo/ /ah/ /ee/ /s/ /sh/ /m/
3 feet	/oo/ /ah/ /ee/ /s/ /sh/ /m/
4 feet	/oo/ /ah/ /ee/ /s/ /sh/ /m/
5 feet	/oo/ /ah/ /ee/ /s/ /sh/ /m/
6 feet	/oo/ /ah/ /ee/ /s/ /sh/ /m/
7 feet	/oo/ /ah/ /ee/ /s/ /sh/ /m/
8 feet	/oo/ /ah/ /ee/ /s/ /sh/ /m/
9 feet	/oo/ /ah/ /ee/ /s/ /sh/ /m/
10 feet	/oo/ /ah/ /ee/ /s/ /sh/ /m/
11 feet	/oo/ /ah/ /ee/ /s/ /sh/ /m/
12 feet	/oo/ /ah/ /ee/ /s/ /sh/ /m/
13 feet	/oo/ /ah/ /ee/ /s/ /sh/ /m/
14 feet	/oo/ /ah/ /ee/ /s/ /sh/ /m/
15 feet	/oo/ /ah/ /ee/ /s/ /sh/ /m/
16 feet	/oo/ /ah/ /ee/ /s/ /sh/ /m/
17 feet	/oo/ /ah/ /ee/ /s/ /sh/ /m/
18 feet	/oo/ /ah/ /ee/ /s/ /sh/ /m/
19 feet	/oo/ /ah/ /ee/ /s/ /sh/ /m/
20 feet	/oo/ /ah/ /ee/ /s/ /sh/ /m/

Note: Taken from Auditory Options; available at http://www.auditoryoptions.org/ling_six_chart.htm; downloaded December 2009. Sounds should be presented in a random order at each distance.

to segmentals. As discussed in Chapter 6, *suprasegmentals* refer to the perception of aspects such as frequency, intensity, rate, and stress or to prosodic elements. *Segmentals* refer to vowels and consonants. The type of discrimination used in this type of task makes use of gross cues, such as differences in sound qualities or duration (Flexer, 1999).

With respect to suprasegmentals, children can discriminate differences in the tone of their parents' voices from excitement and happiness to sadness and anger. They also discover that different people and objects have different sounds or make different sounds. According to Bader (2001): "Discrimination allows children to tell whether auditory patterns are the same or different from others. How sounds differ and what the sounds mean come later in the developmental schema" (p. 118). Luetke-Stahlman and Luckner (1991) remarked, "The primary purpose of assessing auditory discrimination is to determine objectives for the student who can detect sounds but who is having difficulty discriminating between two or more stimuli" (p. 206). This information may be useful in a number of ways, including programming hearing aids, mapping a cochlear implant processor, and developing goals for aural rehabilitation.

With discrimination tasks, children evaluate whether a particular sound is the same as or different from another sound. We have already mentioned that the Six Sound Test of Ling (1976, 2002) can be used as a discrimination task. In this case, children discriminate among the six sounds, presented in pairs as an example (not an easy task!). Other examples include beating on an object, such as a drum, for a number of times and requiring children to tell you the number of beats they heard.

Erber (1982) details the elements of the GASP Subtest 2, which can be utilized as both a detection and discrimination assessment. The items on this test are vocabulary words that are known by children being tested. It should be ensured that children are familiar with the set of words, especially because this is not a vocabulary test. For example, there may be pictures of items or objects in children's environment, such as a shoe, pencil, airplane, elephant, ball, table, popcorn, and so on. The examiner or teacher presents the known words in a random order. Standing behind the child, the examiner or teacher requests the child to repeat the word.

IDENTIFICATION

The task of identification requires memory, but not necessarily an understanding of the word. The child may identify animals associated with the sounds they make—for example, *cow–moo*; *pig–oink*; *sheep–baa*. Luetke-Stahlman (1999) provides good procedures for the use of the GASP Subtest 2 (Erber, 1982), mentioned previously, in identification tasks. Luetke-Stahlman (1999) has included adaptations so that this can be used with students who speak and sign for communicative interactions. We include two adaptations here:

1. The adult holds up or points to the stimulus items and says and/or signs the names of each of the items, allowing the student full access to all auditory and visual cues.

2. The adult says the names of each of the items (without holding up or pointing to the stimulus items), allowing the student to use both auditory and speechreading cues to make an auditory and visual match for each item. (p. 76)

In essence, identification tasks involve the use of suprasegmental and segmental aspects of speech, with more fine perception of cues required than for discrimination tasks (Flexer, 1999).

COMPREHENSION

Being the highest and most important stage of auditory development, children need to not only repeat or identify stimuli (e.g., set of sounds, words, etc.), but also demonstrate an understanding of the sounds. Obviously, such understanding is reflective of children's knowledge of their language and the communicative situations (e.g., see discussions in Crystal, 1997, 2006). In addition, as noted by Erber (1982), the skills described in this chapter are in a hierarchy, and comprehension is the scaffold for the skills of detection, discrimination, and identification—these skills must be mastered in order for this higher level of auditory processing to occur. Comprehension or understanding can be demonstrated via nonverbal cues, appropriate actions, or with the use of language.

In general, the procedures for comprehension assessments are somewhat similar to identification assessments. If we stay with Erber's approach (1982), then we can see the similarities with the use of the GASP Subtest 3. Initially, the therapist or teacher should ensure that the child can repeat each sentence appropriately and should be given permission to speechread. The child should be familiar with all vocabulary used in the sentences and should be familiar with the task. Then the actual test begins in which the therapist or teacher stands behind the child (or uses a blocking element such as a screen) and presents sentences in random order. The therapist or teacher requests a response to each question. A scoring guide is used to record the child's response.

This task can be modified to fit the demands and requirements of the school day. With some ingenuity, teachers can create questions that pertain to instructions or directions of worksheets or classroom dialogue. This provides teachers with additional information, particularly related to their children's language skills. No formal scoring guide is needed.

Similar to speechreading, auditory training/learning is also complex and difficult. With the advances in amplification, it is assumed that this development will become easier for children. **Table 8-4** provides major points on the components of auditory development.

 ## *General Summary of Auditory Activities*

It is interesting to track the development and use of auditory activities from the early training manuals to those focusing on listening or development. For example, the early auditory training manuals emphasize activities or conditions such as "wearing a hearing aid; participating in auditory exercises; having attention drawn to meaningful sounds; using sound for warning and arousal; modifying your own behavior so that the student must understand all or part of what you say through hearing alone; advising parents of the use of hearing and hearing aids" (Clarke School for the Deaf, 1971, p. vii).

The beginning activities require children to focus on tasks such as discriminating nonverbal sounds (e.g., bells and drums). After much practice in this area, the next step was

Table
8-4

The Nature and Components of Auditory Development

Auditory Development

- The development of audition in children who are d/Deaf or hard of hearing proceeds through stages that are similar to children who have typical hearing. This is similar to the qualitative-similarity hypothesis, which has been applied to the development of language and literacy.

- The facilitation, assessment, and remediation of audition can be discussed with respect to the chronological age periods of children and adolescents such as birth to 3, 3 to 5, and so on.

- If access to the auditory signal is limited or distorted, then many children will have difficulty with the development of speech perception and speech discrimination abilities.

- The development of audition has been labeled *auditory training* or *auditory learning.*

- The model of Erber (1982) has been used (and elaborated on) to assess and facilitate auditory development. This model focuses on four concepts: detection, discrimination, identification, and comprehension.

- Detection is the first stage and refers to the awareness or absence of a sound.

- Discrimination refers to the ability to distinguish between different sounds.

- The task of identification requires memory, but not necessarily an understanding of the word.

- Comprehension is the highest and most important stage of auditory development. Children need to not only repeat or identify stimuli (e.g., set of sounds, words, etc.), but also demonstrate an understanding of the sounds.

for children to discriminate among speech sounds, words, and sentences. Although these early training manuals have been criticized (e.g., see discussions in Cole & Gregory, 1986), it should be remembered that these activities were based on the relations between suprasegmentals and segmentals, which are sometimes neglected, as mentioned previously.

With the advent of digital hearing aids and cochlear implants, much of the current emphasis is on developing listening or comprehension skills (e.g., see Harrison, 2006).

This does not preclude the development of and attention to suprasegmental aspects. In essence, the alluring maxim is to teach the child to learn to listen and learn by listening, rather than to learn to hear (e.g., see discussions in Harrison, 2006; Ling, 1986; Osberger, 1990; see also the reviews in Paul, 2009; Spencer & Marschark, 2006).

This current process has been labeled *auditory learning* or *auditory development*. There are activities for developing spoken language, and these activities are related to the child's real-life experiences (e.g., see activities discussed in Luetke-Stahlman, 1999; Luetke-Stahlman & Luckner, 1991). Auditory learning or development stresses the comprehension of meaningful sounds, words, and sentences (e.g., Erber, 1982; Luetke-Stahlman, 1999; Sanders, 1982). The use of relevant activities in classrooms and even in clinical settings has been influenced by pragmatics, the language component that addresses the uses and functions of language (e.g., see Owens, 2004).

Several widely used programs, manuals, and curricula are available that contain development and assessment components (e.g., see Erber, 1982; Stout & Van ert Windle, 1992; Thies & Trammel, 1983; Van ert Windle & Stout, 1984). Thies and Trammel (1983) developed a model called the Auditory Skills Instructional Planning System. A section of this model that has had some appeal and use is the Test of Auditory Comprehension (TAC), which has components for placement. There is also the Auditory Skills Curriculum, which contains activities with sequenced objectives across four areas: discrimination, memory-sequencing, feedback, and figure-ground.

The Developmental Approach to Successful Listening-Revised (DASL) (Stout & Van ert Windle, 1992) highlights three types of hierarchical auditory skills: sound awareness, phonetic listening, and auditory comprehension. The hierarchy is based on the developmental stages of audition in young children (e.g., Bader, 2001).

During the sound awareness stage (also analogous to a general phonological awareness stage), the child becomes aware or is tuned in to amplified sounds. The activities for developing phonetic listening are based on major principles of the speech training program associated with Ling (1976). Ling (1976; see also 1989, 2002), as have others (e.g., see discussions in Bader, 2001; Crystal, 1997, 2006), asserted that children need to perceive both nonsegmental and segmental features of speech, especially for developing skills in language use. With respect to Stout and Van ert Windle (1992) and the development of auditory comprehension skills, it is remarked that children should engage in activities that focus on the discrimination and identification of common phrases. Stout and Van ert Windle (1992) recommend a progression from simple phrases to the comprehension of connected discourse.

Additional curricula are available that are either variations on the same themes or extensions with applications to classroom settings (e.g., Graham, 1992; Maxwell, 1981; Toomey, 1991). Nearly all curricula and programs are essentially related to the aspects of Erber's model (1982) involving detection, discrimination, identification, and comprehension. The issue now is to conduct more rigorous research paradigms to measure the effectiveness of either the programs or aspects or components.

With auditory learning or development, there is, obviously, a strong focus on the development of residual hearing. A few programs emphasize lessons that develop children's auditory skills for discriminating phonemes in syllables and words in phrases. There are also activities for the development of auditory memory skills. For example, with infants and toddlers, Simser (1993) suggested the following activities (only a sample of items of increasing difficulty are presented here):

- begin with repeated sound-word associations, e.g., tic-toc, tic-toc vs. moo-oo-oo, moo-oo-oo.
- identify known single items at the end of a sentence, e.g., "Give me the *car*," and then in the middle of a sentence "Put the *car* in the water."
- identify objects by listening to descriptive phrases, e.g., "It flies up in the sky, it has wings and you ride in it"—in closed and then open set.
- follow conversation of known topic.
- listen to a story and answer pertinent questions.
- follow conversation of undisclosed but familiar topic. (pp. 228–229)

With a greater emphasis on early identification of hearing loss, there has been an increase in developmental auditory curricula for infants and preschoolers. The John Tracy Clinic, founded in 1942 by actor Spencer Tracy and his wife Louise, was based on principles that the Tracys used in teaching their deaf son, John, auditory development and lip reading skills. The John Tracy Clinic has offered free correspondence courses for parents to support the development of listening and language skills for children birth to 5 years of age. Initially, these courses were offered by mail; however, parents can now complete the courses online. Another example is a curriculum designed for children as young as 3 years of age—the Speech Perception Instructional Curriculum and Evaluation (SPICE) (Moog, Biedenstein, & Davidson, 1995).

We need to borrow from the extensive work of Luetke-Stahlman (1999) again. This scholar promotes an integrated approach with auditory development that involves the use of speechreading and other cues such as fingerspelling, tactile, kinesthetic, print, and so on. She proposes that effective auditory facilitation activities embellish the following characteristics:

1. Assessment to establish stimuli that are slightly challenging to the student who is D/HH.

2. The use of spoken stimuli rather than noise or musical instruments if the outcome for the student is to comprehend auditory information. This does not preclude the inclusion of meaningful environmental sounds (the microwave buzzer, the telephone ringing, etc.).

3. Integration of speech, speechreading, and audition employed:
   - To encourage spoken interchanges
   - To verify auditory reception
   - To practice speech production

4. Expectation that speech and audition skills will be integrated daily into the academic areas.

5. Use of the adapted Cummins model to set targets and provide systematic facilitation in this communication area.

6. In addition to continued facilitation of speech articulation, possible instruction in musical instruments such as cello or piano for students who are ready for fine discrimination of sound. (pp. 80–81)

In addition, Luetke-Stahlman (1999), again adhering to Erber's (1982) model, proposes facilitation activities in all four areas of auditory development: detection, discrimination, identification, and comprehension.

The activities described by Luetke-Stahlman (1999) are certainly not exhaustive, but it requires the imagination of the clinician or teacher to create opportunities throughout the day for embedding auditory development activities. For the clinician, this can be related to language activities. For the teacher, students can use their auditory skills across the content areas in response to questions, discussing topics, or collaborating on a project.

In essence, the various auditory development approaches share many common features, especially those that stress auditory–verbal activities. Samples of activities for specific goals can be found in a number of sources (e.g., Erber, 1982; Sanders, 1982; see also the discussions in Luetke-Stahlman, 1999; Moog, Biedenstein, Davidson, & Brenner, 1994; Simser, 1993).

Current auditory development approaches seem to be similar to the use of natural methods for teaching speech and language, which have been in use for many years (e.g., Moores, 1996, 2001; Rose, McAnally, & Quigley, 2004). As mentioned previously, most of the approaches have been influenced by the use of pragmatics in language development (e.g., see discussion in Owens, 2004). These influences can be seen in both clinical and school settings.

A brief useful discussion of methods and approaches to develop and evaluate auditory and speech perception skills in children and adolescent can be found in Luetke-Stahlman (1999) and Osberger (1990). Past programs have become the foundation for the future of aural rehabilitation programs, integrating computer-based models and principles of an adaptive program, which challenges the person with a hearing loss to improve his or her listening skills in a progressive manner. As discussed in Chapter 4, the Listening and Communication Enhancement (LACE) program is a self-guided program that uses interesting and relevant stimuli, presented in a variety of situations, including with background noise, to develop listening skills in older children and adults (Sweetow & Henderson-Sabes, 2004). A renaissance of interest in aural rehabilitation in children started with cochlear implant protocols; however, models such as LACE have set the stage for successful implementation of systematic and intensive programs focusing on auditory development and integrating other types of skills such as speechreading and communication repair strategies, as outlined by Elfenbein (1992).

Kricos and McCarthy (2007) have suggested that programs that address auditory development into the twenty-first century will take into account collaborative approaches based on neuroscience, cognitive science, and auditory science in addition to the traditional therapy approaches adopted historically. These programs will be augmented by the creativity and imagination of clinicians and teachers and will capitalize on the new knowledge of auditory plasticity and cognitive neuroscience.

This chapter has highlighted that both auditory development (training/learning) and speechreading are important processes that can be, and perhaps must be, learned to maximize communication success for children with hearing loss. Despite even better technologies on the horizon, there "is a growing awareness and acceptance that devices and products have limitations dictated by our own sensory and neural systems. Auditory training may fill that gap" (Kricos & McCarthy, 2007, p. 96).

Summary of Major Points

In this chapter, our goal was to provide basic information on the concepts of speechreading and auditory development (i.e., training/learning). We hope that we were able to answer a few of your questions that you developed prior to and during your reading of the chapter. We have no doubt that you will need to read further on these topics.

The overall intent of this chapter was to provide a brief introduction to the *Key Concepts*, as follows:

- The nature and study of speechreading

- The nature and study of auditory development

- Implications for instruction and further research

With respect to speechreading, we highlighted that

- Speechreading refers to the process of understanding a spoken message.

- Traditionally, the label *lip reading* has been used to describe this process. However, the comprehension of the spoken message seems to involve more than just reading the lips, although the lips do provide a substantial or the overwhelming bulk of the information.

- It is often argued that there should be a continuing understanding of the process of speechreading with or without the aid of amplification.

- Speechreading has been investigated in relation to four broad areas: speaker-sender, environment, lip reader-receiver, and code-stimulus.

- The findings on adults cannot be generalized indiscriminately to younger populations such as adolescents and children.

- Children can speechread short, syntactically simple sentences more easily than long complex sentences, especially those that involve embedded elements such as relative clauses (e.g., *The boy who kissed the girl ran away*). In fact, children seem to have fewer difficulties with subject-verb-object (S-V-O) constructions (e.g., *The girl is happy*).

- Because there seems to be a wide gap between knowledge of speechreading and how this translates into practice, there has been a call for more sophisticated research designs. Multidisciplinary and multifaceted approaches are needed that take into account the interactive effects of numerous variables, especially those delineated within the O'Neill and Oyer framework, that have been studied in previous speechreading studies.

With regard to auditory development, we stated that

- The development of audition in children who are d/Deaf or hard of hearing proceeds through stages that are similar to children who have typical hearing.

- If access to the auditory signal is limited or dysfunctional, then many children will have difficulty with the development of speech perception and speech discrimination abilities.

- The development of audition has been labeled *auditory training* or *auditory learning*. Regardless of how it is labeled and despite the differences of opinions in educators and researchers, auditory training/learning refers to the use of techniques to assist children in their development of audition or use of residual hearing.

- The model of Erber (1982) has been used (and elaborated on) to assess and facilitate auditory development. This model focuses on four concepts: detection, discrimination, identification, and comprehension.

- With the advent of powerful amplification systems such as digital hearing aids and cochlear implants, much of the current emphasis is on developing listening or comprehension skills.

- Several widely used programs, manuals, and curricula are available that contain development and assessment components.

- Current auditory development approaches seem to be similar to the use of natural methods for teaching speech and language, which have been in use for many years. Most of the approaches have been influenced by the use of pragmatics in language development.

With respect to implications for instruction and further research, it was stated that

- It is not feasible to provide clear, unambiguous guidelines for the development of speechreading skills, even in classroom situations.

- Suggestions for improving or developing speechreading skills are often proffered with respect to the four domains of O'Neill and Oyer (1981).

- Formal and informal assessments of speechreading should be administered in a variety of settings and such assessments should provide strengths and areas of improvement, similar to criterion-referenced or diagnostic tests.

- More complex, comprehensive paradigms are needed, but such research is hampered by the availability of good speechreading tests. There is also a need to investigate speechreading in conjunction with other domains such as auditory development and speech.

- With respect to auditory development, more rigorous research needs to be conducted to measure the effectiveness of either the programs or aspects or components.

It is hoped that you understand the value of developing speechreading and auditory training/learning skills in children who are d/Deaf or hard of hearing. The virtues of combining such development with the use of current amplification or assistive devices have also been touted. This developmental process should commence during the child's early years. This brings up the topic of early intervention, which is covered in the next chapter.

Chapter Questions

Note: *Some answers to the questions can be found in the chapter; however, others have a variety of possible responses based on the students' backgrounds and experiences.*

1. Describe the following terms:
    a. Speechreading
    b. Auditory development

2. The authors state that there is a difference between speechreading and lip reading. Discuss this difference.

3. Label and discuss the four areas of speechreading for research and development purposes, as offered by O'Neill and Oyer (1981). Which ones seems to be the most difficult to investigate? Why?

4. What do we know about speechreading development, according to research? Do we know enough to proffer instructional implications, especially for developing speechreading skills? Why or why not?

5. Why is it difficult to measure or assess speechreading skill?

6. According to the authors, what are future research endeavors in the area of speechreading?

7. With respect to auditory development, what are the four major components with respect to Erber's (1982) model? Describe each component.

8. What are a few common elements across curricula or programs involving auditory training/learning?

9. Explain the significance of a listening attitude or a listening consciousness in auditory development.

10. A child who points to a pig when a parent says "oink" is demonstrating:

   a. Detection

   b. Discrimination

   c. Identification

   d. Comprehension

   Explain why you selected this answer.

11. If you had an opportunity to converse with the authors, what burning questions would you ask them? Share and discuss these questions with your instructor and classmates.

Challenge Questions

Note: *Complete answers are not in the text. Additional research/reading is required. In some cases, reading further or elsewhere in the text might provide some information to guide the response to a particular question.*

1. Do you think speechreading should be investigated with or without audition? Why or why not? On what did you base your response?

2. This chapter briefly mentions the qualitative-similarity hypothesis. How does this hypothesis relate to the development of the English language (i.e., oral language ability)? Do you think that this hypothesis applies to children who are learning English as a second language? Why or why not?

3. How is it possible for children to develop the foundations for aural habilitation or auditory development in English if they do not have the capacity (despite modern technological advances) to access the sounds of English? [Note: This was discussed in the earlier chapters of this book, particularly in Chapter 7.]

Suggested Activities

1. Interview teachers of d/Deaf or hard of hearing students in your area and obtain their views on the value and practice of speechreading and auditory learning in their programs. Did they take courses as part of their educational preparation? If yes, were these courses helpful in their careers? If no, why not? Share your findings with your instructor and your classmates.

2. Observe the teachers or clinicians in their settings as they work on developing or rehabilitating (for adults) the skills of speechreading and/or auditory learning. Describe their lessons or practices. Are these descriptions similar to the information presented in this chapter? Share your findings with your instructor and your classmates.

3. Select a partner (or two) and develop lessons on speechreading and auditory learning. Do the contents and goals of your lessons vary according to the age and ability of your students/clients? Are there any guidelines to follow for developing such lessons? Share your findings with your instructor and your classmates.

References

Anastasi, A., & Urbina, S. (1997). *Psychological testing* (7th ed.). Upper Saddle River, NJ: Prentice Hall.

Bader, J. (2001). Development of auditory skills in children who are hearing impaired. In R. Hull (Ed.), *Aural rehabilitation: Serving children and adults* (4th ed.; pp. 115–128). San Diego, CA: Singular/Thomson Learning.

Berger, K. (1972). *Speechreading: Principles and methods.* Baltimore, MD: National Educational Press.

Black, J., O'Reilly, P., & Peck, L. (1963). Self-administered training in lipreading. *Journal of Speech and Hearing Disorders, 28,* 183–186.

Borg, W., & Gall, M. (1983). *Educational research* (4th ed.). White Plains, NY: Longman.

Cain, K., & Oakhill, J. (2007). *Children's comprehension problems in oral and written language: A cognitive perspective.* New York: The Guilford Press.

Clarke School for the Deaf. (1971). *Auditory training.* Northampton, MA: Author.

Cole, E., & Gregory, H. (Eds.). (1986). Auditory learning. *Volta Review, 88*(5), September.

Crawford, J., Dancer, J., & Pittenger, J. (1986). Initial performance level on a speechreading task as related to subsequent improvement after short-term training. *Volta Review, 88,* 101–105.

Crystal, D. (1995). *The Cambridge encyclopedia of the English language.* New York: Cambridge University Press.

Crystal, D. (1997). *The Cambridge encyclopedia of language* (2nd ed.). New York: Cambridge University Press.

Crystal, D. (2006). *How language works.* London, England: Penguin Books.

Dancer, J., Krain, M., Thompson, C., Davis, P., & Glenn, J. (1994). A cross-sectional investigation of speechreading in adults: Effects of age, gender, practice, and education. *Volta Review, 96,* 31–40.

De Filippo, C., & Sims, D. (Eds.). (1988). New reflections on speechreading. *Volta Review, 90*(5), September.

Dodd, B., & Campbell, R. (Eds.). (1987). *Hearing by eye.* London, England: Erlbaum.

Elfenbein, J. (1992). Coping with communication breakdown: A program of strategy development for children who have hearing losses. *American Journal of Audiology, 1*(7), 25–29.

Erber, N. (1982). *Auditory training.* Washington, DC: Alexander Graham Bell Association for the Deaf.

Farwell, R. (1976). Speechreading: A research review. *American Annals of the Deaf, 121,* 13–30.

Flexer, C. (1999). *Facilitating hearing and listening in young children* (2nd ed.). San Diego, CA: Singular.

Gagne, J. P., & Jennings, M. B. (2000). Audiologic rehabilitation intervention services of adults with acquired hearing impairment. In M. Valente, H. Hosford-Dunn, & R. Roeser (Eds.), *Audiology treatment* (pp. 547–579). New York: Thieme.

Graham, T. (1992). *Listening is a way of loving.* Atlanta: Humanics Publishing Group.

Harrison, M. (Ed.). (2006). Early hearing detection and intervention: Trends, progress, and challenges. *The Volta Review, 106*(3) (monograph).

Israel, S., & Duffy, G. (2009). *Handbook of research on reading comprehension.* New York: Routledge.

Jeffers, J., & Barley, M. (1971). *Speechreading (lipreading)*. Springfield, IL: Thomas.

Kricos, P. B., & McCarthy, P. (2007). From ear to there: A historical perspective on auditory training. *Seminars in Hearing, 28*(2), 89–98.

Ling, D. (1976). *Speech and the hearing-impaired child: Theory and practice*. Washington, DC: Alexander Graham Bell Association for the Deaf.

Ling, D. (1986). Devices and procedures for auditory learning. *Volta Review, 88*(5), 19–28.

Ling, D. (1989). *Aural habilitation: The foundation of verbal learning in hearing-impaired children* (2nd ed.). Washington, DC: Alexander Graham Bell Association for the Deaf.

Ling, D. (2001). Speech development for children who are hearing impaired. In R. Hull (Ed.), *Aural rehabilitation: Serving children and adults* (4th ed.; pp. 145–165). San Diego, CA: Singular/Thomson Learning.

Ling, D. (2002). *Speech and the hearing-impaired child: Theory and practice* (2nd ed.). Washington, DC: Alexander Graham Bell Association for the Deaf.

Luetke-Stahlman, B. (1999). *Language across the curriculum: When students are deaf or hard of hearing*. Hillsboro, OR: Butte Publications.

Luetke-Stahlman, B., & Luckner, J. (1991). *Effectively educating students with hearing impairments*. White Plains, NY: Longman.

Marschark, M., Lang, H., & Albertini, J. (2002). *Educating deaf students: From research to practice*. New York: Oxford University Press.

Maxwell, M. (1981). *Listening games for elementary grades*. Washington, DC: Acropolis Books.

Moog, J. S., Biedenstein, J., & Davidson, L. (1995). *Speech perception instructional curriculum and evaluation (SPICE)*. St. Louis, MO: Central Institute for the Deaf.

Moog, J., Biedenstein, J., Davidson, L., & Brenner, C. (1994). Instruction for developing speech perception skills. *Volta Review, 96*(5), 61–73.

Moores, D. (1996). *Educating the deaf: Psychology, principles, and practices* (4th ed.). Boston, MA: Houghton-Mifflin.

Moores, D. (2001). *Educating the deaf: Psychology, principles, and practices* (5th ed.). Boston, MA: Houghton-Mifflin.

Nation, K. (2005). Connections between language and reading in children with poor reading comprehension. In H. Catts & A. Kamhi (Eds.), *The connections between language and reading disabilities* (pp. 41–54). Mahwah, NJ: Erlbaum.

Nitchie, E. (1902/1979). *How to read lips for fun and profit*. New York: Hawthorn.

O'Neill, J., & Oyer, H. (1981). *Visual communication for the hard of hearing: History, research, methods* (2nd ed.). Englewood Cliffs, NJ: Prentice-Hall.

Osberger, M. (1990). Audition. *Volta Review, 92*, 34–53.

Owens, R. (2004). *Language disorders: A functional approach to assessment and intervention* (4th ed.). Boston, MA: Pearson Education.

Paul, P. (1988). The effects of viewing angle and visibility on speechreading comprehension ability. *Hearsay: The Journal of the Ohio Speech and Hearing Association*, Fall, 100–103.

Paul, P. (2001). *Language and deafness* (3rd ed.). San Diego, CA: Singular/Thomson Learning.

Paul, P. (2008). Introduction: Reading and children with disabilities. *Reading and children with disabilities. Balanced Reading Instruction, 15*(2), 1–12.

Paul, P. (2009). *Language and deafness* (4th ed.). Sudbury, MA: Jones & Bartlett.

Pearson, P. D., & Stallman, A. (1994). Resistance, complacency, and reform in reading assessment. In F. Lehr & J. Osborn (Eds.), *Reading, language, and literacy: Instruction for the twenty-first century* (pp. 239–251). Hillsdale, NJ: Erlbaum.

Pichora-Fuller, M. K., & Benguerel, A. (1991). The design of CAST (Computer-aided speechreading training). *Journal of Speech and Hearing Research, 34*(2), 202–212.

Robbins, A., Svirsky, M., Osberger, M., & Pisoni, D. (1996). *Beyond the audiogram: The role of functional assessment.* Paper presented at the Fourth International Symposium on Childhood Deafness, Kiawah Island, South Carolina.

Rose, S., McAnally, P., & Quigley, S. (2004). *Language learning practices with deaf children* (3rd ed.). Austin, TX: Pro-Ed.

Samar, V., & Sims, D. (1983). Visual evoked response correlates of speechreading performance in normal-hearing adults: A replication and factor analytic extension. *Journal of Speech and Hearing Research, 26,* 2–9.

Sanders, D. (1982). *Aural rehabilitation: A management model* (2nd ed.). Englewood Cliffs, NJ: Prentice-Hall.

Shepherd, D. (1982). Visual-neural correlate of speechreading ability in normal-hearing adults: Reliability. *Journal of Speech and Hearing Research, 25,* 521–527.

Silverman, S. R., & Kricos, P. (1990). Speechreading. *Volta Review, 92,* 21–32.

Simser, J. (1993). Auditory-verbal intervention: Infants and toddlers. *Volta Review, 95,* 217–229.

Spencer, P., & Marschark, M. (Eds.). (2006). *Advances in the spoken language development of deaf and hard of hearing children.* New York: Oxford University Press.

Spradlin, K., Dancer, J., & Monfils, B. (1989). Effects of verbal encouragement on self-ratings of lipreading performance. *Volta Review, 91,* 209–216.

Squires, S., & Dancer, J. (1986). Auditory versus visual practice effects in the intelligibility of words in everyday sentences. *Journal of Auditory Research, 26,* 5–10.

Sticht, T., & James, J. (1984). Listening and reading. In Pearson, P. D., Barr, R., Kamil, M., & Mosenthal, P. (Eds.), *Handbook of reading research* (pp. 293–317). New York: Longman.

Stoker, R., & Ling, D. (Eds.). (1992). Speech production in hearing-impaired children and youth: Theory and practice. *Volta Review, 94*(5).

Stout, G., & Van ert Windle, J. (1992). *Developmental approach to successful listening-Revised (DASL).* Englewood, CO: Resource Point.

Sweetow, R.W., & Henderson-Sabes, J. (2004). The case of LACE, individualized listening and auditory communication enhancement training. *Hearing Journal, 57*(3), 32–40.

Thies, T., & Trammel, J. (1983). Development and implementation of the auditory skills instructional planning system. In I. Hochberg, H. Levitt, & M. Osberger (Eds.), *Speech of the hearing impaired* (pp. 349–366). Baltimore, MD: University Park Press.

Toomey, M. (1991). *Defining and describing.* Marblehead, MA: Circuit.

Trezek, B. J., Wang, Y., & Paul, P. (2010). *Reading and deafness: Theory, research, and practice.* Clifton Park, NY: Delmar/Cengage Learning.

Tye-Murray, N., Tyler, R., Bong, B. & Nares, T. (1988). Using laser videodisc technology to train speechreading and assertive listening skills. *Journal of the Academy of Rehabilitative Audiology, 21*(1), 143–152.

Van ert Windle, J., & Stout, G. (1984). *Developmental approach to successful listening.* San Diego, CA: College-Hill Press.

Wang, Y., Trezek, B., Luckner, J., & Paul, P. (2008). The role of phonology and phonological-related skills in reading instruction for students who are deaf or hard of hearing. *American Annals of the Deaf, 153*(4), 396–407.

Weikum, W. M., Vouloumanos, A., Navarra, J., Soto-Faraco, S., Sebastián-Gallés, N., & Werker, J. F. (2007, May 25). Visual language discrimination in infancy. *Science 316*(5828), 1159.

Further Readings

Beebe, H. (1953). *A guide to help the severely hard of hearing child.* New York: Karger.

Berg, F. (2008). *Speech development guide for children with hearing loss.* San Diego, CA: Plural.

Calvert, D., & Silverman, S. (1983). *Speech and deafness.* Washington, DC: Alexander Graham Bell Association for the Deaf.

Cole, E. B., & Flexer, C. A. (2007). *Children with hearing loss: Developing listening and talking—birth to six.* San Diego, CA: Plural.

Goldstein, M. (1939). *The acoustic method.* St. Louis, MO: Laryngoscope Press.

Ling, D. (Ed.). (1984). *Early intervention for hearing-impaired children: Oral options.* San Diego, CA: College-Hill Press.

EARLY INTERVENTION

Ye Wang
Karen S. Engler

Identification of hearing loss in infancy, followed by appropriate inter-vention by age 6 months, can result in normal language development, regardless of degree of hearing loss. As the average age of identifica-tion of hearing loss moves downward toward 2 months, children with hearing loss will enter the educational system earlier and with lan-guage skills commensurate with those of their hearing peers. In order to provide appropriate services to children with hearing loss and their families, early interventionists will need to forge links to health care providers involved in universal newborn hearing screening programs, to have specialized training in deafness and hearing loss, and to have expertise in providing services to very young children and to children with hearing loss in the broad range from mild to profound.

—Arehart & Yoshinaga-Itano (1999, p. 19)

Key Concepts

After completing this chapter, you should have a basic understanding of:

- Early identification (universal newborn screening)
- Early amplification
- Parent–professional cooperative partnerships

- Early intervention assessments

- Early intervention techniques and strategies

It is estimated that out of every 1000 births in the United States 2 to 3 babies are born d/Deaf or hard of hearing (National Institute on Deafness and Other Communication Disorders [NIDCD], 2008). When adding significant, permanent, unilateral hearing loss data, the number increases to approximately 8 per 1000 births (Stach & Ramachandran, 2008). Prior to newborn hearing screening, the average age of identification in the United States was roughly 2 and one-half years of age, with some milder hearing losses remaining undetected until school age (National Center for Hearing Assessment and Management [NCHAM], 2008).

Because they are in the process of learning language, even a slight or mild hearing loss (between 15 dB and 40 dB) may adversely affect the development of infants and young children. Infants, toddlers, and young children typically do not have the linguistic competence or attending skills of older individuals (Flexer, 1994). On the contrary, an older individual with linguistic competence who misses communication due to a slight or mild hearing loss should have more skills at his or her disposal to gain access to the parts of the communication that were missed through the utilization of contextual cues, linguistic knowledge, and communication repair strategies.

The passage at the beginning of this chapter seems to highlight and promote a few of the benefits and issues related to early intervention. In fact, Arehart and Yoshinaga-Itano (1999) concluded that the contributing factors for the late identification of children are: (1) the limitation of the high-risk registry method historically used in early identification of children who are d/Deaf or hard of hearing, because only 50% of children have high-risk factors (see further discussion on the high-risk factors later in this chapter); (2) hearing loss is virtually invisible to the naked eye, because concerns about the hearing abilities of children without significant medical issues or concurrent disabilities often do not emerge until observation of language development delays (see also Diefendorf, 2002; Northern & Downs, 1991, 2002); and (3) the majority of children with hearing loss are hard of hearing and do not have obvious multiple disabilities.

Currently, 44 states and the District of Columbia have enacted universal newborn hearing screening legislation (NCHAM, 2008). By the end of 2001, all states, including those without legislative mandates, had initiated an early hearing detection and intervention program (White, 2008). However, early identification of hearing loss is only the first step; appropriate and immediate intervention must follow to ensure successful outcomes of children (Arehart & Yoshinaga-Itano, 1999).

This chapter starts with an introduction on early identification of hearing loss (i.e., universal newborn hearing screening/early hearing detection and intervention). Next, it discusses the importance of early amplification for many infants, especially those who were not born into a Deaf family. Then, several components of early intervention are introduced with details: (1) parent–professional cooperative partnerships, (2) formal and informal assessments leading to reflective decisions, and (3) the techniques and strategies used in early intervention. Finally, we conclude with the implications for the training of professionals and recommended directions for future research and practice.

As you read along, think of a few questions that you expect to be answered after completing the chapter. Here is a list to get you started, based on the *Key Concepts* mentioned previously:

- What are the major components of early intervention?
- What is early amplification?
- What is or should be the involvement of parents?
- What assessments, strategies, and techniques are crucial for early intervention?

Early Identification

One of the most important components of early intervention is the use of universal newborn hearing screening (UNHS), which is a systematic means of screening the hearing of all newborns in an effort to decrease the age at identification for infants with hearing losses. Screening for hearing loss is the first, critical step toward providing early intervention services to infants and their families. For many, the terminology has shifted to early hearing detection and intervention (EHDI) to better reflect the significance of the total package—screening, diagnosis, early intervention services, family support, and long-term goal setting—in meeting the needs of infants and their families (White, 2008).

Very young children who lack suitable language stimulation during the first 2 to 3 years of life are likely to fail to reach their true language potential. Whether the lack of language stimulation is due to hearing loss or deprivation of quality language opportunities, the result remains the same (Northern & Downs, 1991, 2002). In addition to language, undetected hearing loss may adversely affect speech and social-emotional development, as well as a child's academic performance and achievement (Joint Committee on Infant Hearing [JCIH], 2007).

Screening the hearing of newborns was first suggested in the 1960s through the research efforts of Marion Downs and in the *1965 Babbidge Report to the Secretary of Health, Education, and Welfare* (Northern & Downs, 1991, 2002). The type of screening advocated in these early programs was based on a *risk-register approach* to hearing loss, suggesting that infants born with certain factors, such as prematurity or craniofacial anomalies, were at a higher risk for hearing loss and should undergo a hearing screening. Screening techniques in these early days used behavioral techniques and were somewhat crude in terms of sensitivity and specificity, which are two measures of the effectiveness of a test.

Nearly 30 years later in 1990, Hawaii became the first state in the United States to initiate legislation for newborn hearing screening (NHS) (White, 2008). Much has occurred from the time of the initial conception of NHS until Hawaii began screening newborns. The Joint Committee on Infant Hearing (JCIH) was instrumental in providing professional leadership in the area of newborn hearing screening (Diefendorf, 2002). In 1972, the JCIH recommended the selective screening of infant's hearing based on high-risk factors that were known to increase the likelihood of an infant having a hearing loss. Initially, the high-risk register had five items, or risk factors. An additional five high-risk factors were added and a few items altered within the registry between 1982 and 1994 (JCIH, 2008).

In 1993, the National Institutes of Health (NIH) recommended that all infants have their hearing screened prior to being discharged from the hospital (NCHAM, 2008). In 1994, JCIH followed suit with the full support of the NIH in the promotion of universal hearing screening of all newborns (JCIH, 2008). In addition, technological advances in hearing screening technology and methods (see Chapter 3), federal government financing, legislative backing, as well as initiatives by individual groups and organizations contributed to the expansion of NHS (White, 2008). A brief history of newborn hearing screening in the United States is provided in **Table 9-1**.

Communication beginning at birth for all children is the vision of the Center for Disease Control and Prevention (CDC) and the JCIH, and is supported by other member organizations of the JCIH, including the American Academy of Audiology (AAA), the American Speech-Language-Hearing Association (ASHA), the Council on Education of the Deaf (CED), and the American Academy of Pediatrics (AAP). Seven goals support this vision.

Table 9-1

History of Newborn Hearing Screening

Year	Events
1960s	The *1965 Babbidge Report to the Secretary of Health, Education, and Welfare.*
1972	The JCIH recommended the selective screening of infants' hearing based on five high-risk factors. An additional five high-risk factors were added and a few items altered within the registry between 1982 and 1994.
1990	Hawaii became the first state in the United States to initiate legislation for NHS.
1993	The NIH recommended that all infants have their hearing screened prior to being discharged from the hospital.
1994	The JCIH followed suit with the full support of the NIH.
2007	94% of newborns were screened for hearing loss in 48 states, 1 U.S. territory, and 1 commonwealth.

The first goal recommends that all infants should have their hearing screened using a physiological method by the age of 1 month, preferably prior to being discharged from the hospital. A pass result indicates no need for further evaluation; however, communicative development should be monitored during well-baby visits in the medical home, which is discussed further in Chapter 10 (JCIH, 2007). An initial screening fail should result in a hearing evaluation completed prior to the age of 3 months (JCIH, 2007). If the results of the audiologic evaluation are consistent with normal hearing acuity, parents should be encouraged to monitor their child's development and schedule an audiometric follow-up. If, however, a hearing loss is diagnosed, considerations for amplification, choices in early intervention, early intervention services, and coordination with the infant's medical home should occur.

Early intervention services should begin prior to the age of 6 months (EHDI, 2008). Infants identified with hearing losses should receive early intervention services by professionals possessing expertise in deafness and hearing loss, such as educators of the d/Deaf and hard of hearing, speech-language pathologists, and audiologists (JCIH, 2007). This model is also known as the *1-3-6 plan*, reflecting the screening, diagnosis, and intervention guidelines in the early months of the infant's life. The decision tree for the 1-3-6 plan is illustrated in **Figure 9-1**.

The fourth goal focuses on the identification of hearing losses that may have been missed through screening or may have occurred later during the first years of life due to late onset, progressive, or acquired nature of the hearing loss. In addition, tracking and monitoring of EHDI programs is critical to ascertain that infants receive appropriate early intervention services. The remaining goals focus on the coordination of services and tracking and monitoring of services within each state to evaluate outcomes of goals and minimize loss of infants' families at points of follow-up (EHDI, 2008).

Forty-eight states within the United States (excluding Georgia, Delaware); one U.S. territory, Guam; and one commonwealth, Commonwealth of Northern Mariana Islands, were included in the 2007 CDC EHDI summary data (EHDI, 2007). The data indicate that 94% of newborns were screened for hearing loss. Of the remaining 6%, 5.6% were missed, undocumented, or unknown. Parent refusal and infant death were the reasons for the final .4% not being screened.

According to EHDI data, 4,016,827 infants were born during 2007, of which 63,269 infants did not pass a newborn hearing screening. Of those that failed, 6.3%, or 3950, were confirmed to have hearing loss (i.e., approximately 2.5 per 1000 births); 44.8% were lost to follow-up and/or documentation; 7.5% were in the diagnostic hearing evaluation process; and 37% had no hearing loss. The remaining 4.3% included 1.6% of infants/families who moved and 2.7% of which families refused follow-up or the infant died (EHDI, 2007). Having nearly 45% of the newborns screened lost to follow-up and/or documentation indicates the need for continued growth and improvement in EHDI programs at the state and national levels.

Early identification is only the first step. For many infants with identification of hearing losses, early amplification is the next crucial step. For many scholars, early identification and early amplification go hand-in-hand. We discuss the issue of early amplification in the following section.

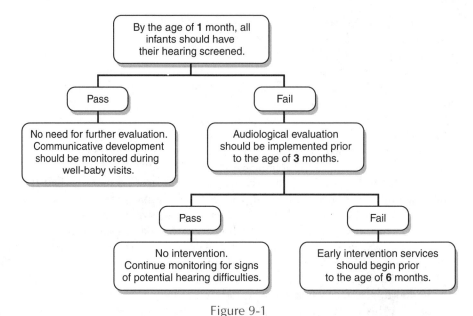

Figure 9-1

The 1-3-6 Plan for Hearing Screening, Diagnostic Evaluation, and Intervention

Sources: *Adapted from EHDI (2008) and JCIH (2007).*

 Early Amplification

The importance of communication is indisputable:

> Communication is at the core of our existence. Individuals thrive on their ability to convey ideas and express feelings. Concepts are formed, vocabulary expanded, values instilled, and educational horizons broadened, all through the channel of communication. For at the heart of expressing oneself lies language—the basic tool that in turn links us to our culture, home, community, and surrounding environment. By being provided with the opportunity to share our thoughts, feelings, and knowledge with others, our lives become enhanced and we are able to transmit our information base to others, thus creating a bond with previous and future generations. (Scheetz, 2001, p. 107)

Acquiring a first language requires ongoing communication exchanges with competent language users, full access to the symbols of the language, and direct feedback through the sensory modality used to communicate to shape the child's efforts in the production of the symbols of that language (Boothroyd, 2008). For an infant who is congenitally deaf born to parents who are also Deaf and utilize American Sign Language (ASL), the language requirements just presented may be met through sign language. Likewise, hearing children born to hearing parents are able to fulfill these language requirements through spoken language (Boothroyd, 2008). However, approximately 5% of babies who are deaf are born to families with one or more d/Deaf parents. The other 95% of infants who are deaf are born to parents who are hearing and utilize spoken communication (Mitchell & Karchmer, 2004).

For an infant with hearing loss, early amplification is crucial to the development of auditory neural pathways in the brain (Flexer, 1994). Current research emphasizes the importance of both heredity and experiences and the intricacies of their interactions in the development of the brain (Shore, 1997). It is recognized that the experiences of the infant and young child play a critical role in the shaping of the way in which their brains develop and that early interactions play a pivotal role in affecting brain development. Consequently, brain development is viewed from a nonlinear perspective, which recognizes critical time periods for developing specific knowledge and skill sets.

At a young age, the developing connections within the brain are critical to the brain's overall development. The connections allow for the processing of information not only during the early years, but throughout adulthood. Furthermore, repeated stimulation/use of the wired connections in the brain reinforces those connections and allows the pathway to become permanent. In short, brain connections develop rapidly and early in life, especially during the first few years.

One framework for understanding these issues is that of Piaget. According to Piaget (1952), the first two years of a child's life is the period of sensorimotor development, during which an infant organizes sensory impressions and begins to create perceptual schema that are the basis for further cognitive development. Acquiring a native language is part of the process in developing a perceptual scheme. It requires that the sense organs deliver reliable, constant information to the brain. The brain detects, identifies, and recognizes specific patterns of sensory impressions, which are then associated with the events that produced them. Consequently, the sensory impressions become meaningful for the infant. "Perceptual development requires sensory stimulation to be accessible and consistent. Inaccessible or intermittent sensory stimulation inhibit its development. Full-time use (i.e., all waking hours) of amplification is required for the brain to develop a perceptual scheme that includes sounds. Intermittent or inconsistent auditory stimulation will not be included in perceptual development" (Gatty, 2003, p. 411). Again, as noted in Chapters 2 and 3 of this book, hearing occurs at the level of the brain and should be developed or utilized early in life.

Learning through audition requires early and appropriate amplification and comprehensive hearing management (Flexer, 1994). In most cases, ideal early intervention programs recognize the importance of pediatric amplification and the consistent, systematic, audiologic follow-along for infants and children (Pollack, Goldberg, & Caleffe-Schenck, 1997). The National Association of the Deaf (NAD) 2000 Position Statement on cochlear implants (see Chapter 5) acknowledged advancements in all forms of technology that may cultivate improvements in the quality of life for individuals who are d/Deaf or hard of hearing, which includes, but is not limited to, hearing technology such as hearing aids and cochlear implants. Examples of other technologies include closed captioning, video relay services, text telephones, and FM systems (NAD, 2000).

Working with infants who are d/Deaf or hard of hearing, audiologists are responsible for the fitting of amplification and ongoing audiologic management (Flexer, 1994; Pollack et al., 1997). Information regarding hearing aids and cochlear implants is provided in Chapters 4 and 5 of this text, respectively. There is also a significant counseling component based on the fact that most families are entering uncharted territory. A diagnosis of deafness is often initially devastating for parents who are hearing. Denial of the hearing loss, concern, feeling an injustice, anger, blaming each other, and many questions abound in the minds of the parents. This process of grieving is normal and expected.

Professionals working with the families of these children should be well versed in providing needed support and, when appropriate, making appropriate referrals. Any family should be given access to information and resources that allow the child to maximize his or her potential (JCIH, 2007). The role of the professionals is to provide parents with the necessary information and resources so that they can develop realistic expectations for the future of their child's development and be confident in the informed decisions they make. Additional information on this issue is provided in Chapter 10.

Effects of Early Intervention and Early Amplification

Early amplification might not be applicable for every infant with a hearing loss—especially the ones born to Deaf families; however, appropriate early intervention must immediately follow the identification of hearing loss. Unfortunately, historically, after a child was identified with hearing loss, a significant amount of time, often as much as a year, elapsed before intervention was implemented (see the review in Arehart & Yoshinaga-Itano, 1999). Based on the 1-3-6 plan discussed previously, ideally, early intervention should follow identification of hearing loss prior to the age of 6 months. The research literature has suggested that no matter which mode of communication is adopted, one of the most effective strategies for the normal language development of children is identification of hearing loss as early as possible, followed by appropriate intervention by age 6 months (Apuzzo & Yoshinaga-Itano, 1995; Arehart & Yoshinaga-Itano, 1999; Yoshinaga-Itano, 2003; Yoshinaga-Itano, Sedey, Coulter, & Mehl, 1998).

In one of the pioneer studies, Yoshinaga-Itano and colleagues (1998) found that children whose hearing losses were identified by 6 months of age followed by early intervention demonstrated significantly better language scores than those identified after 6 months of age. When cognitive abilities were controlled, this language advantage was independent of all other factors, including test age, communication mode, degree of hearing loss, socioeconomic status, gender, minority status, and the presence or absence of additional disabilities.

In another well-cited study, Moeller (2000) showed that children who were enrolled earliest (e.g., by 11 months of age) achieved scores significantly higher on language outcome measures, such as vocabulary and verbal reasoning skills, at 5 years of age than did later-enrolled children. Furthermore, early-enrolled children with various degrees of hearing losses performed approximately equally as well as their hearing peers on these measures. Among the various factors influencing performance, only two factors explained a significant variance in the scores measured at age 5: family involvement and age at enrollment, and family involvement explained the most variance after all other factors were controlled. Finally, the results revealed an interaction between the factors of family involvement and age at enrollment. Although all children benefited from early enrollment, those with high levels of family involvement were the most successful children in the study.

In a recent study, Nittrouer (2010) investigated the factors related to the variability in developmental outcomes, particularly language. Developmental data on behavior, personality, and cognition, as well as various data on language development were collected on the participants every 6 months between 12 and 48 months of age. Children with hearing loss were no different from hearing children on behavioral, psychosocial, or cognitive measurements, except for classification, a cognitive task associated with language processing. However, the children's rate of language acquisition was significantly influenced simply by virtue of having a hearing loss. And the critical factor on language development was how responsive parents were to their children's communicative attempts instead of language models used or modes of communication (e.g., signing, oral, etc.). Furthermore, children with better performance in language measurements all had been identified with hearing loss before the age of 1 year.

In sum, early identification followed by early amplification and parental involvement have been constantly identified as critical factors on the language development of a child who is d/Deaf or hard of hearing. The importance of family involvement leads to our first component topic in early intervention: parent–professional cooperative partnerships.

Parent–Professional Cooperative Partnerships

After years of studying the development of typical children, White (1975) concluded: "the informal education that families provide for their children makes more of an impact on a child's total educational development than the formal educational system" (p. 4). Although parents are the first and most important teachers of their children, many *hearing* families are often initially ill-equipped with knowledge of hearing loss and its ramifications on the developing infant. Therefore, the parent–professional cooperative partnership is critical. The concept of interdisciplinary teams is discussed in detail in Chapter 10.

Since the 1970s, federal and state legislations have encouraged family-centered service delivery in early childhood special education. For example, parental involvement in educational planning for children with disabilities was mandated by the Education for All Handicapped Children Act of 1975. Then, the Education of the Handicapped Act Amendments of 1986 required states to provide early intervention services for children with special needs from birth to kindergarten. Later, the Individuals with Disabilities Education Amendments of 1997 specified that early intervention services should be provided in settings where children would be if they were not in early intervention; that is, in the home and the community, including childcare settings (Allen & Petr, 1996). A brief summary of the history and legislations related to family-centered early intervention service is provided in **Table 9-2**.

Early intervention for infants and toddlers focuses on two primary goals. The first goal is to assist the baby and family in establishing communication, capitalizing on the infant's residual hearing, and supporting early social interactions. The second goal is to support the baby and family so that the baby becomes fully integrated within the family unit (Boys Town National Research Hospital, 2009). A cooperative parent–professional partnership is critical in serving the various needs of infants and toddlers and their families.

Early intervention providers may work with parents and families who are very diverse in terms of family make-up, culture, race, education level, and socioeconomic level. For example, in American culture parents are typically the decision makers in most parts of their child's life (Gatty, 2003). However, in many other cultures, such as Asian or African cultures, "parents may see themselves as nurturers and caregivers of young children but view education as the responsibility of teachers, habilitation as the responsibility of the therapists, or deafness as a medical disability in which advice from the doctor is valued above that of other professionals" (Gatty, 2003, p. 418). Furthermore, some traditional cultures might rely on supernatural explanations of problems and consider the practice of inter-

Table 9-2

Summary of the History and Legislation Related to Family-Centered Early Intervention Service

Year	Events
1950s	The term *family-centered* was coined by the Family-Centered Project of St. Paul, Minnesota.
1975	*Education for All Handicapped Children Act:* Parental involvement in educational planning for children with disabilities was mandated.
1986	*Education of the Handicapped Act Amendments:* States were required to provide early intervention services for children with special needs from birth to kindergarten.
1997	*Individuals with Disabilities Education Amendments:* Early intervention services were required to be provided in settings where children would be if they were not in early intervention; that is, in the home and the community, including childcare settings.

vention as futile. Therefore, an open discussion between the professionals and the family on empowerment is critical.

Parents may be at different places within the grieving process, from denial to acceptance and anywhere in between. Although there is always the opportunity for an exception, it may be beneficial to consider some underlying beliefs about parents:

- Parents know their child best.

- Parents want what is best for their child.

- Parents want to communicate with their child.

- Parents want their child to be happy.

- Parents want their child to have friends.

- Parents have choices (e.g., communication and technology).

Having a positive belief set about parents and working from where the family is rather than where professionals believe the family should be appears to be a winning combination. It offers early intervention providers the opportunity to build on family strengths and to organize around parent concerns (Ostrosky, 2002). Furthermore, research on collaborative partnerships between parents and professionals has yielded some consistent successful themes: communication, commitment, equality, skills, trust, and respect (Blue-Banning, Summers, Frankland, Nelson, & Beegle, 2004). Both parents and professionals should be equal partners, and parent input should be valued and respected. In addition, parents want professionals to be competent and skilled.

For communication to happen, at least two entities need to be involved. Communication may take place between the parent and child, the child and his or her sibling, the professional and parent, and so on. In the case of parent–professional exchanges, it is very important for the early intervention provider to really listen, not only to what the parent says, but also to what goes unsaid. For example, a parent may verbalize the importance of the baby wearing hearing aids, yet when the early intervention provider (e.g., Deaf Education Parent-Infant Specialist) arrives for home visits the baby may be generally without his or her hearing aids.

Related to the above scenario, questions to consider include the following: Could it be that brainstorming about ways to keep the hearing aids on might be helpful? Is it possible that the early intervention provider needs to find a way to better explain the importance of amplification in the development of auditory pathways to the brain? Could it also be possible that the early intervention provider is imposing his or her beliefs about amplification, when the family's primary focus is on the development of a visual language such as ASL? Or still yet, could it be that the parent is simply exhausted, both physically and mentally, because the family is so strapped for money, that surviving to keep food on the table and heat in their home is their primary goal at this time? And what about the family whose infant has additional disabilities, and hearing loss appears to be the least of the parent's concern at the time? There are so many possibilities, yet really listening and caring for the child and family should allow the interventionist to obtain a glimpse into how he or she might best serve the family at a particular time, including recognizing when an outside referral is appropriate (e.g., counseling, respite care, support services, etc.).

Ultimately, the success of any EHDI program depends on the collaborative integration of families and a variety of professionals (JCIH, 2007). Within the families, early intervention programs should strive to involve fathers and other family members (Moeller, 2002).Within the field of communication sciences and disorders, each discipline—audiology, education of the d/Deaf and hard of hearing, and speech-language pathology—brings valuable expertise to serving young children with hearing losses and their families.

 ## Formal and Informal Assessments

One of the most challenging parts of early intervention starts with assessment. "*Assessment* refers to the ongoing procedures used to identify the child's unique strengths and needs, as well as the family's concerns, priorities, and resources regarding the child's development in order to plan intervention services" (Woods & Wetherby, 2007, p. 8). As indicated by the quote, assessment is a *process* rather than a series of *snapshots* of a child in isolated situations. It is a *means* to provide information regarding future intervention rather than an *end*. It is a parent–professional *team* rather than the professional's *one-man show*.

Woods and Wetherby (2007) proffered three trends in early childhood assessment: family-guided, naturalistic, and team-based collaboration. A comprehensive assessment should encompass all areas of a child's development, including cognition, language and communication, social-emotional, perceptual-fine motor, gross motor, and adaptive skills; and for preschoolers, pre-academic skills, such as early literacy skills (Sass-Lehrer, 2003).

Hafer and Stredler-Brown (2003) suggested five best practices in assessments of young children who are d/Deaf or hard of hearing:

1. Use multiple perspectives including the ones from parents, the early interventionist, and primary care physician and, whenever applicable, the perspectives from a d/Deaf or hard of hearing adult;

2. Use multiple techniques and instruments, particularly videotapes;

3. Assess on multiple occasions such as when the child is with hearing children or when he or she is with other d/Deaf or hard of hearing children, and in multiple settings including home, child care facility, and clinic;

4. Use functional item content and apply accommodations based on the child's communication mode whenever possible; and

5. Make collaborative decisions and have the parents play the key role in the decision making process.

A variety of formal and informal assessments are available to collect data leading to reflective decisions for intervention. Informal assessments such as discussions with parents to identify their concerns and needs not only can strengthen the equal participation of professionals and parents, but also can provide a guide for immediate intervention activities

(Spencer, 2003). Formal assessments such as checklists and scales are useful in organizing observations and making them objective.

Two caveats must be kept in mind: (1) the role of the interventionist is to identify and reinforce the positive behaviors occurring during an interaction, rather than being "the expert" to judge the parents or caregivers; and (2) the reason for the assessment is to use it as a basis for future interventions instead of using it for assessment purposes only (Spencer, 2003). Two examples of formal assessments and the necessary accommodations for young children with hearing loss are discussed in the following two sections.

MacArthur-Bates Communicative Development Inventories (CDIs)

Parents possess knowledge of their child's language development. The *MacArthur-Bates Communicative Development Inventories* (CDIs) (Fenson, Marchman, Thal, Dale, Reznick, & Bates, 2007) capitalize on this knowledge through inventories that are completed by the parents. For example, parents are able to observe their child in a variety of settings and situations; therefore, the language information reported more closely represents their child's actual language skills. The CDIs have been adapted for young children who use sign language (Watkins, 2004).

Each inventory consists of two primary forms. The first inventory, CDI: Words and Gestures, is designed for infants and toddlers within 8 to 18 months of age. The second inventory, CDI: Words and Sentences, is designed for use with children aged 16 to 30 months. Both inventories take approximately 20 to 40 minutes to complete. Shortened forms exist for both levels and may be used in situations such as when the literacy of the parents is limited or when the child is learning two languages and the professional is gathering information about the child's proficiency in both languages (Fenson et al., 2007). A CDI-III form is available for use with children aged 30 to 37 months of age.

The CDI: Words and Gestures form focuses on what the child understands as well as what the child says. Fewer than 400 words are included in the inventory. The early signs of language comprehension (i.e., understanding his or her own name and "no-no") are addressed, as are common phrases. Furthermore, inventory questions entail early communicative gestures (i.e., extending arms to indicate "pick me up"; waving bye-bye; shaking head "no") along with early games and routines, actions with objects (e.g., child puts on a hat; throws a ball; drinks from a cup), and demonstration of parenting routines (e.g., rocking a doll; brushing a baby's hair) and other adult activities (e.g., watering a plant; putting on glasses).

The CDI: Words and Sentences form focuses only on the child's expressive language. It includes 680 vocabulary words. The inventory explores sentence length, the child's use of grammar, and the complexity of the child's language.

Professionals and families may be interested in utilizing the normative data from the CDIs as a comparison with children who are hearing. Although the data must be interpreted with caution, comparisons may provide added insight into strengths and gaps for a particular child. Some young children who are d/Deaf or hard of hearing will attend school in a typical classroom within their public school districts. These children will be competing with children who are hearing within the classroom and throughout life. Professionals and parents alike should have high expectations for the child who is d/Deaf or hard of hearing and give strong consideration to a goal of performing in the areas of language, academics, and life commensurate with peers who are hearing.

An adaptation to the method of recording data on the CDIs for a child who is transitioning from sign language to spoken English may provide additional information to parents and professionals. Parents may be instructed to mark items that are understood or expressed in spoken language and use another symbol to indicate those items in which the child is able to perform successfully only if sign language is presented for language comprehension or if sign language is only used by the child to express particular words or phrase. This provides data on differences in the child's communication with and without sign language in the areas of receptive and expressive language. Furthermore, it may indicate, at a point in time, the child's primary mode of communication or a shift in his or her primary mode.

COTTAGE ACQUISITION SCALES FOR LISTENING, LANGUAGE & SPEECH (CASLLS)

"The goal of the CASLLS is to encourage the use of an integrated approach to language intervention by providing professionals with a single set of instruments for following the development of language, listening, cognition and speech" (Wilkes, 2001, p. 1). The role and interrelatedness of cognition and social language in language acquisition provided some of the theoretical basis for the Cottage Acquisition Scales for Listening, Language & Speech, or CASLLS. The design of the CASLLS encompasses a variety of uses, for example, assessment, selection of targeted objectives, and charting of an individual child's progress (Wilkes, 2001).

The CASLLS are based on the stages of the typically developing child across the age ranges, birth to 3 months through 6 to 8 years of age. There are five separate CASLLS forms. Four of the forms are distinguishable by the following levels: Pre-Verbal, Pre-Sentence, Simple Sentence, and Complex Sentence, as well as by age ranges and contents in various categories. The fifth CASLLS form includes the following aspects of phonology: sound awareness, sound discrimination, and articulation (Wilkes, 2001).

Tracking of skill development is available on each CASLLS form under three letter headings: E, M, and G. E stands for *emerging*. This may be marked if the child has demonstrated the behavior on at least one occasion. M indicates *mastery* within at least one context or setting. Lastly, G represents that the child has *generalized* the selected item across settings with little to no errors present (Wilkes, 2001).

Wilkes (2001) suggested utilizing a complete language sample analysis of the child's language for initially determining and completing the appropriate CASLLS form. Subsequent data may be collected through random, frequent samplings of the child's language within different settings. A language sampling form that includes spaces for the language used by the communication partner(s), the context (social, linguistic, and cognitive) in which the exchange occurred, and the child's exact language used or observable behaviors is located in the appendix of the manual.

For children who are d/Deaf or hard of hearing and are learning spoken English, the CASLLS entails a succinct set of tools that provides age ranges and a method of tracking the child's development in the areas of cognition, listening, pragmatics, semantics, syntax, and phonology. In addition, the CASLLS Companion may be ordered to supplement the tool. The CASLLS Companion contains detailed information about the different grammatical forms as well as suggested activities to work on these forms.

A comparison of the two formal assessments discussed in this chapter is presented in **Table 9-3**.

Table 9-3	Comparison of MacArthur-Bates Communicative Development Inventories (CDIs) and Cottage Acquisition Scales for Listening, Language & Speech (CASLLS)	
	CDIs	**CASLLS**
Targets	*CDI: Words and Gestures:* Children aged 8 to18 months. *CDI: Words and Sentences:* Children aged 16 to 30 months. *CDI-III form:* Children aged 30 to 37 months.	Deaf or hard of hearing children aged birth to 3 months through 6 to 8 years of age.
Subtests	*CDI: Words and Gestures:* Focuses on what the child understands as well as what the child says; fewer than 400 words are included. *CDI: Words and Sentences:* Focuses only on the child's expressive language. Includes 680 vocabulary words.	Pre-Verbal. Pre-Sentence. Simple Sentence. Complex Sentence. Phonology: Sound awareness, sound discrimination, and articulation.
Time to complete	20 to 40 minutes for each inventory.	Varies.

(continues)

	CDIs	CASLLS
Table 9-3	**Comparison of MacArthur-Bates Communicative Development Inventories (CDIs) and Cottage Acquisition Scales for Listening, Language, & Speech (CASLLS) (continued)**	
Data collection	Parent questionnaires.	A complete language sample analysis of the child's language for initially determining and completing the appropriate CASLLS form. Subsequent data may be collected through random, frequent samplings of the child's language within different settings.
Normative data	Available for hearing children and children who are d/Deaf or hard of hearing. Adaptations are made for children who use sign language.	Not applicable.

In a nutshell, a variety of tools are available for assessing young children. Care should be taken when selecting tools for children who are d/Deaf or hard of hearing. The selection should consider the child's primary mode of communication, parent goals, additional disabilities, and the strengthening of auditory perceptual skills. In addition, professionals should be knowledgeable of assessment tools that are and are not normed on children who are d/Deaf or hard of hearing, share rationale relative to tool use, and report results with caution, especially for those tools not normed on children who are d/Deaf or hard of hearing.

 ## Techniques and Strategies

A number of techniques and strategies have been used in early intervention situations or programs. Only the following ones are discussed in detail here: the family-guided routine-based approach, parent-implemented language intervention, and other strategies to ensure high-quality service delivery.

FAMILY-GUIDED ROUTINE-BASED APPROACH

An infant's daily life consists of many routines, such as feeding, dressing, bathing, and diaper changing. These routines provide the infant with a sense of comfort and predictability, and, most important, the opportunities for language learning (Pence & Justice, 2008). Many research studies on early intervention have emphasized the importance of selecting family-guided, predictable, and positive routines that occur on a recurrent, regular basis to offer multiple opportunities for teaching and learning (e.g., Bricker & Cripe, 1992; Prizant & Bailey, 1992; Venn & Wolery, 1992).

Cripe and Venn (1997) suggested a six-step early intervention procedure: (1) identify the common schedule of the day, including normal routines; (2) select preferred daily routines for intervention; (3) build upon natural strategies or intuitive parenting behaviors used by parents or care providers; (4) implement and discuss plans with service providers; (5) teach parents or care providers new strategies and models, when appropriate; and (6) monitor progress, revise, modify, and collect feedback. Such a family-guided routine-based approach requires the early interventionist to observe and respect the family's natural interaction strategies. In addition, it "enhances the competence of the care providers, increases the likelihood that the teaching and learning opportunities will occur frequently, and respects the uniqueness of each care provider and child dyad" (Cripe & Venn, 1997, p. 22).

The principles of the parent–professional partnership are equality, mutuality, and teamwork (Allen & Petr, 1996). "Equal partners does not mean that parents and professional assume each other's roles, but rather that they respect each other's roles and contributions. While professionals bring technical knowledge and expertise to this relationship, parents offer the most intimate knowledge of their children and often special skills" (Nelkin, 1987, p. 9). A family-guided routine-based approach should ensure that the families, whenever possible, are the primary and ultimate decision makers in the intervention process. Professionals are working *for* families instead of working *with* them (Allen & Petr, 1996).

Another important characteristic of a family-guided routine-based approach is that the service should be individualized to reflect needs and strengths. From assessment selection and goal setting to intervention planning and implementation, the process should be fitted to the needs, coping strategies, and resources of each particular family, rather than expecting every family to match the preformulized approach decided by the professionals (Allen & Petr, 1996). This sensitivity to each family's needs and strengths is particularly important when considering the communication mode of a child who is d/Deaf or hard of hearing.

PARENT-IMPLEMENTED LANGUAGE INTERVENTION

In a landmark study, Hart and Risley (1999) confirmed that the first three years of a child's life is the most important period for learning languages. Before a hearing child produces his or her first word at an average age of 11 months, he or she has been listening to an average of 700 to 800 utterances per hour, half of which are results of "overhearing" conversations not directed to the child. Unfortunately, for a lot of d/Deaf and many hard of hearing children born to hearing parents, most of these valuable *incidental language-learning moments* are lost forever. Hart and Risley (1999) concluded that a significant factor in the child's cognitive development was the amount of parent–child interactions per hour. Furthermore, what mattered was not only the quantity of the interactions, but also the quality of the interactions, such as language diversity, affirmative feedback, responsiveness, and so on.

In a study on deaf children of hearing parents, Calderon (2000) found that, instead of direct school-based parental involvement, maternal communication skill was significantly associated with the child's language development, early reading skills, and social-emotional development. An effective language intervention for children has to involve the parents.

The two primary models of parent-implemented language intervention are direct instruction and activity-based instruction. *Direct instruction* is a behavior model, in which parents use didactic language instruction based on stimulus-response associations and operant conditioning principles to teach children new linguistic forms (e.g., Gersten, Woodward, & Darch, 1986; Miller & Sloane, 1976; Salzberg & Villani, 1983). It is teacher-directed, fast-paced, and highly structured.

Studies on direct instruction have constantly supported significant academic gains of the children. Nevertheless, the positive results have been shown mostly with school-age children; the generalizability of the findings to younger children has yet to be determined (Losardo & Bricker, 1994). Meanwhile, the direct instruction model has been criticized because of limited evidence to support parents' transferred use of the intervention strategies into a novel setting and children's generalized use of new linguistic forms to noninstructional time, especially for children with language impairments and/or children younger than 36 months of age (Hemmeter & Kaiser, 1994; Losardo & Bricker, 1994; McWilliam, 2000). Fey (1986) characterized it as a lack of *ecological validity*.

In contrast, *activity-based instruction* is a transactional model in which the mutual effect between the child and the social environment is emphasized. It is a naturalistic language intervention in that the topic of intervention and the reinforcement for communication are typically identified by the child's immediate interest in the environment. It is also referred to as *milieu teaching* (Alpert & Kaiser, 1992; Hemmeter & Kaiser, 1994; Laski, Charlop, & Schreibman, 1988). Activity-based instruction has been reported to better assist parents in generalizing their use of the strategies to other settings and maintaining their use (Alpert & Kaiser, 1992) as well as to increase children's vocalizations (Laski et al., 1988).

In essence, parent-implemented language intervention should not be an *either-or* choice between direct instruction and activity-based instruction. As suggested by McWilliam (2000), many research studies supporting naturalistic, activity-based interventions have simply shown that natural interventions can work instead of comparing "natural" versus "unnatural." An effective intervention should be a balanced intervention, and, most important, the intervention should be provided by parents or caregivers rather than the professionals. "It is important to remember that the amount of a service is not what's important, because *all the child's learning occurs between sessions*"(McWilliam, 2000, p. 20).

OTHER STRATEGIES TO ENSURE HIGH-QUALITY SERVICE DELIVERY

Research shows that much of what families in the early intervention programs expect is *being normal*; that is, they would like to interact in the community that is typical of others with similar interests and/or backgrounds (McGonigel, 1991). A high-quality service delivery should ensure that the normalcy of a family's life is disrupted at a minimum.

Allen and Petr (1996) suggested the following six strategies for a user-friendly service delivery in early intervention: (1) maximized accessibility; (2) flexibility and individualizing services in as many areas as possible; (3) noncategorical service delivery and funding; (4) comprehensiveness in capacity; (5) coordination of the service delivery team; (6) and the integration and expansion of a wide variety of community-based supports and resources that include both informal/formal networks and services. Working with families of children who are d/Deaf or hard of hearing, professionals need to have the moral and ethical responsibility to ensure that service delivery and funding are noncategorical or unbiased. Services and available funding for the families should not be limited to methodological affiliations or technological preferences of the professionals or clinics.

Allen and Petr (1996) further recommend family-sensitive information-sharing processes in which professionals communicate with the family in their primary language without the use of jargon, on a regular basis, in a variety of formats. "Within this model, the family generally maintains control over what information is shared, with whom, and in what manner, and confidentiality of family information is important" (p. 66). Trust, respect, communication, shared vision, and cultural sensitivity are five critical factors in high-quality early intervention service delivery (Blue-Banning et al., 2004).

A summary of the major principles of various techniques and strategies that have been used in early intervention for children who are d/Deaf or hard of hearing is provided in **Table 9-4**.

Conclusion

In sum, infant development is often compromised by the presence of an undetected hearing loss (Diefendorf, 2002). By its very nature, hearing loss provides incomplete access to spoken language that may result in a negative effect on its acquisition (Flexer, 1994). Furthermore, undetected, and therefore unmanaged, hearing loss may also negatively interfere with a child's social, emotional, and cognitive development as well as academic achievement (NCHAM, 2008). Early identification of hearing loss followed by immediate early intervention is one of the most important predictors of later normal development in a child's language, as well as academic and social life. Early amplification is critical for the development of auditory neural pathways for a child who is d/Deaf or hard of hearing.

UNHS programs typically are related to health systems rather than education systems. Therefore, a link between health and education services should be developed for educators of children who are d/Deaf or hard of hearing to be involved in early identification and intervention for infants (Arehart & Yoshinaga-Itano, 1999). Furthermore, the

Table
9-4

Major Principles of Techniques and Strategies in Early Intervention for Children Who Are d/Deaf or Hard of Hearing

Family-Guided Routine-Based Approach

- Select family-guided, predictable, and positive routines to offer multiple opportunities for teaching and learning.
- Follow the six-step early intervention procedure suggested by Cripe and Venn (1997).
- Observe and respect the family's natural interaction strategies.
- Enhance mutual respect and cooperation between the care provider and professional by joint problem-solving practice.
- The parent–professional partnership should be equal, mutual, and teamwork.
- The families, whenever possible, are the primary and ultimate decision makers in the intervention process. Professionals are working *for* families instead of working *with* them.
- The service should be individualized to reflect family needs and strengths.

Parent-Implemented Language Intervention

- A significant factor in the child's cognitive development, including language development, is the quantity and quality of parent–child interaction, including language diversity, affirmative feedback, and responsiveness.
- Parent-implemented language intervention should not be an either-or choice between direction instruction and activity-based instruction. An effective intervention should be a balanced intervention.
- The intervention should be provided by parents or caregivers rather than the professionals.

Other Strategies to Ensure High-Quality Service Delivery

- Ensure that the normalcy of a family's life is disrupted at a minimum.
- Follow the six strategies for a user-friendly service delivery in early intervention suggested by Allen and Petr (1996).
- Have the moral and ethical responsibility to ensure that service delivery and funding are noncategorical or unbiased.
- Communicate with the family following the family-sensitive information-sharing processes; that is, in their primary language without the use of jargon, on a regular basis, in a variety of formats.
- Five critical factors in high-quality early intervention service delivery are trust, respect, communication, shared vision, and cultural sensitivity.

developmental opportunities and challenges confronting young children are diverse, and the range of early intervention services and supports needed is extensive. Thus, an interdisciplinary practice, which is sometimes referred to as *professional pluralism* (Shonkoff & Meisels, 2000), should incorporate a wide range of professional disciplines, such as education, speech-language pathology, audiology, psychology, medicine, social work, occupational and physical therapy, child care, nursing, and public health. Professional preparation programs should train the professionals to work in a multidisciplinary team and prepare them to facilitate parent–child interaction.

One reminder for all professionals (and future ones!): families and young children who are d/Deaf or hard of hearing are not homogeneous groups, but are often different from each other on virtually every dimension. One intervention program is not appropriate for all children and families. The IFSP should be truly individualized instead of *one size fits all.*

We conclude the chapter with the following passage from the Committee on Integrating the Science of Early Childhood Development:

> The time has come to stop blaming parents, communities, business, and government—and to shape a shared agenda to ensure both a rewarding childhood and a promising future for all children. Central to this agenda is the importance of matching needs and capabilities. Families, for example, are the best vehicle for providing loving and caring relationships and for creating safe and nurturing environments that promote healthy physical, cognitive, linguistic, social, emotional, and moral development. (Shonkoff & Philips, 2000, p. 414)

Summary of Major Points

We hope that we have answered a number of your questions that you may have developed at the beginning of this chapter. If not, we encourage you to do further reading and to dialogue with your instructor and classmates. Now that you have completed this chapter, we also hope that you understand the importance of early intervention for young children who are d/Deaf or hard of hearing and are acquainted with some basic techniques and strategies used to deliver high-quality early intervention services.

The general intent of this chapter was to present a brief introduction on early intervention. The *Key Concepts* were as follows:

- Early identification (universal newborn screening)

- Early amplification

- Parent–professional cooperative partnerships

- Early intervention assessments

- Early intervention techniques and strategies

With respect to early intervention, we remarked that

- Universal newborn hearing screening (UNHS) is a systematic means of screening the hearing of all newborns in an effort to decrease the age at identification for infants with hearing losses.

■ To meet the needs of infants with hearing losses and their families, UNHS has shifted to early hearing detection and intervention (EHDI) programs to reflect the significance of the total package, which includes screening, diagnosis, early intervention services, and family support.

■ In a collaborated effort among several organizations, a 1-3-6 plan has been suggested for hearing screening, diagnostic evaluation, and intervention. All infants should have their hearing screened by the age of 1 month, preferably prior to being discharged from the hospital. An initial failed screening should result in implementation of the evaluation component prior to the age of 3 months. If hearing loss is diagnosed, early intervention services should begin prior to the age of 6 months.

■ Based on the 2007 CDC EHDI summary data, approximately 45% of newborn screenings were lost to follow-up and/or documentation, which indicates the need for continued growth and improvement in EHDI programs at the state and national levels.

With respect to early amplification, it was stated that

■ 95% of infants who are deaf are born to one or two parents who are hearing and utilize spoken communication. For most of these infants, early amplification is crucial to the development of auditory neural pathways in the brain for spoken-language development.

■ Based on Piaget's (1952) theory, the first two years of a child's life is the period of sensorimotor development, during which an infant will organize sensory impressions and begin to create perceptual schema, such as acquiring a native language. Full-time use (i.e., all waking hours) of amplification as early as possible is required for the brain to develop a perceptual scheme that includes sounds.

In the section on parent–professional cooperative partnerships, the following points were made

■ Early intervention refers to the planning and executing of actions by caregivers and professionals designed to assist children in the acquisition and use of target skills.

■ The research literature has suggested that the most effective strategy for normal language development of children who are d/Deaf or hard of hearing is identification of hearing loss as early as possible, followed by appropriate intervention by age 6 months.

■ Family-centered service delivery recognizes the centrality of the family in the lives of the individuals. It is guided by fully informed choices made by the family and focuses on the strengths and capabilities of these families.

■ Since the 1970s, federal and state legislation have encouraged family-centered service delivery in early childhood special education. Examples include the Education for All Handicapped Children Act of 1975, the Education of the Handicapped Act

Amendments of 1986, and the Individuals with Disabilities Education Amendments of 1997.

- Early intervention for infants and toddlers who are d/Deaf or hard of hearing focuses on two primary goals: (1) to assist the baby and family in establishing communication, capitalizing on the infant's residual hearing and supporting early social interactions; and (2) to support the baby and family so that the baby becomes fully integrated within the family unit.

- Early intervention providers should prepare to work with parents and families who are very diverse in terms of family make-up, culture, race, education level, and socioeconomic status. Having a positive belief set about parents and working from where the family is rather than from where professionals believe the family should be appears to be a winning combination.

In the section on early intervention assessments, it was highlighted that

- Assessment refers to the ongoing procedures used to identify the child's unique strengths and needs, as well as the family's concerns, priorities, and resources regarding the child's development in order to plan intervention services.

- The three trends in early childhood assessment are family-guided, naturalistic, and team-based collaboration.

- A variety of formal and informal assessments are available to collect data leading to reflective decisions for intervention. Two formal assessments for young children who are d/Deaf or hard of hearing are the MacArthur-Bates Communicative Development Inventories (CDIs) and the Cottage Acquisition Scales for Listening, Language & Speech (CASLLS).

Regarding early intervention techniques and strategies, the following points were made

- A family-guided routine-based approach is widely used to offer multiple teaching and learning opportunities for young children who are d/Deaf or hard of hearing.

- Hart and Risley (1999) concluded that a significant factor in the child's cognitive development was the amount of parent–child interactions per hour; moreover, what mattered was not only the quantity of the interactions, but also the quality of the interactions.

- A parent-implemented language intervention should not be an either-or choice between direction instruction and activity-based instruction. An effective intervention should be a balanced intervention and, most important, the intervention should be provided by parents or caregivers rather than the professionals.

- Additional techniques and strategies in delivering a high-quality service delivery are: (1) ensure the normalcy of a family's life is disrupted to a minimum; (2) be user-friendly; and (3) involve family-sensitive information-sharing processes.

Now that you have an understanding of how to work with young children who are d/Deaf or hard of hearing in the early intervention process, you are ready for speech, hearing, and language collaborations in the schools, which is the topic of Chapter 10.

Chapter Questions

Note: Some answers to the questions can be found in the chapter; however, others have a variety of possible responses based on the students' backgrounds and experiences.

1. How do UNHS and EHDI programs differ?

2. Discuss the 1-3-6 plan.

3. What are the two primary goals in early intervention for infants and toddlers who are d/Deaf or hard of hearing?

4. What is assessment? What are three trends in early childhood assessment?

5. What are the strengths of formal and informal assessments?

6. What considerations should be taken into account when selecting an assessment tool for children who are d/Deaf or hard of hearing?

7. When discussing the family-guided routine-based approach in early intervention, the authors suggest that professionals are working *for* families instead of working *with* them. What does this mean?

8. What are the two primary models of parent-implemented language interventions? Which one should be used in working with children who are d/Deaf or hard of hearing?

9. If you had an opportunity to converse with the authors, what burning questions would you ask them? Share and discuss these questions with your instructor and classmates.

Challenge Questions

Note: Complete answers are not in the text. Additional research/reading is required. In some cases, reading further or elsewhere in the text might provide some information to guide the response to a particular question.

1. This chapter suggests that early amplification might not be appropriate for every infant identified with a hearing loss. Do you agree? Why or why not?

2. The family-based early intervention model emphasizes the empowerment of the parents of a child who is d/Deaf or hard of hearing. Can over-empowerment become an issue? Why or why not? [This question will be asked again in Chapter 10.]

3. At the end of the chapter, the authors discuss *professional pluralism* in the early intervention services and supports provided for infants who are d/Deaf or hard of hearing and their families. What are the concerns that we should have about professional pluralism?

Suggested Activities

1. Develop one protocol of four to five questions that you would like to ask professionals who work with infants and toddlers who are d/Deaf or hard of hearing and their families. Here are a couple of sample questions to get you started:

   - What is your philosophy of educating young children who are d/Deaf or hard of hearing?

   - What role do you believe the parents should have within early intervention sessions?

   Using the protocol, conduct interviews with the following individuals:

   a. Audiologists who work with very young children with hearing losses

   b. Educators of the d/Deaf and hard of hearing who are early intervention providers

   c. Speech language pathologists who also work with the birth-to-3 age group, including children who are d/Deaf or hard of hearing.

   Discuss the results of your interviews with your instructor and classmates.

   a. Did you observe any particular patterns (similarities and/or differences) in the responses by type of profession? If yes, what were the similarities and/or differences? Why do you believe this may have occurred?

   b. What did you learn from this experience? Any "aha" moments? Any surprises? Did this experience alter your perceptions? If yes, how?

2. As you know, parent–professional cooperative partnerships have been identified as a critical component in the provision of early intervention services. Based on the research findings within this section of the chapter, determine five character traits that you believe would be important for an early intervention provider to possess. What characteristics did you most frequently select? Put yourself in the role of a professional, how might a session look if you possess these character traits? Share your ideas with your instructor and classmates.

References

Allen, R., & Petr, C. G. (1996). Towards developing standards and measurements for family-centered practice in family support programs. In G. Singer, L. Powers, & A. Olson (Eds.), *Redefining family support: Innovations in public-private partnerships* (pp. 57–86). Baltimore, MD: Brookes.

Alpert, C. L., & Kaiser, A. P. (1992). Training parents to do milieu language teaching with their language-impaired preschool children. *Journal of Early Intervention, 16*, 31–52.

Apuzzo, M., & Yoshinaga-Itano, C. (1995). Early identification of infants with significant hearing loss and the Minnesota Child Development Inventory. *Seminars in Hearing, 16*(2), 124–139.

Arehart, K., & Yoshinaga-Itano, C. (1999). The role of educators of the deaf in the early identification of hearing loss. *American Annals of the Deaf, 144*, 19–23.

Blue-Banning, M., Summers, J. A., Frankland, H. C., Nelson, L. L., & Beegle, G. (2004). Dimensions of family and professional partnerships: Constructive guidelines for collaboration. *Exceptional Children, 70*(2), 167–184.

Boothroyd, A. (2008). The acoustic speech signal. In J. Madell & C. Flexer (Eds.), *Pediatric audiology diagnosis, technology, and management* (pp. 159–167). New York: Thieme.

Boys Town National Research Hospital. (2009, July 25). Retrieved July 25, 2009, from http://www.babyhearing.org.

Bricker, D., & Cripe, J. (1992). *An activity-based approach to early intervention.* Baltimore, MD: Brookes.

Calderon, R. (2000). Parental involvement in deaf children's education programs as a predictor of child's language, early reading, and social-emotional development. *Journal of Deaf Studies and Deaf Education, 5*(2), 140–155.

Cripe, J. W., & Venn, M. L. (1997). Family-guided routines for early intervention services. *Young Exceptional Children, 1*(1), 18–26.

Diefendorf, A. O. (2002). Detection and assessment of hearing loss in infants and children. In J. Katz, R. Burkard, & L. Medwetsky (Eds.), *Handbook of clinical audiology* (pp. 469–480). Baltimore, MD: Lippincott Williams & Wilkins.

Early Hearing Detection & Intervention (EHDI) Program. (2007). *Summary of 2007 National CDC EHDI data: Version 1.* Retrieved June 14, 2009, from http://wonder.cdc.gov.

Early Hearing Detection & Intervention (EHDI) Program. (2008). *National EHDI goals.* Retrieved June 14, 2009, from http://www.cdc.gov/NCBDDD/ehdi/nationalgoals.htm.

Fenson, L., Marchman, V. A., Thal, D. J., Dale, P. S., Reznick, J. S., & Bates, E. (2007). *The MacArthur Communicative Development Inventories: User's guide and technical manual* (2nd ed.). Baltimore, MD: Brookes.

Fey, M. E. (1986). *Language intervention with young children.* San Diego, CA: College-Hill Press.

Flexer, C. (1994). *Facilitating hearing and listening in young children.* San Diego, CA: Singular.

Gatty, J. C. (2003). Technology: Its impact on education and the future. In B. Bodner-Johnson & M. Sass-Lehrer (Eds.), *The young deaf or hard of hearing child—A family-centered approach to early education* (pp. 127–149). Baltimore, MD: Brookes.

Gersten, R., Woodward, J., & Darch, C. (1986). Direct instruction: A research-based approach to curriculum design and teaching. *Exceptional Children, 53*, 17–31.

Hafer, J. C., & Stredler-Brown, A. (2003). Family-centered developmental assessment. In B. Bodner-Johnson, & M. Sass-Lehrer (Eds.), *The young deaf or hard of hearing child—A family-centered approach to early education* (pp. 127–149). Baltimore, MD: Brookes.

Hart, B., & Risley, T. R. (1999). *The social world of children learning to talk.* Baltimore, MD: Brookes.

Hemmeter, M. L., & Kaiser, A. P. (1994). Enhanced milieu teaching: Effects of parent-implemented language intervention. *Journal of Early Intervention, 18*(3), 269–289.

Joint Committee on Infant Hearing (JCIH). (2007). Year 2007 position statement: Principles and guidelines for hearing detection and intervention programs. *American Academy of Pediatrics, 120*, 898–921.

Joint Committee on Infant Hearing (JCIH). (2008). *History of the joint committee on infant hearing.* Retrieved June 14, 2009, from http://www.jcih.org/history.htm.

Laski, K. E., Charlop, M. H., & Schreibman, L. (1988). Training parents to use the Natural Language Paradigm to increase their autistic children's speech. *Journal of Applied Behavior Analysis, 21,* 391–400.

Losardo, A., & Bricker, D. (1994). Activity-based intervention and direct instruction: A comparison study. *American Journal on Mental Retardation, 98*(6), 744–765.

McGonigel, M. J. (1991). Philosophy and conceptual framework. In M. J. McGonigel, R. K. Kaufman, & B. H. Johnson (Eds.), *Guidelines and recommended practices for the individualized family service plan* (2nd ed., pp. 7–14). Bethesda, MD: Association for the Care of Children's Health.

McWilliam, R. A. (2000). It's only natural . . . to have early intervention in the environments where it's needed. In S. Sandall & M. Ostrosky (Eds.), *Young Exceptional Children Monograph Series No. 2: Natural Environments and Inclusion* (pp. 17–26). Denver, CO: The Division for Early Childhood of the Council for Exceptional Children.

Miller, S. J., & Sloane, H. M. (1976). The generalization effects of parent training across stimulus settings. *Journal of Applied Behavior Analysis, 9,* 355–370.

Mitchell, R. E., & Karchmer, M. A. (2004). Chasing the mythical ten percent: Parental hearing status of deaf and hard of hearing students in the United States. *Sign Language Studies, 4,* 138–163.

Moeller, M. P. (2000). Early intervention and language development in children who are deaf and hard of hearing. *Pediatrics, 106*(3), e43.

Moeller, M. P. (2002). Intervention and outcomes for young children who are deaf and hard of hearing and their families. In E. Kurtzer-White & D. Luterman (Eds.), *Early childhood deafness* (pp. 109–138). Timonium, MD: York.

Moeller, M. P., & Condon, M. (1994). A collaborative, problem-solving approach to early intervention. In J. Roush & N. D. Matkin (Eds.), *Infants and toddlers with hearing loss: Identification, assessment and family-centered intervention* (pp. 163–192). Timonium, MD: York.

National Association of the Deaf (NAD). (2000). *NAD position statement on Cochlear Implants.* Retrieved June 15, 2009, from http://www.nad.org/issues/technology/assistive-listening/cochlear-implants.

National Center for Hearing Assessment (NCHAM). (2008). *Background of the national center for hearing assessment & management.* Retrieved June 14, 2009, from http://www.infanthearing.org.

National Institute on Deafness and Other Communication Disorders (NIDCD). (2008). *Quick statistics.* Retrieved June 22, 2009, from http://www.nidcd.nih.gov/health/statistics/quick.htm.

Nelkin, V. (1987). *Family-centered health care for medically fragile children: Principles and practices.* Washington, DC: Georgetown University Child Development Center.

Nittrouer, S. (2010). *Early development of children with hearing loss.* San Diego, CA: Plural Publishing.

Northern, J. L., & Downs, M. P. (1991). *Hearing in children.* Baltimore, MD: Williams & Wilkins.

Northern, J., & Downs, M. (2002). *Hearing in children* (5th ed.). Baltimore, MD: Lippincott Williams & Wilkins.

Ostrosky, M. (2002). *Assessment: Gathering meaningful information (Young exceptional children).* Frederick, CO: Sopris West.

Pence, K. L., & Justice, L. M. (2008). *Language development from theory to practice.* Upper Saddle River, NJ: Pearson Education.

Piaget, J. (1952). *The language and thought of the child.* London: Routledge & Kegan.

Pollack, D., Goldberg, D., & Caleffe-Schenck, N. (1997). *Educational audiology for the limited-hearing infant and preschooler: An auditory-verbal program* (3rd ed.). Springfield, IL: Thomas.

Prizant, B., & Bailey, D. (1992). Facilitating the acquisition and use of communication skills. In D. B. Bailey & M. Wolery (Eds.), *Teaching infants and preschoolers with disabilities* (2nd ed., pp. 299–362). New York: Merrill.

Salzberg, C. L., & Villani, T. V. (1983). Speech training by parents of Down syndrome toddlers: Generalization across settings and instructional contexts. *American Journal of Mental Deficiency, 87,* 403–413.

Sass-Lehrer, M. (2003). Programs and services for deaf and hard of hearing children and their families. In B. Bodner-Johnson & M. Sass-Lehrer (Eds.), *The young deaf or hard of hearing child—A family-centered approach to early education* (pp. 153–180). Baltimore, MD: Brookes.

Scheetz, N. A. (2001). *Orientation to deafness* (2nd ed.). Needham Heights, MA: Allyn & Bacon.

Shonkoff, J. P., & Meisels, S. J. (Eds.). (2000). *Handbook of early childhood intervention.* New York: Cambridge University Press.

Shonkoff, J. P., & Philips, D. A. (Eds.). (2000). *From neurons to neighborhoods.* Washington, DC: National Academy Press.

Shore, R. (1997). *Rethinking the brain: New insights into early development.* New York: Families and Work Institute.

Spencer, P. E. (2003). Parent–child interaction: Implications for intervention and development. In B. Bodner-Johnson & M. Sass-Lehrer (Eds.), *The young deaf or hard of hearing child—A family-centered approach to early education* (pp. 333–368). Baltimore, MD: Brookes.

Stach, B. A., & Ramachandran, V. S. (2008). Hearing disorders in children. In J. Madell & C. Flexer (Eds.), *Pediatric audiology diagnosis, technology, and management* (pp. 3–12). New York: Thieme.

Venn, M. L., & Wolery, M. (1992). Increasing day care staff members' interactions during caregiving routines. *Journal of Early Intervention, 16,* 304–319.

Watkins, S. (2004). *SKI-HI Curriculum: Family-centered programming for infants and young children with hearing loss.* Logan, UT: Utah State University Press.

White, B. L. (1975). *The first three years of life.* New York: Avon Books.

White, K. R. (2008). Newborn hearing screening. In J. Madell & C. Flexer (Eds.), *Pediatric audiology diagnosis, technology, and management* (pp. 31–41). New York: Thieme.

Wilkes, E. M. (2001). *Cottage Acquisition Scales for Listening, Language, and Speech.* San Antonio: TX: Sunshine Cottage School for Deaf Children.

Woods, J., & Wetherby, A. M. (2007). Considerations for family-guided communication assessment of infants and toddlers in natural environments. In A. G. Kamhi, J. J. Masterson, & K. Apel (Eds.), *Clinical decision making in developmental language disorders* (pp. 3–22). Baltimore, MD: Brookes.

Yoshinaga-Itano, C. (2003). From screening to early identification and intervention: Discovering predictors to successful outcomes from children with significant hearing loss. *Journal of Deaf Studies and Deaf Education, 8*(1), 11–30.

Yoshinaga-Itano, C., Sedey, A. L., Coulter, D. K., & Mehl, A. L. (1998). The language of early- and later-identified children with hearing loss. *Pediatrics, 102,* 1161–1171.

Further Readings

Bagnato, S. J., & Simeonsson, R. J. (2008). *Authentic assessment for early childhood intervention: Best practices.* New York: Guilford Press.

Coleman, J. G. (2006). *The early intervention dictionary: A multidisciplinary guide to terminology.* Bethesda, MD: Woodbine House.

Karoly, L. A., Kilburn, M. R., & Cannon, J. S. (2005). *Early childhood interventions: Proven results, future promise.* Santa Monica, CA: RAND Corporation.

Rossi, K. (2003). *Learn to talk around the clock: A professional's early intervention toolbox.* Washington, DC: Alexander Graham Bell Association for the Deaf and Hard of Hearing.

The Royal National Institute for Deaf People. (2001). *Effective early intervention for deaf children 0–5 and their families.* London, UK: The Royal National Institute for Deaf People.

ROLE OF INTERDISCIPLINARY TEAMS

Some of the early literature on interdisciplinary . . . teams now seems somewhat idealistic and categorical. Teams were espoused on ideological rather than on pragmatic grounds. As we have come to see, the issue is not "team versus no team," but rather what kind of team, for what purpose, and under what conditions. Interdisciplinary . . . teams are not an end in themselves, but a means for more effective communication and cooperation . . . .

—Baldwin (2007, p. 33)

Synergy is the highest activity of life; it creates new untapped alternatives.

—Covey (2004, p. 261)

Key Concepts

After completing this chapter, readers should have a basic understanding of:

- Nature of teams and team members
- Types of team-based approaches
- Family-centered and family-directed types of care
- Medical, educational, and cultural care models

Much of what we have written in this book thus far has stressed the need for interdisciplinary support for children and adolescents who are d/Deaf or hard of hearing. A number of issues have added to the complexities of decision making for families of children with hearing loss, including advances in early identification and intervention (as discussed in

Chapter 9), changes in educational politics and policies, and innovations in technology (as discussed in Chapters 4 and 5). In the past, it was not unusual to hear horror stories from families about the *professional behavior* (or lack thereof) of professionals such as audiologists or otolaryngologists. For instance, a number of these professionals either apologized to the parents (e.g., "I'm so sorry to tell you that your child has a hearing loss, and he will need to wear a hearing aid, which we know is stigmatizing"), chided them for technology choices (e.g., choosing an implant over hearing aids), or criticized them for communication choices (e.g., total communication over auditory-oral). Often, these decisions were based on professional biases, and, in many cases, parents were placed in the middle between professionals who had differing opinions or approaches.

More recently, the trite expression of TEAM as an acronym for "Together Everyone Achieves More" may signify a new period for children and adolescents who are d/Deaf or hard of hearing. DesGeorges (2003) describes a "new era of hope" for families of all children with hearing loss. Early identification and intervention has been the key to changing some abysmal outcomes of the past. There may be a positive change or improvement in reading, given that many d/Deaf and a number of hard of hearing still graduate with an average third- or fourth-grade reading level (Marschark, 1997, 2007; Paul, 2009).

This "new era of hope" has improved outcomes regardless of communication mode or educational philosophy, but it is predicated on decisions made early in the child's life and education. A significant aspect of this "new era of hope" is how professionals work together to support children and their families.

The team approach discussed in this chapter has been one of the foundations for this text. For example, we, the authors, have presented our viewpoints based on our professional and personal experiences, the research in our respective fields, and the standards for our professions. We hope that our team approach has provided you with a greater breadth and understanding of information than if the book had been written by a single author from a single professional viewpoint.

Analogously, a similar type of team approach can be of benefit in supporting the child or adolescent with a hearing loss. A team approach should involve addressing alternate philosophies, methods, and ideas that help to provide the best outcomes for the child and his or her family. A common theme in both health care and education is that diverse perspectives lead to better decision making, because no one discipline can provide everything that a child and his or her family needs (Kilgo et al., 2003).

As you read this chapter, we encourage you to think of questions that will or should be answered. As we stated in previous chapters, your questions should be motivated by the *Key Concepts*. A sample group of questions might be as follows:

- What is the nature of the concept of a team?

- What is/are the role(s) of the interdisciplinary team? What about the individual members of the team? Who are members of a team?

- What are the types of team approaches?

- What is the role of the family in team-based approaches?
- Are there specific team models or philosophies?

Given that this is the last content chapter of this book, we expect you to keep in mind what you have learned from previous chapters. Try to imagine the need to apply information about issues such as amplification, the development of reading and writing, the development of speech, and so on. We do not intend to address the specifics of a particular discipline area such as mathematics or reading; however, it is clear that such knowledge needs to be brought to the table. Let us begin with a discussion of teams and team members.

Teams and Team Members

Interdisciplinary teams are obviously made up of more than one team member. The family and child are always members of any team. The other team members depend on a number of factors, including the age of the child, if the child has medical issues in addition to hearing loss, and educational placement, to name a few. When a child is first identified as having a hearing loss, the focus may be on diagnosing and determining the etiology; therefore, the team members may include the parents, audiologist, pediatrician, and otolaryngologist.

The concept of *medical home* is introduced here and described in more detail later in the chapter. This medical home may be an active aspect of the team for a young child with hearing loss, because medical considerations may be critical during this early stage. With advances in understanding the genetic aspects of hearing loss, it is not unusual for families of young children to be referred to a geneticist or medical genetics team, which often coordinates information as part of this medical home. Genetic counseling can help to provide the family with information about the nature of the hearing loss, inheritance patterns, and implications of genetic conditions in order to make informed decisions (Rehm & Madore, 2008).

When an early intervention program is initiated, other members may join the team, including an early intervention specialist, a teacher of the d/Deaf/hard of hearing, a speech-language pathologist, an occupational and/or physical therapist, and others. In some cases, a social worker and psychologist are also involved in the team. As the child progresses through school, new audiologists may join the team, including an educational audiologist and/or an implant audiologist. Team membership may vary if the child is identified as having a severe disorder or an additional low-incidence type of disability, such as deaf-blindness (Mascia & Mascia, 2003).

As adolescents who are d/Deaf or hard of hearing transition from school to higher education or work, other community resource persons may become part of the team, including the office of disability services coordinator at a university or a vocational rehabilitation counselor. Teams may have a case coordinator, and that role may vary based on the child's age and needs of the family and child.

Interdisciplinary, Multidisciplinary, and Transdisciplinary Approaches

The idea of working in teams is not a new one in either patient care or education. Madell and Flexer (2008) suggest that the "goal of team management is to have all involved professionals provide services in a coordinated way to a child with a hearing loss and his family" (p. 210). When on a team, professionals need to balance responsibilities, values, knowledge, skills, and even goals about patient care against their role as a team member in shared decision making (Interdisciplinary Team Issues, 2009).

The terms *multidisciplinary*, *interdisciplinary*, and *transdisciplinary* are often used interchangeably, and although the terms are similar, they are not the same. You may think this is antics with semantics; however, there are subtle yet substantive differences in how teams are organized that may influence how they function and their potential outcomes. Because you are reading this book, it is likely that you will be part of one of these types of teams at some point in your career; thus, a brief discussion to address the varying concepts is included here.

Historically, team approaches often focused on a multidisciplinary approach to services. A multidisciplinary team approach incorporates a number of different disciplines or professionals viewing the child with hearing loss from their own perspectives. Each profession provides its own consultation, although this may be done in the same place, such as a hospital or school, on the same day. The team may have a case conference to coordinate findings and make recommendations. Multidisciplinary teams provide more knowledge and experience than disciplines operating in isolation (Jessup, 2007).

Interdisciplinary or transdisciplinary models take the best of the multidisciplinary team function to the next level. As noted by Jessup (2007), interdisciplinary team approaches integrate separate discipline approaches into a single consultation. Case history, assessment, intervention, and goal setting are done with the team working together as a group. This model also focuses on involving the child and his or her family as equal team members.

The concept of interdisciplinary teams in relation to childhood hearing loss started to gain popularity with the early intervention of hearing loss and the advent of the Individuals with Disabilities in Education Act (IDEA). Prior to this time, parents had little input into decision making for their children and were often told what type of communication mode or educational program in which the child would participate, regardless of their preferences. As interdisciplinary teams have become more common, the idea of *family-centered* or *family-directed care/education* has become prevalent and is discussed in more detail later.

This holistic view of understanding the child or adolescent should result in better goal setting and outcomes than when professionals are working independently of each other. Jessup (2007) points out that one of the strengths of the interdisciplinary team is the fact that professionals from different disciplines are encouraged to question each other and explore alternate avenues, stepping out of what she describes as "discipline silos" to work toward the best outcome for the patient.

A transdisciplinary team approach may be considered as even more honed than an interdisciplinary model. The differences between interdisciplinary and transdisciplinary are subtle and often focus on case coordination and collaboration. As noted by Kilgo and colleagues (2003), transdisciplinary models provide the opportunity for disciplines to work together while the family has one primary contact, which is the professional who coordinates the team. This transdisciplinary approach views the child's development in a holistic manner, while avoiding duplication of services (Kilgo et al., 2003; McWilliam, 2000).

One of the most obvious advantages of the interdisciplinary approach described here is the patient-centered aspect of care. Both interdisciplinary and transdisciplinary teams reject traditional hierarchies (e.g., the concept that the physician is the "captain" of the team) in favor of situational leadership, collaboration, and communication. In addition, team members develop transferable skills in areas of problem solving, conflict resolution, and team building (Kilgo et al., 2003).

As noted by Rabidoux (2005), the current best practice suggests the need for a transdisciplinary approach. This team-based orientation has been recommended for addressing specific aspects of children who are hard of hearing or d/Deaf, including assessment, team meetings and program planning, related services, intervention activities, and service coordination, a concept that permeates both the medical and educational models, which are discussed later (Miller & Stayton, 2000).

Differences in knowledge and experience among team members are both a challenge and a benefit in the team process. It has been recommended that professionals need to work together in order to best utilize the expertise and insights of each member (Interdisciplinary Team Issues, 2009). Although disagreements between professionals would be expected, these differences in opinion are part of the strength of teams—again, recommendations and decisions from this team process are superior to those made by individual professionals or when professionals may be of the same experience or viewpoint. However, mutual respect must govern the team process, and professionals are expected to behave in a professional manner. The team approaches are summarized in **Table 10-1**.

Family-Centered and Family-Directed Types of Care

A more recent approach moves away from a focus on the "patient"; rather, there is an emphasis on the family, not just as a focus, but as an integral member of the team (see also the discussion in Chapter 9). Historically, most educational, communication, and even medical decisions about children with hearing loss were made by someone other than parents. Decisions were often made by well-meaning professionals, such as a physician or audiologist, or an educator, such as a teacher or a principal. In many cases, these "decision makers" purported to be acting in the best interest of the child and helping the parent. These decisions makers brought their own biases and beliefs to the process, and, in some cases, these differed significantly from the parents' values.

Table 10-1	Team Models	
Type of Team	**Major Components**	
Multidisciplinary	• Different professions see child separately through their own professional "eyes."	
	• May be a series of consultations that happen in the same physical location by separate professionals; can save time for the family.	
	• May have case conference.	
	• Superior to professionals working in isolation.	
Interdisciplinary	• Integrates individual components into one team.	
	• Professionals are encouraged to step outside of their individual disciplines and question, challenge, and learn from each other.	
	• Parents are considered to be equal partners on the team.	
Transdisciplinary	• May co-evaluate or co-treat.	
	• Any discipline can be case coordinator; case coordination and collaboration are keys.	
	• Holistic approach to child development.	

Many changes have occurred, resulting in a shift from parents being told what they should do to parents directing the care, service delivery, and communicating options for their children. Sass-Lehrer (2004) stated that the shift from a professionally centered service of the past to the current family-directed model has been driven by evidence-based research and practices, new theoretical perspectives, and changing forces in the social and political climate. As noted by Sass-Lehrer and Bodner-Johnson (2003), family-centered care is the foundation for early intervention and the best practice for working with families of children with hearing loss.

Family-directed care is mandated as part of legislative policy in early intervention for all children with special needs (see also the discussion of related aspects in Chapter 9). This approach requires an understanding of child development and the role that the family plays in this development. An example of this is early identification of hearing loss, the approach now available with UNHS programs in nearly every state (again, see Chapter 9).

Roush and Kamo (2008) point out that, historically, hearing loss was confirmed after weeks, months, or sometimes years of parental suspicion that the child had a hearing loss. Fortunately, this is now an issue of the past, because hearing loss is now identified in early infancy. However, this presents a new group of challenges and concerns. Roush and Kamo (2008) suggest that this early identification "puts parents in the difficult position of needing to accept the diagnosis without the benefit of direct observation" (p. 269).

The "old school" view of the benevolent professional or educator dictating choices to the parent has been replaced by the parents being active members of the team, growing into the role of leading the team for their child. It is critical that professionals working with the family have knowledge of general development, the role of the family dynamics, and the family's social and cultural background in order to facilitate service delivery to a child. It is important that the impact of the hearing loss on the family is considered, along with the family's role in the life of a child.

Family-directed care is a tenet of an early hearing loss detection and intervention (EHDI) program, as outlined by the Joint Committee on Infant Hearing (JCIH, 2007). The JCIH recommends parent participation in the development of a hearing care system, because parents are able to recognize what is most important for their families (JCIH, 2000). This approach suggests that parents should be involved in serving in advisory groups, assist with the development of educational materials, and provide support to other families in the process of early identification of their child's hearing loss.

One of the major issues in the early identification of hearing loss, and one in which both family involvement and systematic family participation may be vital, is that of providing unbiased information regarding communication and educational options. In some cases, provincial views and biases may be offered based on a geographic location.

A number of excellent organizations have the goal of providing unbiased information to professionals and families. One of the best examples, Beginnings for Parents of Children who are Deaf or Hard of Hearing (2009), is a nonprofit organization incorporated in 1987 in North Carolina. Beginnings provides impartial information based on the premise that parents, given accurate, objective information about hearing loss, will make sound decisions for their child.

Another organization, developed by parents of children with hearing loss, is Hands and Voices (2009), a group dedicated to providing parents and professionals unbiased information regarding communication modes and methods. Contact information for several organizations that focus on presenting unbiased information to parents and families is listed in the Appendix of this book.

Medical, Educational, and Cultural Models

In this section, we shall consider several groups of models that can be categorized as medical, educational, or cultural. These models have evolved since their inception. Many factors have influenced this evolution, such as mandates for universal newborn hearing screening, the development of early intervention programs, the enactment of the Americans with Disabilities Act (ADA), and the implementation of the Individuals with Disabilities in Education Act (IDEA), just to name a few.

Sorkin (2008) remarked that there is a new model for "disability" that stipulates that there is no shame or pity in having a disability. Individuals with a disability, instead of hiding, have developed pride in their abilities and have celebrated their differences. This is an alternative viewpoint, and considering the tenets of Deaf culture as well, it is clear that the United States has become a more culturally and linguistically diverse nation, with educators stating a commitment to cultural proficiency through multicultural education, which may also be a factor in this transition (Johnson & Nieto, 2007).

These issues underscore the multifaceted nature of addressing the needs of d/Deaf and hard of hearing children, particularly in building a team-based initiative. The current movement has engendered many models; however, only three are discussed here: hearing loss as a medical issue, hearing loss as an educational matter, and hearing loss as part of the culture of deafness. Each model has implications for the lives of children and adolescents and certainly has influenced the nature of the team process.

MEDICAL HOME (I.E., MEDICAL MODEL)

The advent of UNHS programs and EHDI services has resulted in the development of models and service delivery systems that address the needs of children who are d/Deaf and hard of hearing and their families (as discussed also in Chapter 9). It has been recommended that all aspects of hearing loss in children be embedded in a system of comprehensive services that include identification of hearing loss, family guidance and support, selection and fitting of technology, and counseling (Jerger, Roeser, & Tobey, 2001).

In most cases, parents have little or no knowledge of hearing loss; however, they may be asked to quickly make decisions related to technology and educational, communicative, and habilitation options. In the past, when information to parents was viewed as fragmented and not coordinated, it affected the process for their child, from diagnosis to intervention. In essence, this situation underlies the importance of providing a coordinated system (Fitzpatrick, Angus, Drieux-Smith, Graham, & Coyle, 2008).

The model of health care in the United States, along with the focus on identification of hearing loss as a medical issue, has resulted in the development of a coordinated team approach of the *medical home*, a concept outlined by the American Academy of Pediatrics (AAP). The medical home is:

> ...an active process, a philosophy of care that emphasizes the role of the primary care physician, particularly for children who have special needs. This physician serves as a focal point not only for the typical primary medical care of the child but also for the support of parents and family, the coordination of specialty medical care, the provision of referrals for various services, the assurance of timely follow-up and the medical interface for educational interventions. (Mehl, 2007, p. 25)

From a team perspective, the medical home has considerable appeal because the child and family benefit from coordination of services, appropriate medical follow-up, and support. Preece (2004) delineates the benefits of a single professional, usually the pediatrician, coordinating care and information flow related to the child's health. There is also benefit in reducing the time and cost redundancies that can occur in health care.

As noted earlier in the chapter, addressing the medical and genetic aspects of childhood hearing loss can provide information about etiology of the hearing loss, which can help to direct management and appropriate services for the child. However, this model can be limited by the view that the hearing loss is a medical problem to be cured and by a lack of knowledge on the part of a physician.

Physicians are often ill-prepared to take a leadership role on a team. For example, it has been reported that pediatricians generally have little knowledge of hearing screening or evaluation techniques in infants. In addition, they do not routinely recommend screening of hearing, even when parents have expressed concern (Colozza & Anastasio, 2009).

The value of the medical home approach is maximized when it is implemented as part of a team. Preece (2004) stated that for the medical home model to work there must be strong communication among the team members. This team model and methods for enhancing communication have been recommended by the JCHI (2007).

In essence, the medical model is only one way of addressing children who are d/Deaf or hard of hearing. It may be an effective approach for a child with a newly identified hearing loss, when the child is an infant or toddler, or when the child has multiple disabilities. Many of the questions that can be answered in the medical-model type of team—what is the etiology of the hearing loss or does the child have any other medical conditions coexisting with the hearing loss, for example—are answered.

EDUCATIONAL TEAM MODEL

The focus in the preschool and school-aged years becomes education for the child who is d/Deaf and/or hard of hearing, with goals for communication mode, educational placement, and class placement, to name a few (Tye-Murray, 2009). This focus provides the rationale for the development and use of the educational team model.

A brief discussion of educational laws addressing children with hearing loss is provided here as a context for this team discussion. As discussed elsewhere, historically, many children with hearing loss have been educated in programs that are "self-contained" (e.g., Marschark, 2007; Moores, 2001). These programs are often not housed in schools in the child's neighborhood or even in her or his school district. In some cases, children lived in a residential program for children with hearing loss or were transported to a centralized program where children from many schools were included in a "day" program.

These educational options often separated children from their siblings and neighborhood friends. The decision on placement was rarely made with, or even based on, parental input. Rather, it was driven by a convenience factor for the district and the conservation of resources. The goal was often to place all children with hearing loss into a homogeneous group. Parents were told "this is what we have to offer" and were given a "take it or leave it" option with regard to their child's education (Sorkin, 2008).

In 1975, the Individuals with Disabilities Education Act (IDEA) was signed into law. IDEA embraced the concept that every child was to be provided with a free and appropriate public education (FAPE) in their least restrictive environment (LRE). The concept of LRE stressed that children with hearing loss must be educated with peers who do not have a hearing loss, to the maximum extent possible. The LRE refers to a continuum that covers several possibilities including self-contained classrooms and mainstreamed classrooms, where students with hearing loss are educated in classrooms with hearing peers.

IDEA is a federal law that provides state and local funding to address all children with disabilities in educational settings, including preschool. Specifically, educational services and support are provided to children between the ages of 3 and 21 years of age, inclusive. Other federal laws related to education that have been enacted include No Child Left Behind (NCLB), which holds schools accountable for academic achievement for all students, and Section 504 of the Rehabilitation Act of 1973, which requires that schools cannot discriminate against children with hearing loss and must provide access to school programs.

One of the cornerstones of IDEA is the concept of a team-based approach to educational planning and goal setting for children with disabilities. The work of the team is reflected in a document known as the *Individualized Education Plan* (IEP) for school-aged children and the *Individualized Family Service Plan* (IFSP) for preschoolers. As noted by Sorkin (2008), the "IEP is a written legal document that provides detail on the special education and related services that a child needs to receive an education" (p. 221). Educators, professionals, parents, and, in some cases, the child, come together to address appropriate goals, how the goals will be achieved, and how progress will be measured. The IFSP is a similar type of document, but addresses both the needs of the child and the needs and goals of the family in the process of early intervention.

The role of the parents in the process is a significant focus of the federal legislation. In contrast to the past, when educational settings and goals were dictated to families, the current landscape assures that parents participate in the direction of their child's educational program. Some educators would argue that perhaps this pendulum has swung too far with parents *directing* or *dictating* their child's education. The process is clearly outlined for parents, including their rights if they disagree with goals or the process for their child, in documents such as *Whose IDEA Is This? A Parent's Guide to the Individuals with Disabilities Education Improvement Act of 2004 (IDEA)* (e.g., the procedural safeguards notice published by the Ohio Department of Education, 2009).

CULTURAL MODELS

Neither the medical model nor the educational model fully addresses the concept of hearing loss or deafness as a culture. The medical model is perceived as seeing the hearing loss as a "problem to be fixed" with the team focused on the "fixing." The educational model is perceived as focusing on educational choice and advocacy; yet, the team is often focused on the concept of disability, and not on ability or difference.

As noted earlier, one of the foci of EHDI programs is to provide unbiased information to parents regarding hearing loss and deafness. The intent is that parents can make decisions based on what is best for their children and families in terms of cultural and societal inclusion. Because most children with hearing loss are born to parents who are hearing, these families might have an automatic knowledge of auditory-oral communication and philosophy, because this is how they communicate as part of the hearing world.

Advocates for a cultural model of deafness insist that appropriate decisions can only be made if families understand their range of options. In addition to providing written information, Web-based options, and recorded information, some EHDI programs include d/Deaf mentors as part of their teams who provide insight into the cultural aspects of hearing loss. In this case, a d/Deaf adult may partner with a family to share his or her personal experiences and to enhance knowledge of the cultural and linguistic heritage of deafness or the DEAF-WORLD (Hyde, 2005). This model promotes the view that deafness is a difference and not a disability (see also the discussion in Paul, 2009). Those who are hard of hearing and/or d/Deaf are part of a minority group, with education being delivered from a "deaf-serving institution" perspective rather than being viewed as needing special education or rehabilitative services (Denzer, 2008).

The team approach in a cultural view provides support for all families of children with hearing loss. This may be especially important if American Sign Language (ASL) is the first language for the child. In this case, resources are provided to support the development of sign both for the child and his or her family.

An Example of a Model of Success for Teams: Cochlear Implants

Regardless of the philosophical model or approach, one of the most effective models for interdisciplinary teams' success has been that of cochlear implantation in working with children with hearing loss. Clearly, as discussed in Chapter 5, cochlear implantation has been successful for at least some children with hearing loss. The implantation processes can be viewed as successful based on a number of factors, including technological advances and evidence-based research that has translated into a standard of care. However, perhaps the most significant aspect of the success has been a team-based service provision to children and their families in the cochlear implantation process.

As noted by Wiley and Meinzen-Derr (2009), cochlear implant candidacy in children is a complex process that requires a team approach. This type of approach provides a comprehensive evaluation of the child and family, not just addressing hearing, but also addressing the "big picture," including communication potential, family expectations, and other factors that contribute to the eventual outcomes.

The greatest successes of cochlear implantation may be more philosophical than technological. Many scholars attribute the success of the implantation process to the technology; however, we, the authors of this text, would contend that the success is just as much related to the information and support of the team approach than by the technology itself. Outcomes are optimized by understanding that the device does not "do the work" and that following the surgery an intense follow-up schedule and therapy program needs to be implemented.

As part of a systematic, integrated approach, these services and support are available to children and their families. The cochlear implantation process can be used as a vehicle for educating families about options, goals, and communication modes. One of the strengths of the team approach to cochlear implantation is to provide information to families, whether or not they ultimately choose to pursue the surgery or whether the child becomes a candidate for cochlear implantation. This is important for the team approach, because very few guidelines exist for individual professionals serving children with hearing loss (Bradham, Snell, & Haynes, 2009).

Wiley and Meinzen-Derr (2009) remarked that something as simple as a team-based informational meeting may address misinformation or augment current knowledge that contributes to better decision making. This type of cochlear implantation model could be implemented for any and all approaches, philosophies, and educational decisions for children with hearing loss to improve outcomes and quality of life for children who are d/Deaf or hard of hearing.

The Future of Teams

We have highlighted that a team approach involves collaboration among professions working with children and adolescents who are d/Deaf or hard of hearing. At the very least, this would involve the professionals targeted by this text: future audiologists, educators, speech-language pathologists, and educational interpreters. Many other professionals may also be involved.

Although not all professionals have the ability to work as part of an interdisciplinary or transdisciplinary team, current best practices certainly support that collaboration and teamwork are the keys to success for children with hearing loss. Challenges are ahead, including issues of consensus building across philosophies, changes in the healthcare funding that limit team options, and developments of technology that change how issues are currently addressed. Regardless of the challenges, it is clear that professionals must be willing to work together to ensure the most positive outcomes for the child.

DesGeorges (2003) states that a team model not only supports the family, but that it also infuses knowledge into the system, improving the process for current families and other families in the future. In addition, as was modeled by early cochlear implantation teams presented previously, in which basic and applied science combined to improve outcomes, it is likely that collaborative and interdisciplinary research by neuroscientists, cognitive scientists, and auditory scientists will change the future landscape of the aural habilitation/rehabilitation process (Kricos & McCarthy, 2007). As new challenges, such as the concept of *telehealth*, are addressed, the roles of teams are likely to increase in addressing the evolving needs of children and adolescents.

Summary of Major Points

In this chapter, our focus was on the nature and role of interdisciplinary teams, including teams that are constructed during the child's formal educational years (i.e., preschool to high school). Some of the information reiterated the major concepts in Chapter 9 on early intervention. However it is stated, it is clear that a variety of professionals need to work together and that families (i.e., parents) should play leading roles in collaborative teams.

Our goal was to present highlights relevant to the following *Key Concepts:*

- Nature of teams and team members

- Types of team-based approaches

- Family-centered and family-directed types of care

- Medical, educational, and cultural care models

With respect to the nature of teams and team members, we stated that

- Interdisciplinary teams are obviously made up of more than one team member. The family and child are always members of any team.

- Members for a team depend on the specific needs of the child and his or her family.

- When an early intervention program is initiated, additional members may join the team, including an early intervention specialist, a teacher of the d/Deaf/hard of hearing, a speech-language pathologist, an occupational and/or physical therapist, and others. In some cases, a social worker and psychologist are also involved in the team.

- Team membership may vary if the child is identified as having a severe disorder or an additional low-incidence type of disability, such as deaf-blindness.

- As adolescents who are d/Deaf or hard of hearing transition from school to higher education or work, other community resource persons may become part of the team.

Considering the types of team-based approaches, it was stated that

- The terms *multidisciplinary*, *interdisciplinary*, and *transdisciplinary* are often used interchangeably, and although the terms are similar, they are not the same.

- A multidisciplinary team approach incorporates a number of different disciplines or professionals viewing the child with hearing loss from their own perspectives.

- Interdisciplinary and transdisciplinary models take the best of the multidisciplinary team function to the next level.

- The concept of interdisciplinary teams in relation to childhood hearing loss started to gain popularity with the EHDI programs and the advent of the Individuals with Disabilities in Education Act (IDEA).

- As interdisciplinary teams have become more common, the idea of *family-centered* or *family-directed care/education* has become prevalent.

- A transdisciplinary team approach may be considered as even more honed than an interdisciplinary model. The current best practice suggests the need for a transdisciplinary approach.

In the section on family-centered and family-directed types of care, it was noted that

- A more recent approach proceeds away from a focus on the "patient"; rather, there is an emphasis on the family, not just as a focus, but as an integral member of the team.

- Many changes have occurred, which has resulted in a shift from parents being told what they should do to parents directing the care, service delivery, and communicating options for their children.

- Family-directed care is mandated as part of a legislative policy in early intervention for all children with special needs.

- It is critical that professionals working with the family have knowledge of general development, the role of the family dynamics, and the family's social and cultural background in order to facilitate service delivery to a child.

With respect to medical, educational, and cultural models, it was stated that

- Care models can be categorized as medical, educational, or cultural.

- There is a new model for "disability" that states that there is no shame or pity in having a disability.

- The model of health care in the United States, along with the focus on identification of hearing loss as a medical issue, has resulted in the development of a coordinated team approach of the medical home.

- The focus in the preschool and school-aged years becomes education for the child who is d/Deaf and/or hard of hearing, with goals for communication mode, educational placement, and class placement, to name a few. This focus provides the rationale for the development and use of the educational team model.

- The cultural model promotes the view that deafness is a difference and not a disability. Those who are hard of hearing and/or d/Deaf are part of a minority group, with education being delivered from a "deaf-serving institution" perspective rather than being viewed as needing special education or rehabilitative services.

- Regardless of the philosophical model or approach, one of the most effective models for interdisciplinary teams' success has been that of cochlear implantation in working with children with hearing loss.

- Although not all professionals have the ability to work as part of an interdisciplinary or transdisciplinary team, current best practices certainly support that collaboration and teamwork are the keys to success for children with hearing loss.

Chapter Questions

Note: *Some answers to the questions can be found in the chapter; however, others have a variety of possible responses based on the students' backgrounds and experiences.*

1. What is the nature of the concept of *team*? How are team members selected? Be sure to discuss the issues of early intervention and transition.

2. Describe briefly the nature and basic tenets of the following team approaches:

   a. Interdisciplinary

   b. Multidisciplinary

   c. Transdisciplinary

   Which approach seems to be supported by research as being the most effective? Explain.

3. What is meant by family-centered or family-directed care? What factors precipitated the shift to this type of care? What was the traditional focus?

4. Discuss the concept of the medical home.

5. Describe the basic tenets of the following models:

   a. Medical

   b. Educational

   c. Cultural

6. What is an IEP? An IFSP? How do they differ?

7. Provide a few major points (at least three) that you have gleaned from the section "An Example of a Model of Success for Teams: Cochlear Implants."

8. Provide a few major points (at least three) that you have learned from the section "The Future of Teams."

9. If you had an opportunity to converse with the authors, what burning questions would you ask them? Share and discuss these questions with your instructor and classmates.

Challenge Questions

Note: *Complete answers are not in the text. Additional research/reading is required. In some cases, reading further or elsewhere in the text might provide some information to guide a response to a particular question.*

1. There is some overlap in information between this chapter and the chapter on early intervention (Chapter 9). Discuss the similarities and differences. [Note: This is a wide-open question, but you might want to focus on the nature of "teams" discussed in both chapters and the concept of family-centered or family-directed care.]

2. Given what was discussed in Chapter 5 regarding the issue of auditory deprivation (i.e., when ears are not stimulated), do you think that parents should really have a choice on whether to implement early amplification (e.g., via digital hearing aids or cochlear implants) for their children? Should laws be passed mandating early amplification? Why or why not?

Suggested Activities

1. Do a review of the literature on the concept of teams in other areas of special education (e.g., children with language/learning disabilities; children with cognitive disabilities, etc.). Do these other areas have similar "teams"? Are there differences? Share your findings with your instructor and classmates.

2. If possible, attend an IEP and an IFSP meeting for a child with hearing loss. Who was present at these meetings? What role did each person play? Can you describe the contributions of each member? Do you feel that all contributions were valued and encouraged? Why or why not? Share your findings with your instructor and classmates.

3. If possible, interview each member of the team in the meetings described in the previous activity (i.e., IEP and IFSP). How does each person feel about his or her role in the "team" meeting? Do these assertions match your observations? Share your findings with your instructor and classmates.

References

Baldwin, D. C. (2007). Some historical notes on interdisciplinary and interprofessional education and practice in health care in the USA. *Journal of Interprofessional Care, 21*(S1), 23–37.

Beginnings for Parents of Children who are Deaf or Hard of Hearing. (2009). Retrieved from http://www.ncbegin.org/about_us/about_us.shtml.

Bradham, T. S., Snell, G., & Haynes, D. (2009). Current practices in pediatric cochlear implantation. *Perspectives on Hearing and Hearing Disorders in Childhood, 19*(1), 32–42.

Colozza, P., & Anastasio, A. (2009). Screening, diagnosing and treating deafness—The knowledge and conduct of doctors serving in neonatology and/or pediatrics in a tertiary teaching hospital. *Sao Paulo Medical Journal, 127*(2), 61–65.

Covey, S. (2004). *The 7 habits of highly effective people: 15th anniversary edition*. New York: Free Press.

Denzer, N. (2008). Deaf-serving institutions as minority settings. In M. Gasman, B. Baez, & C. S. V. Turner (Eds.), *Understanding minority-serving institutions* (pp. 57–70). Albany, NY: State University of New York Press.

DesGeorges, J. (2003). Family perceptions of early hearing, detection, and intervention systems: Listening to and learning from families. *Mental Retardation and Developmental Disabilities Research Review, 9*(3), 89–93.

Fitzpatrick, E., Angus, D., Durieux-Smith, A., Graham, I. D., & Coyle, D. (2008). Parents' needs following identification of childhood hearing loss. *American Journal of Audiology, 17*(6), 38–49.

Hands and Voices (2009). Retrieved from http://www.handsandvoices.org.

Hyde, M. (2005). Newborn hearing screening programs: Overview. *The Journal of Otolaryngology, 34* (Suppl 2), S70–S78.

Interdisciplinary Team Issues. (2009). *Ethics in medicine*. University of Washington School of Medicine. Retrieved from http://depts.washington.edu/bioethx/topics/team.html.

Jerger, S., Roeser, R. J., & Tobey, E. A. (2001). Management of hearing loss in infants: The UTD/Callier Center position statement. *Journal of the American Academy of Audiology, 12*, 329–336.

Jessup, R. (2007). Interdisciplinary versus multidisciplinary care teams: Do we understand the difference? *Australian Health Review, 31*(3), 330–331.

Johnson, R. J., & Nieto, J. (2007). Towards a cultural understanding of the disability and deaf experience. A content analysis of introductory multicultural textbooks. *Multicultural Perspectives, 9*(3), 33–43.

Joint Committee on Infant Hearing. (2000). Year 2000 position statement: Principles and guidelines for early hearing detection and intervention programs. *Pediatrics, 106*(4), 798–817.

Joint Committee on Infant Hearing. (2007). Year 2007 position statement: Principles and guidelines for early hearing detection and intervention programs. *Pediatrics, 120*(4), 898–921.

Kilgo, J. K., Aldridge, J., Denton, B., Vogtel, L., Vincent, J., Burke, C., & Unanue, R. (2003). Transdisciplinary teaming: A vital component of inclusive services. *Focus on Inclusive Education, 1*(1), 1–4.

Kricos, P. B., & McCarthy, P. (2007). From ear to there: A historical perspective on auditory training. *Seminars in Hearing, 28*(2), 89–98.

Madell, J. R., & Flexer, C. (2008). Collaborative team management of children with hearing loss. In J. R. Madell & C. Flexer (Eds.), *Pediatric audiology: Diagnosis, technology, and management* (pp. 210–217). San Diego, CA: Plural Publishing.

Marschark, M. (1997). *Raising and educating a deaf child: A comprehensive guide to the choices, controversies, and decisions faced by parents and educators*. New York: Oxford University Press.

Marschark, M. (2007). *Raising and educating a deaf child: A comprehensive guide to the choices, controversies, and decisions faced by parents and educators* (2nd ed.). New York: Oxford University Press.

Mascia, J., & Mascia, N. (2003). Methods and strategies for audiological assessment of individuals who are deaf-blind with developmental disabilities. *Seminars in Hearing, 24*(3), 211–221.

McWilliam, R. A. (2000). Recommended practices in interdisciplinary models. In S. Sandall, M. McLean, & B. Smith (Eds.), *DEC recommended practices for early intervention/early childhood special education* (pp. 47–54). Longmont, CO: Sopris West.

Mehl, A. (2007). A medical home for infants who are deaf or hard of hearing. *Volta Voices*, (March/April), 24–27.

Miller, P., & Stayton, V. (2000). Recommended practices in personnel preparation. In S. Sandall, M. McLean, & B. Smith (Eds.), *DEC recommended practices for early intervention/early childhood special education* (pp. 77–88). Longmont, CO: Sopris West.

Moores, D. (2001). *Educating the deaf: Psychology, principles, and practices* (5th ed.). Boston: Houghton-Mifflin.

Ohio Department of Education. (2009). *Whose IDEA is this? A parent's guide to the Individuals with Disabilities Education Improvement Act of 2004 (IDEA)*. Retrieved from http://education.ohio.gov/GD/Templates/Pages/ODE/ODEDetail.aspx?Page=3&TopicRelationID=968&Content=69801.

Paul, P. (2009). *Language and deafness* (4th ed.). Sudbury, MA: Jones & Bartlett.

Preece, J. P. (2004). Issues in family-centered pediatric audiology: An overview. *Seminars in Hearing, 25*(4), 291–293.

Rabidoux, P. (2005). Early identification of autism: Roles of the speech-language pathologist and audiologist on a transdisciplinary team. *Seminars in Hearing, 26*(4), 210–216.

Rehm, H. L., & Madore, R. (2008). Genetics of hearing loss. In J. R. Madell & C. Flexer (Eds.), *Pediatric audiology: Diagnosis, technology, and management* (pp. 13–24). San Diego, CA: Plural Publishing.

Roush, J., & Kamo, G. (2008). Counseling and collaboration with parents of children with hearing loss. In J. R. Madell & C. Flexer (Eds.), *Pediatric audiology: Diagnosis, technology, and management* (pp. 269–277). San Diego, CA: Plural Publishing.

Sass-Leher, M. (2004). Early detection of hearing loss: Maintaining a family-centered perspective. *Seminars in Hearing, 25*(4) 295–307.

Sass-Lehrer, M., & Bodner-Johnson, B. (2003). Early intervention: Current approaches to family-centered programming. In M. Marschark & P. Spencer (Eds.), *Deaf studies, language and education* (pp. 65–81). New York: Oxford University Press.

Sorkin, D. L. (2008). Education and access laws for children with hearing loss. In J. R. Madell & C. Flexer (Eds.), *Pediatric audiology: Diagnosis, technology, and management* (pp. 218–231). San Diego, CA: Plural.

Tye-Murray, N. (2009). *Foundations of aural rehabilitation: Children, adults, and their family members*. Clifton Park, NY: Delmar.

Wiley, S., & Meinzen-Derr, J. (2009). Access to cochlear implant candidacy evaluations: Who is not making it to the team evaluations? *International Journal of Audiology, 48*(2), 74–79.

Further Readings

Brown, W., Thurman, S. K., & Pearl, L. F. (1993). *Family-centered early intervention with infants and toddlers: Innovative cross-disciplinary approaches*. Baltimore, MD: Brookes.

Garner, H. G. (1995). *Teamwork models and experience in education*. New York: Allyn & Bacon.

Kumar, S. (Ed.). (2000). *Multidisciplinary approach to rehabilitation*. Woburn, MA: Elsevier Health Sciences.

McGreevey, M. (Ed.). (2006). *Patients as partners*. Oakbrook Terrace, IL: Joint Commission Resources.

Vargas, C. M., & Prelock, P. (2005). *Caring for children with neurodevelopmental disabilities and their families: An innovative approach to interdisciplinary practice*. Philadelphia, PA: Routledge.

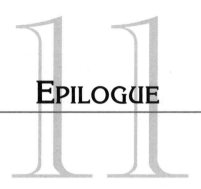

EPILOGUE

What students think they are doing is much more important than what we think we want to teach them. With sustained engagement, they will come to believe that inquiry and argument offer the most promising path to resolving conflicts, solving problems, and achieving goals. They will become convinced that there are things to find out, that analysis is worthwhile, that unexamined beliefs are not worth having.

—Kuhn (2005, pp. 198–199)

The above passage is the other "bookend" to the beginning one by Alexander Pope, which was presented in the Preface. Engaging in inquiry and argument and other similar critical-thinking processes should minimize the negative implications of Pope's message in "A little learning...." If you want a grandiose phrase, here is one of Socrates'—"The unexamined life is not worth living." In any case, we strongly encourage you to engage in intensive and extensive reflective thinking, reading, and writing processes. This will come in handy for your ongoing professional development and accords nicely with the points that shall be proffered in this epilogue.

An epilogue is actually the bookend to a *foreword*; it is similar to an *afterword*. It is supposed to be short and sweet, and typically it offers future trends and patterns. Our goal here is to highlight three salient themes from this book, to proffer a few recommendations for university preparation programs, and to provide our perspectives.

These three themes are:

- The importance of hearing
- The brave new world of technology
- Collaboration among professionals and with parents

In short, our three themes can be briefly labeled as *hearing*, *technology*, and *collaboration*.

The first theme revolves around the concept of *hearing*. It is axiomatic, and actually quite obvious, that audition (i.e., hearing) is critical for the development of speech, language, and literacy. This is the case for the development of English and even other spoken languages. And, as you might have discovered in this book, children and adolescents who are d/Deaf or hard of hearing have many, some almost insurmountable, challenges in this area. In addition, it should be clear that English is somewhat of a special case because it is an opaque, phonemic language. Briefly, this means that some letters have more than one sound, and some sounds have more than one letter.

It should not be surprising that there is a relationship between degree of hearing loss and the ability to not only produce and perceive speech sounds accurately, but also in even reaching a proficient level with speaking, reading, and writing English. We suspect that it is not earthshaking to learn that there are strong interrelations among hearing, speech, language, and literacy. In short, hearing is critical.

Lest you think that we have stated the obvious, and perhaps killed one tree too many to put this on paper, these comments need to be reiterated because of what seems to be a negative stigma associated with a concept such as hearing and its related cousin, speech. This controversy is situated in the long-standing debates between clinical (medical) proponents and cultural proponents, which was mentioned at the beginning of and sporadically throughout the book (see also the discussions in Lane, 1992; Marschark, 2007; Moores, 2001; Paul, 2009).

Moreover, this controversy has spilled over into university preparation programs. Despite the lack of adequate research support for our assertions, it is possible that many programs for the education of d/Deaf or hard of hearing students, for example, do not require more than one course or *any* courses in speech and hearing science (this is certainly the case at Ohio State University, but we are working to change that!). You have also seen vestiges of this controversy in the discussion of digital hearing aids, cochlear implants, and early amplification in this book.

We shall state this one more time, emphatically: we are not belittling the values and mores of cultural proponents. There is a place for such ideas in both schools and clinics. Nevertheless, with respect to the development of English language and literacy, we believe that more attention needs to be paid to hearing (and speech) in university preparation programs. *Hearing* is not a seven-letter word (we'll let you figure out our puny attempt to proffer an analogous metaphor!).

By now, you should understand why we devoted one chapter to the anatomy and physiology of the ear (Chapter 2), one to the assessment of hearing (Chapter 3), and one to the use of rehabilitation techniques (Chapter 8). Of course, we demonstrated the interrelations among hearing, speech, language, and literacy in two other chapters (Chapters 6 and 7). Our crystal ball tells us that hearing will become even more critical in the future with the advent of new technologies, the next theme to be discussed.

Repeat after us: analog is past; digital is now. All right—we won't get carried away. However, it is pretty hard not to become overly excited about the future of technology, which—as you suspected—should enhance (and, perhaps, glorify) the virtues of hearing.

We might not ever achieve the status of *The Six Million Dollar Man*, but research is producing amazing new products.

Will technology ever make a child or adolescent with hearing loss "exactly like" a child with hearing? In this book, we have repeatedly emphasized that digital hearing aids or cochlear implants are not a panacea or a miracle cure. Nevertheless, miracles do happen, and professionals should not rule out the possibility of a new product or technique that might restore hearing completely.

In the interim, there might be competition between the merits of digital hearing aids against those of cochlear implants. The benefits of each device will be increased to match the needs of specific individuals. It is difficult to predict which amplification device will outlast the other; perhaps, this is the wrong focus or an inappropriate way to view the situation. It is hoped that the cost of cochlear implants go down and access to services to maximize benefits from the device increase so that these do not become an impediment to implant candidacy.

We also suspect that there will be additional connections between these amplification devices and other aspects of technology, similar to the revolution going on now with mobile devices (e.g., the iPhone) and so on. We have already seen this trend with wireless capabilities for hearing aid programming and accessing Bluetooth technology to connect hearing aids to a range of gadgets. It would be nice to turn on the coffee maker with our amplification device!

Previously, it was mentioned that technology is going to emphasize the salience of hearing. We should add that it is also going to highlight even more the negative effects of the absence of hearing. In other words, if you do not use your hearing, you will lose it, or, more specifically, lose the ability to use it. To put it professionally: if the ear is not stimulated, there will be a deprivation that might not be overcome. The longer the period of deprivation, the more difficult the recovery, and the recovery probably never reaches the original potential of hearing as it exists in typical ears. It might be helpful to revisit our main points in Chapters 4 and 5.

Before leaving our good friend, technology, we feel the urge to delve into what is perhaps the greatest controversy of them all, namely, the assertion that technology will eradicate the DEAF-WORLD (see Lane, 1992; Lane, Hoffmeister, & Bahan, 1996). To put it another way, technology looks, feels, and smells like audism.

It is hoped that our treatment of this controversy (especially in Chapter 5) has convinced you that this should not be or will be no longer the case, especially in the near future. Yes, the National Association of the Deaf (NAD) has attempted to dispel the negativity associated with a few products of technology. Yes, researchers, scholars, and educators have stressed the need to consider both clinical and cultural aspects. Yes, it is suspected that we will all learn to get along.

Nevertheless, there is something that seems to be left unsaid—at least, according to the peek into our crystal ball. It is entirely possible that technology will minimize or reduce drastically the condition of hearing loss or eventually even prevent it. Our crystal ball, however, does not lead us to believe that technology will eliminate hearing loss completely.

Analogously, we have not eliminated all of our worst diseases—nor will we ever be able to perform this task.

It is shortsighted to interpret our remarks as meaning that deafness is a disease or that the DEAF-WORLD *ought to be* eradicated. We think it is foolish and dangerous to turn back the fast-ticking clock of technology. More important, similar to debates in the professional literature (e.g., see the Paul–Lane debates in Paul, 1996, and synthesized in Paul, 2009), it is important to separate the condition of deafness/hearing loss/and so on from the existence of the DEAF-WORLD.

We admit that this proposed "separation" might be perceived as splitting hairs. However, it can be argued that working to minimize, reduce, or eliminate the effects of deafness or even deafness or hearing loss itself does not equate to eliminating the DEAF-WORLD, or even American Sign Language. In our view, this is not the way that science, medicine, or technology works. No doubt, our rendition here of this complex topic is not adequate, given the brevity of the discussion and our limited space.

Perhaps, we can entice you to read further by starting with an eye-opening article by Cooper (2007), who proffers the idea that "deafness" can be either a good or a bad thing, depending on its relation to other variables (e.g., the development of particular beneficial skills, an unawareness of dangers in the environment, etc.). In a brief email exchange with the first author, Cooper related that her article produced unintended negativism with several members of the Deaf community in England. As a philosopher, Cooper was simply doing her job—exploring a range of views and drawing logical conclusions. We sincerely hope that you do what was suggested previously in the passage by Kuhn at the beginning of this chapter.

We have reached the last theme of this epilogue—*collaboration*. Collaboration was covered in two chapters of this book (Chapters 9 and 10). It does not matter to us whether you think of this concept as analogous to *team work, team teaching, coteaching, interdisciplinary approach,* or *transdisciplinary approach.* One major point made in both chapters is that collaboration contributes to the success of the development of children and adolescents during early intervention and during their school years.

With respect to John Donne, it is true that "No man is an island, entire of itself." In fact, this has become a prevalent trend in research endeavors, namely, that problems are often complex and are better addressed from a multiperspective approach (e.g., in the area of literacy, see Israel & Duffy, 2009). Or, to state it differently, professionals and others need to engage in what the philosopher Wittgenstein has advocated: "Criss-crossing the landscape from multiple directions" (see discussions in Israel & Duffy, 2009; Paul, 2009). The current emphasis on translational research, a "bench-to-bedside" approach, provides hope that, in addition to interdisciplinary clinical and/or educational teams, basic scientists and clinicians will be working together to improve outcomes for children and adolescents with hearing loss (National Institutes of Health, 2009).

We suspect that we have made our points about collaboration. But, we are not done yet. It should be highlighted, underlined, stressed, emphasized—okay, this is enough—that parents should be partners in any collaboration process. The challenge for parents, indeed for all members of the team, is to feel that there is parity in the decision-making process.

Parity means that all members of the team have something important to contribute and that their contributions are valued. When something goes wrong, the entire collaboration team should receive the blame; when something goes right, the entire collaboration team should receive the blame (i.e., credit). Better yet, as mentioned in Chapter 9, let us avoid the blame game entirely.

We are still not done. Parental involvement is so critical that we will go so far as to suggest that all school and clinical meetings should have a *parent advocate* present. This individual can encourage parents to participate and can even speak on behalf of those parents who are reluctant due to the tenets of their culture (see Chapter 9). We recognize that there is always the danger of "parent power" overwhelming the collaboration process. Nevertheless, we shall err on the side of parents. Professionals only spend a few hours a day, at most, with children and adolescents. There is nothing as devastating as uninvolved, uninformed parents.

There is more to say about collaboration—not to mention that this should be a salient component in university preparation programs, that parents should be made aware of the major perspectives to inform their role in the decision-making process. We think we better get off the stage; in fact, it is time to conclude this epilogue.

In closing, it is hoped that we have convinced you of the importance of *hearing, technology,* and *collaboration.* More important, we hope that you have become inspired to do further reading and thinking and, maybe, a little writing as well. It is critical to possess a questioning, inquiring spirit, especially with respect to the complex and controversial topics as mentioned in this book.

We do not claim to have the best answer or perspective, and we do want to encourage other voices. Nevertheless, we agree with Plack (2005) that hearing (i.e., audition) should be studied as much as seeing (i.e., vision). There are, of course, quite a few unanswered questions about hearing, especially if one considers the operations of the central auditory system; but we have come a long way. We shall end with a passage from Plack (2005) to exemplify this message:

> The good news is that progress is being made, and as the reference section demonstrates, many important discoveries have been made in the last few years. As we uncover the ear's remaining secrets, I like to think that there will be a few surprises in store. (p. 239)

References

Cooper, R. (2007). Can it be a good thing to be deaf? *Journal of Medicine and Philosophy, 32,* 563–583.

Israel, S., & Duffy, G. (Eds.). (2009). *Handbook of research on reading comprehension.* New York: Routledge.

Kuhn, D. (2005). *Education for thinking.* Cambridge, MA: Harvard University Press.

Lane, H. (1992). *The mask of benevolence: Disabling the Deaf community.* New York: Vintage.

Lane, H., Hoffmeister, R., & Bahan, B. (1996). *A journey into the DEAF-WORLD.* San Diego, CA: DawnSign Press.

Marschark, M. (2007). *Raising and educating a deaf child: A comprehensive guide to the choices, controversies, and decisions faced by parents and educators* (2nd ed.). New York: Oxford University Press.

Moores, D. (2001). *Educating the deaf: Psychology, principles, and practices* (5th ed.). Boston: Houghton-Mifflin.

National Institutes of Health. (2009). *NIH roadmap for medical research*. Retrieved from: http://nihroadmap.nih.gov/clinicalresearch/overview-translational.asp.

Paul, P. (1996). Is there a psychology of deafness?: A reply to Harlan Lane. *BRIDGE: Bridging Research in Deafness and General Education, 15*(2), 5–7.

Paul, P. (2009). *Language and deafness* (4th ed.). Sudbury, MA: Jones & Bartlett.

Plack, C. (2005). *The sense of hearing.* Mahwah, NJ: Erlbaum.

Further Readings

Beveridge, W. (1980). *Seeds of discovery.* New York: W. W. Norton & Company.

Flage, D. (2004). *The art of questioning: An introduction to critical thinking.* Upper Saddle River, NJ: Pearson/Prentice Hall.

Phillips, D., & Soltis, J. (2004). *Perspectives on learning.* New York: Teachers College Press.

Appendix

A BRIEF LIST OF ORGANIZATIONS

Alexander Graham Bell Association for the Deaf and Hard of Hearing

3417 Volta Place, NW
Washington, DC 20007
Phone: (202) 337-5220
Web site: www.agbell.org

The focus is on helping families, healthcare providers, and educators understand childhood hearing loss, with an emphasis on the importance of early diagnosis and intervention. AG Bell is noted for promoting oral options and emphasizing the development of speech, speechreading, and auditory training/learning.

American Academy of Audiology

11730 Plaza America Drive, Suite 300
Reston, VA 20190
Phone: (800) AAA-2336
Web site: www.audiology.org

Described as the "world's largest professional organization of, by, and for audiologists," the American Academy of Audiology has information about the profession of audiology and also offers consumer information.

American Sign Language Teachers Association

P.O. Box 92445
Rochester, NY 14692-9998
Web site: www.aslta.org

This organization promotes American Sign Language (ASL) and Deaf culture through excellent teaching. It has established standards for the evaluation of effective teaching of ASL as a second language in educational programs.

American Society for Deaf Children

800 Florida Ave., #2047
Washington, DC 20002-3695
Phone: (866) 895-4206
Web site: www.deafchildren.org

A nonprofit organization designed to support and educate families of children who are deaf or hard of hearing. The organization also addresses advocacy for high-quality educational services for children with hearing loss. The organization is supportive of the wide range of options for families of children.

American Speech-Language-Hearing Association

2200 Research Boulevard
Rockville, MD 20850-3289
Phone: (800) 638-8255
Web site: www.asha.org

A professional, scientific, and credentialing association for speech-language pathologists, audiologists, and speech, language, and hearing scientists. Information about careers in speech and hearing fields is provided, and consumer information is also available.

Association of Late Deafened Adults

8038 MacIntosh Lane
Rockford, IL 61107
Phone: (815) 332-1515
Web site: www.alda.org

This organization supports adults who are d/Deaf or hard of hearing. The focus is on adults who have lost their hearing later in life.

Audiology Online

Phone: (800) 753-2160
Web site: www.audiologyonline.com

Online learning source for audiology, with a broad range of information related to hearing loss and related topics.

Baby Hearing

Web site: www.babyhearing.org

A Web site sponsored by the Boys Town National Research Hospital with information about newborn hearing screening, pediatric hearing loss identification, and early intervention for parents and professionals.

Better Hearing Institute

1444 I Street, NW, Suite 700
Washington, DC 20005
Phone: (202) 449-1100
Web site: www.betterhearing.org

A nonprofit corporation that educates the public about hearing loss and what can be done to address it.

Dangerous Decibels

Web site: www.dangerousdecibels.org

A public health campaign designed to reduce the incidence and prevalence of noise-induced hearing loss (NIHL) by changing knowledge, attitudes, and behaviors of school-aged children. Provides fun educational materials about the function of the ear and also how to protect hearing.

Hands and Voices

P.O. Box 3093
Boulder, CO 80307
Phone: (303) 492-6283
Web site: www.handsandvoices.org

Organization made up of people who have common interests connected through the community of deafness that provides unbiased options and support for children who have hearing loss.

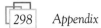

Hearing Loss Association of America

7910 Woodmont Ave, Suite 1200
Bethesda, MD 20814
Phone: (301) 657-2248
Web site: www.hearingloss.org

Described as the nation's leading organization representing people with hearing loss. Focus is on helping people to learn to live with hearing loss.

Marion Downs Hearing Center

1793 Quentin Street, Unit 2
Aurora, CO 80045
Phone: (720) 848-3042
Web site: www.mariondowns.com

The Downs Center provides services, resources, education, and research to support the needs of individuals who are d/Deaf or hard of hearing, their families, and professionals. The Center provides good information on the early identification of hearing loss.

National Association of the Deaf

8360 Fenton Street
Silver Springs, MD 20910
Phone: (301) 587-1788
Web site: www.nad.org

The nation's premier civil rights organization of, by, and for d/Deaf or hard of hearing individuals, NAD provides information about issues and resources for people who are d/Deaf.

National Institute on Deafness and Other Communication Disorders

31 Center Drive, MSC 2320
Bethesda, MD 20892
Web site: www.nidcd.nih.gov/health/hearing

NIDCD provides information regarding hearing, hearing loss, hearing aids, and protecting hearing.

Raising Deaf Kids

Web site: www.raisingdeafkids.org

Developed by the Deafness and Family Communication Center (DFCC) at Children's Hospital of Philadelphia, the Web site provides information for parents of children of all ages who are d/Deaf or hard of hearing.

INDEX